The Omentum

Basic Research and Clinical Applications

The Omentum

Basic Research and Clinical Applications

Edited by
Harry S. Goldsmith, MD

Ciné-Med®

Ciné-Med Publishing, Inc.

Woodbury, CT

Cine-Med, Inc.
127 Main Street North
Woodbury, CT 06798
(203) 263-0006
www.cine-med.com

ISBN 978-0-9823868-0-4

Printed in Canada

CONTENTS

CONTRIBUTORS

Editor

Harry S. Goldsmith, MD
University of California-Davis, PO Box 493,
Glenbrook, NV 89413

Contributors

Mitchel S. Berger, MD
Chair, Department of Neurosurgery
University of California – San Francisco,
San Francisco, CA 94143-0112

Mathias Brandt, MD
Bathildiskrankenhaus, Maulbeeralle 1, Bad Pyrmont, 31812, Germany

Jack de la Torre, MD, PhD
Senior Scientist
Banner Sun Health Research Institute, Sun City, AZ

Jiang Feng, MD
Department of Neurosurgery, Xin-Hua Hospital, Shanghai Second
Medical University, 1665 Kong Jiang Road, Shanghai 200092,
People's Republic of China

R. Lawrence Ferguson, MD
2515 North Clark Street, Suite 800, Chicago, IL 60614-2720

Junko Hara, PhD
Director of Research
Shankle Clinic, Irvine, CA

R.A. Gettleman, MD
2515 North Clark Street, Suite 800, Chicago, IL 60614-2720

Robert S. Hattner, MD
Professor Emeritus, Radiology
University of California – San Francisco, San Francisco, CA

S. Hendryk, MD, PhD
Associate Professor of Neurosurgery
Department of Neurosurgery and Neurotraumatology
Silesian University of Medicine
Katowice, Poland

Xu-ming Hua, MD
*Department of Neurosurgery, Xin-Hua Hospital, Shanghai Second
Medical University, 1665 Kong Jiang Road, Shanghai 200092,
People's Republic of China*

Jun Karasawa, MD
*Department of Neurosurgery, Osaka Neurological Institute, 2-6-23 Shonai- Takara-Machi,
Toyonaka, Osaka 561-0836, Japan*

C. Everett Koop, MD, ScD
The C. Everett Koop Institute at Dartmouth, Hanover, NH 03755-3862

D. Latka, MD
*Department of Neurosurgery and Neurotraumatology, Silesian Medical
Academy, Aleka Legionow 10, Byrom 41-902, Poland*

Jeffrey A. Lee, MD
*Department of Neurosurgery, Kaiser Permenente,
San Diego, CA*

Bo Levander, MD, PhD, MA
*Professor, Department of Neuro-Orthopedic Surgery, Karolinska Institute,
Center for Brain and Cord Research, Stockholm, Sweden*

Dorothea Liebermann-Meffert, MD
*Chirurgische Klinik, Klinikum R.D. Isar Technische Universitat,
Ismaningerstr. 22, Munich D-81675, Germany*

Natalia O. Litbarg, MD
University of Illinois Medical Center, Hektoen Institiute for Medicine, Chicago, IL

Ming Liu, MD
*Department of Neurosurgery, Xin-Hua Hospital, Shanghai Second
Medical University, 1665 Kong Jiang Road, Shanghai 200092,
People's Republic of China*

E.Z. Longa, MD
*Instituto de Cirugia Experimental, Facultadde Medicine, Universidad
Central de Venezuela, Caracus, Venezuela*

Martin G. Luken III, MD
Private Practice, Harvey, IL

Christlane H. May, MD
*Department of Neurosurgery, St. Gertrauden Hospital, Paretzer Str. 12,
Berlin 10713, Germany*

R. Mrówka, MD, PhD
*Department of Neurosurgery and Neurotraumatology, Silesian Medical
Academy, Aleja Legionow 10, Bytom 41-902, Poland*

Chicao Nagashima, MD
*Saitama-Nagashima Clinic, 3-1-14 Ogose-Higashi, Ogose, Saitama
3500414, Japan*

B. Perira, MD
Neurovascular Laboratory, Department of Neurosurgery, University of California–San Francisco, CA 94143

W. Regalson, MD
Medical College of Virginia (VCU), PO Box 980273, Richmond, VA 23298

William R. Shankle, MS, MD
Medical Director/Program Director, Shankle Clinic/Memory and Cognitive Disorders Program, Hoag Neurosciences Institute, Irvine, CA

Yoshihito Shimada, MD
Department of Neurosurgery, Kurosawa Hospital, 3-19-2 Nakai-Machi, Takasaki City, Gumma 370-0852, Japan

Ashok K. Singh, PhD
John Stroger Jr Hospital of Cook County, Chicago, IL

Gary K. Steinberg, MD, PhD
Stanford University Medical Center, Department of Neurosurgery, Stanford, CA

Hajime Touho, MD
Department of Neurosurgery, Osaka Neurological Institute, 2-6-23 Shonai-Takara-Machi, Toyonaka, Osaka 561-0836, Japan

Sigfreld Vogel, MD, PhD
Department of Neurosurgery, St. Gertrauden Hospital, Paretzer Str. 12, Berlin 10713, Germany

Thomas Walz, MD
Bathildiskrankenhaus, Maulbeeralle 4, Bad Pyrmont 31812, Germany

Phillip R. Weinstein, MD
Professor of Neurological Surgery, Department of Neurosurgery, University of California – San Francisco, San Francisco, CA

Wei-Lie Wu, MD
Department of Neurosurgery, Xin-Hua Hospital, Shanghai Second Medical University, 1665 Kong Jian Road, Shanghai 200092, People's Republic of China

Shun-quing Xu, MS
Department of Neurosurgery, Xin-Hua Hospital, Shanghai Second Medical University, 1665 Kong Jiang Road, Shanghai 200092, People's Republic of China

J. Zong, MD
Department of Neurosurgery, Xin-Hua Hospital, Shanghai Second Medical University, 1665 Kong Jiang Road, Shanghai 200092, People's Republic of China

TRIBUTE TO DENIS BURKITT

Not long before he died, I had the pleasure of giving to Denis Burkitt the Bower Award of the Franklin Institute in Philadelphia. The reason he was awarded the prize and what he did with it are the measures of the man.

The Bower Award is given annually, in the form of a substantial financial award, to a scientist whose research embodies the high-minded, low-tech approach of Benjamin Franklin to electricity when he made that discovery with nothing but a kite, some string, and a key.

Denis Burkitt's mind was much like that of Franklin—innovative and creative—but his experiments were simple, with far-reaching implications. His studies that propelled fiber into its significant role in modern nutrition were done with plastic bags, paper clips, and records kept on a clipboard in African villages.

His discovery of Burkitt's lymphoma combined observation, correspondence with missionaries throughout a large section of Africa, tabulation of cases with map tacks on a wall-mounted map of the continent, and a hair-raising adventure in a Land Rover, visiting all of the sightings of what was eventually to be known as Burkitt's lymphoma.

The last communication I had from Denis was the second one after the Bower Award ceremony in Philadelphia, where he brought down the house with his combination of simple science and Irish wit. He wrote to inform me that he and his wife, Olive, never well-off financially, had completed the list of recipients of his prize money. He gave it all away.

There were volumes that could be written about Denis Burkitt, but these anecdotes are the measure of the man.

C. Everett Koop

DEDICATION

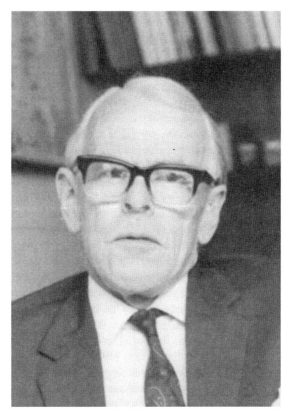

This book is dedicated to the memory of Denis P. Burkitt.

Denis Parsons Burkitt was born in 1911 in the small town of Inniskillin, Northern Ireland. He was the oldest son of James Parsons Burkitt, a civil engineer, and Gwendolyn (Hill) Burkitt, the daughter of William Hill, a well-known architect in the city of Cork. He had an idyllic childhood, except for the unfortunate loss of an eye at a young age due to a stone-throwing incident in school. He was educated in England, during which time he himself acknowledged that he was a poor student.

Burkitt entered the engineering school at Trinity College, Dublin, in 1929 at age 18 without any conviction as to his future career. He had been brought up in a loving Christian home and during his first year of college, he was introduced into the College Christian Union, which had a profound influence on his subsequent career. By the end of his first year in college, he had decided to pursue medicine as his career. From then on, he pursued his studies with dedication and success.

In 1938, he obtained the Fellowship of the Royal College of Surgeons in Edinburgh. At that time, he wished to work overseas before starting his surgical practice, but the British Colonial Office refused his services because of the loss of his eye. He subsequently spent 6 months as a cargo ship's surgeon sailing to Manchuria, where he further reflected on his desire to work somewhere in the Third World. On his return, the Second World War broke out and Burkitt joined the Royal Army Medical Corps, where he served for the next 4 years in East Africa and Asia. When the war ended and he was demobilized in 1946, he applied again to the British Colonial Office, requesting service in Uganda, a country he had visited during his military service and a place to which he felt drawn. Within 6 months, he sailed for that country.

Although Burkitt was a surgeon, he felt that to be true to his calling as a medical missionary he had to be willing to take any position to which he was assigned. Consequently, he was assigned to an isolated and unhealthy station in northern Uganda where he was the only qualified doctor for a population of 300,000. He had to deal with every branch of medicine and commonly was required to operate by the light of a lamp with an untrained assistant giving anesthesia. Because of his insufficient background in orthopedic surgery, he took a short leave back to England to become more proficient in orthopedics.

After 18 months working in the bush, he was transferred to Kampala, the capital of Uganda, where he became head of the surgical service in the city's main teaching hospital. While serving at the Mulago Hospital, he noticed a group of children who had developed huge tumors of the jaw. He studied this disease by buying a used car for several hundred dollars and driving throughout central Africa in order to trace the development of the tumor at various altitudes and latitudes. He reported these tumors, which were successfully treated with chemotherapy. These types of tumors were subsequently labeled Burkitt's lymphoma, which later gained him worldwide interest and the acclaim of the medical profession. However, personal glory never held any interest for Burkitt, who always felt that he was merely a vehicle for God's work.

Following his initial success with Burkitt's lymphoma, he began to notice that African patients did not suffer from many of the common Western gastrointestinal diseases such as appendicitis, colon cancer, diverticulitis, etc. In trying to reason the cause of this, Burkitt began to take into account the large volume of stool produced daily by his African patients. Further study showed that the increased stool volume resulted from the high fiber level that is standard in the African diet. Based on these observations, Burkitt spent the rest of his life crusading for increased fiber content to be incorporated into the diet of individuals in the Western world. He was initially thought to be wrong in his conclusions, but eventually his theories were confirmed. Practically everyone in the Western world today has had his diet affected in some manner by the work of Denis Burkitt.

The political upheaval in Uganda in 1966 forced Burkitt, after 20 years in that country, to relinquish surgery and return to England. He continued to work full time in medical research, studying the epidemiology of cancer and Western diseases. He retired from the British Medical Council in 1976 and, until his death in 1993, he was in great demand as a lecturer all over the world.

Above are a few of the professional facts of the life of Denis Burkitt, but one had to know him as a person to realize the uniqueness of his personality. He was blessed in life with his marriage to Olive Rogers who supported him in every way throughout his life and, together with their three daughters, provided him with a loving and relaxing home. Burkitt said his marriage was the greatest blessing he received on earth.

I was truly fortunate in having the magnificent opportunity of having Denis Burkitt as a friend. I had been in his home and he had spent time in mine over the years. It was not long after our first meeting that I realized I had encountered a truly great individual. He was the only person I have ever met who had neither hard feelings nor jealousy towards others. He gave more than he ever took. An example of this is a personal incident that I have told of on many occasions to highlight the character of this man. At sometime in the mid-1970s, Dr. Burkitt and I were at a meeting of the Pan-Pacific Surgical Association in Honolulu. He told me that he felt the reason his African patients didn't develop Western-style gastrointestinal problems was due to the high concentration of bran in their diet, which accelerated their stool transit time, thus decreasing the opportunity for toxic material in the stool to cause trouble. Burkitt had measured the stool transit time in the black African, which was very rapid, and in the white English population, which was very slow. What he felt he needed was the measurement of the stool transit times in white and black Americans since he believed a difference in the transit times between these two groups would indicate a genetic basis for the discrepancy between the stool transit times. But if the transit times proved to be comparable in both the white and black groups, this he believed would indicate that diet was the major factor in any difference between the transit times. Dr. Burkitt said he needed this information and I simply said I would get it for him. Years later, he sent me a copy of a letter that he sent his wife that night telling her that he had at last found an American doctor who would measure the stool transit times that he needed. Upon returning from the meeting, Burkitt later sent me instructions on how to conduct the study. It involved the swallowing of barium pellets by volunteers who over the next days collected their stools in plastic bags, which were then x-rayed for the presence of a set number of barium pellets. Burkitt later laughed when I told him that if I had known the procedure of the study, I probably would have not been so eager to help him. After gathering the data from the study, I sent the information to Dr. Burkitt. He wrote and thanked me, and I heard nothing further until approximately a year later, when I learned that Dr. Burkitt had submitted the data for publication. He not only put my name on his paper, but he had placed it as first author. Anyone in academic medicine knows the significance of such an act.

This book is dedicated to the memory of Dr. Burkitt. To have known him was indeed a privilege. He was an unpretentious and brilliant man who left this earth better than the way he found it. The strength of his character was based on a strong Christian faith, which was the dominating force of his entire life. When major honors were being heaped upon him, he always remained humble and was truly an inspiration to many. He was a surgeon, a scientist, and a family man who cherished the ideals of his faith and showed to all those around him an aura of spirituality that was truly perceptible.

In 1988, the First International Congress of Omentum was held in Raleigh-Durham, North Carolina, and Dr. Burkitt was the guest speaker at this conference. He concluded his speech, which resulted in a 3-minute standing ovation, with these remarks: "We are each and all of us dependent on others. I have often affirmed and do so again that I would gladly lay all the trophies that have been given to me at the feet of my wife and my mother to whom I owe so much." He ended by quoting the words of St. Paul, which are on the wall of his study: "What do you possess that was not given to you? If then you really received it all as a gift, why take the credit to yourself?"

All who were ever touched by Dr. Burkitt will forever remember his contributions and above all, his rare spiritual quality. To Denis P. Burkitt: hail and farewell.

Harry S. Goldsmith

AN OVERVIEW OF OMENTAL APPLICATION

W. REGELSON

INTRODUCTION

It should not be surprising that the omentum possesses trophic developmental roles involving neural and vascular responses. Developmentally, the omentum is derived from the embryologic yolk sac and plays a role in neural, lymphatic, and gastrointestinal organization. The yolk sac also gives rise to the spleen and blood islands critical to hematopoiesis and angiogenesis. It is also the yolk-sac–derived splanchnic mesoderm between the endoderm of the gut and the pericardial cavity that contributes to the development of the heart and circulatory system[1-5] and, in addition, gives rise to the spleen and peritoneal omental "milky spots."[1-5]

In our 1988 review,[5] we summarized the broad physiologic role of the omentum, speaking of its proven and potential clinical value.

The omentum as a "hose" delivers blood or neurotransmitters, and it also delivers angiotrophic, neurotrophic, or other regulating substances because it is a physiologic delivery system—a delivery system that brings in blood or trophic stimulation to an area in need. In addition to it being utilized as a "hose," it is also a "sucker" where we have excess fluid, i.e., traumatic or congenital hydrocephalus, or the edema of injury, where the omentum can act as a lymphatic conduit to remove edema or cerebral spinal fluid. In omental clinical utilization, we can have access to it as either a "hose" or a "sucker," as it can act as a physiologic controlling system wherein it can both deliver oxygenated blood and remove metabolic "waste" and edema fluid and/or be used to modulate the volume of spinal fluid.

Another aspect of omental physiology is that it is a trophic "generator." It is a generator because, as has been shown by Goldsmith and Vineberg's earlier observations, there is an omental glycolipid present in the omentum that stimulates angiogenesis. It is thus not surprising that the omentum as a transposition not only carries supplemental arterial blood from the aorta, but also, wherever it is placed, stimulates the growth of new blood vessels into the brain, spinal cord, or myocardium.

The omentum, like its yolk sac embryonic precursor, is trophic in its action because it not only provides for the balance of vascular perfusion and differentiating cytokines, but also provides for fluid return. In addition, through its complement of omental lymphoid organs (milky spots) and peritoneal macrophages, it is involved in host defense.[2,3]

Vineberg et al.[6] showed that the omentum has a vascular tropism similar in action to the chronic epithelium of the early embryo.[7] They felt that the "blood-hungry free omental graft seeks its own blood supply in contrast to fatty tissue derived from alternative sources." However, the omentum is uniquely different from the chorion as it induces penetration of new blood vessels from the host in similar fashion to that seen in tumor tissue. It stimulates vascularization of the embryonic type wherein vessels from the graft anastomose to those of the host.[7]

In regard to the angiogenic role of the omentum, it has great relevance to problems of aging wherein the loss of effective blood supply is not just due to a decrease in perfusion pressure due to arteriosclerosis but related to a decrease in tissue capillary ratios that can interfere with perfusion and wound healing.[8,9]

In support of the above, Goldsmith and Castimpoolas[10] and Goldsmith et al[11] showed that they could increase vascular perfusion[10] by administration of a lipid angiogenic factor obtained from the omentum.[11] This glycolipid angiogenic omental factor apparently works in areas distant from local sites on systemic injection.

It is obvious that if we can adequately maintain the formation of new blood vessels at sites of ischemic injury or repair, it may serve to preserve the youthful state of our tissue. This is pertinent not only to cerebral or spinal cord ischemia, but also to coronary disease and the problems of peripheral vascular disease as seen in thromboangitis obliterans, diabetes, arteriosclerosis, and Buerger's disease.[12] In Russia, free autologous omental graft has been used successfully to treat thromboangitis obliterans of the extremity.[13]

In regard to the above, patents were issued for the omental angiogenic glycolipid,[14] which showed angiogenic stimulation on systemic administration. Of interest, this porcine omental angiogenic fraction enhanced the action of gangliosides on wound healing.[14] This is of particular interest in that the GM1 ganglioside has been shown to stimulate neuronal regeneration in central nervous system (CNS) injury.[15,16]

The porcine omental extract developed commercially by Angio-Medical Corporation was shown to clinically stimulate wound healing[14,15] but was marketed as a "cosmetic" hair growth factor,[17,18] which led bureaucratically to U.S. Food and Drug Administration (FDA) closure and the disappearance of this omental glycolipid from clinical studies despite proven activity in topical hair restoration.

In addition to angiogenic factors, the omentum was shown to possess inhibitors of fibronolytic activity that abetted homeostasis.[18,19]

More recently, Takada et al.[20] have used an omental lipid fraction to enhance rat skin flap survival on local injection into the flap.

Neovascularization and vasodilatation were reported in the injected flap. In addition, regeneration of an autotransplanted spleen was enhanced when placed in an omental pouch when the angiogenic omental lipid fraction was given both intramuscularly and into autografted spleen "chips."[21]

This text focuses largely on the role of the omental transposition in the treatment of neuropathology. Clinical studies describing the value of this technique in brain and spinal cord injury, stroke, Moyamoya disease, encephalitis, and communicating hydrocephalus are well represented. In both animal experimentation and in clinical trial, the omentum, as a transposed pedicle with its aortic blood supply intact, or as a free autologous implant, has also served to augment cardiac blood supply in conditions of ischemia. As this text is focused on the role of the omental transposition in the treatment of CNS disease, we feel it appropriate to review the omentum's value in other areas, particularly in coronary insufficiency, where its past clinical value has recently been almost totally ignored.

MYOCARDIAL REVASCULARIZATION

The vast bulk of the approximately 600,000 coronary artery bypass graft (CABG) procedures done each year are primarily for the symptomatic relief of anginal pain with hope for the extension of cardiac survival. Thus, it is appropriate to review current and past procedures utilizing the omentum as a vascular source or as a stimulus to angiogenesis that have a bearing on both clinical cardiac ischemia and survival.

The first study of the omentum in coronary disease was that of O'Shaughnessy,[22] who pioneered using cardiac omentopexy to supplement myocardial blood supply in dogs. In O'Shaughnessy's technique, the omentum was still attached to the stomach and its vascular supply was intact.

Knock[23] and Knock et al.[24] expanded on O'Shaughnessy's procedure, removing the epicardium to produce firm adhesions between the omentum and heart muscle. They tunneled omental strips into the left ventricle for stimulation of deep vascularization. To augment superficial implantation of the omentum, the surface of the left ventricle was abraded with talc or other scarifying agents applied within the pericardial sac. Following the procedure, dogs with ameriod-induced coronary occlusion demonstrated a protective vascular dependence on the new blood supply derived from this omental procedure.

Vineberg[26-32] conducted numerous dog and clinical studies using autologous free omental grafts alone or combined with internal mammary arterial implants that were positioned directly within the myocardium. Vineberg's omental homografts, free of vascular attachments, showed dramatic angiogenesis-inducing action[6] when in contact with adjacent areas of the heart. Vineberg[6] was the first to show that a free graft of omental fat placed in the anterior eye chamber generated new blood vessel formation. Fat from other sources was without effect. Clinical reports of the relief of angina were described by Vineberg, and a significant number of patients were treated combining free graft omental cardiac placement to the pericardial free

surface of the heart with internal mammary implantation.[31,32]

In regard to the above, arteriolar injection techniques in both dog and man showed clear-cut arteriolar communication between the omental graft, heart, and adjacent great vessels in contact with the omental free graft.[32] Vineberg and Lwin[32] showed that the omental graft with aortic attachment could maintain coronary needs and substitute for occluded vessels 18 days after the procedure. Vineberg, in his text,[30] stressed the ease with which the procedure could be done for the treatment of post-infarct patients with a failing heart.

Goldsmith,[33] in early work, examined omental transposition vs. the autologous omental free graft in a study of myocardial revascularization in dogs. This was before CABG and the Vineberg procedure of implanting the internal mammary artery into the myocardium became available, with omental free grafts applied to the myocardial surface being the only clinical approach involving coronary intervention at that time. Clinical experience with the use of omental grafts or transpositions have been lost as the technology for heart/lung machines have led to overwhelming clinical enthusiasm for CABG.

Goldsmith's[33] technique improved on the potential of previous omental to cardiac placement. In Goldsmith's application, the detached lengthened omentum was moved through the diaphragm and applied directly to the myocardium. Vascular connections between the omentum and the heart were demonstrated by dye injection. Unfortunately, the application of this technique for treatment or prevention of coronary insufficiency has never been clinically attempted. However the technique to extend the omentum into a large pedicle that could completely envelop the heart and still preserve its abdominal aortic vasculature is well defined for application of this technique to brain and spinal cord as described in this and Goldsmith's previous text.[34]

More recently, Galajda et al.[35] have repeated aspects of Vineberg's use of the free omentum with confirmation of enhanced vascularization around the internal mammary graft.

THE OMENTUM AS A SOURCE OF STEM CELL PRODUCTION AND/OR CELL DIFFERENTIATION

Siek, Marquis, and Goldsmith[36] have described the effect of an omental glycolipid on neural growth and differentiation. They described the effects of their omental glycolipid derivative on *in vitro* neural growth and differentiation. They used neuroblastoma and pheochromocytoma tumor cell lines that, when exposed to the omental glycolipid, were stimulated to put out neurite extensions. However, even though these tumor cells appeared morphologically differentiated, they continued to divide and they were not committed to neurotransmitter production. These omental glycolipid exposed neural tumor cells continued to divide without synthesizing acetylcholine or catecholamines. In summary, what occurred under the influence of this omental factor was the conversion of an undifferentiated tumor cell to a cell with embryonic qualities of pre-differentiation, i.e., morphologic differentiation, but the absence of end-stage functional differentiation that precludes cell division.

The importance of the above is relative to research indicating that embryonic cells have clinical usefulness when transplanted into adults.[37,38]

While the projected clinical use of human embryonic transplants is in difficulty because of the ethical issues involved in obtaining embryos, if we could transform adult or cancer cells to the pre-differentiated embryonic state, it would give us the opportunity to develop resources for fetal cell transplantation. Could the omental glycolipid affect this process?

In more practical terms, because of the growing dependency on tissue culture for peptide and monoclonal antibody production, the question has to be asked, can the omental glycolipid(s) or other omental factors act in tissue culture to sustain cell survival? We must ask if the omental glycolipid factor(s) influence the growth of characteristics or other cells lines to prevent senescence. We must answer the question as to whether there are a wide range of growth factors present in the omentum that could control differentiation and cell division. That there will be a variety of omental factors is supported by the observation that the omental milky bodies stimulate bone marrow targets to exclusively produce macrophage colonies.[39]

McCluer et al.[40] have characterized a feline omental lipid that includes gangliosides and glycolipids that possess growth factor modulating action with particular relevance to angiogenesis and wound healing. This work in regard to omental glycolipid growth and differentiating factors needs renewed activity.

The value of Goldsmith's heart model[33] and the Vineberg clinical experience[30] is self-evident and provides an intelligent synergy or alternative to CABG, angioplasty, laser myocardial puncture, or the local and systemic use of angiogenic factors. The omental transposition, going back to O'Shaughnessy in 1938,[19] provides for both angiogenesis and major blood flow augmentation from an aortic source. Omental capillaries depend on pressure gradients[30,41,42] in the right direction to maintain perfusion in relation to the omental transposition's aortic arterial source.

Pertinent to the above is Goldsmith's observation that in both the *in situ* omentum and in the long-term placement of the transposition for the treatment of stroke, there is complete absence of any evidence of arteriosclerosis in omental vessels up to 10 years later. This observation is supported by Speiser et al,[45] and others, who have shown that cultured endothelial cells from human omentum contain 100 times the quantity of human plasminogen activator as compared to that seen in umbilical vein endothelial cells.[44]

It should not be surprising that glycolipids have neurotrophic or angiogenic properties. Brunelli et al.[45] reported clinical improvement in radiation-induced brachial plexus injury using omental grafts.

In regard to mechanisms, fat is under sympathetic control, which is particularly true of thermogenic brown fat. Fat can also be very vascular where its mobilization and storage must respond rapidly to environmental changes effecting heat generation or calorie intake. In addition, fat solubility characterizes steroid hormones that are stored in fat and thus the omentum as a peritoneal buffer may also be a key to steroid, as well as catechol action, governing systemic energentics based on fat mobilization and the generation of heat or inflammation.

In regard to the above, the omentum is also found in birds and salamanders.[2,46] As vascular and neurotrophic factors are present in the omentum, one must ask if this can influence the salamander's capacity for limb-bud regeneration, which is based on innervation and vascularization. At the first Omental Conference organized by Goldsmith,[34] Huber et al.[47] showed that an omental chloroform/methanol fraction clearly stimulated bone repair.

BONE REPAIR

Huber et al.[47] showed that their omental angiogenesis fraction used in bone repair resulted in an 80% increase in bone density, and significant higher rates of bone strength and healing. Unfortunately, this work disappears from the literature in 1989, with the demise of the Angio-Medical Corporation[48] Could an omental graft or the omental transposition be used to help in bone repair or fracture repair? Could omental angiogenic lipid fractions stimulate bone morphogenic proteins that stimulate *de novo* bone formation?[48-50] Is there

a place for omental glycolipids in the systemic or local treatment of osteoporosis or fractures?

IMMUNOLOGY

The omentum and spleen have a common origin embryologically.[1,2,46] Lymphatic development is present in the omentum.[1-4] We also have Dux's observations[4] regarding the role of the omentum in the maintenance of immunity, which has clinical relevance to the use of bioresponse modifiers (BRMs) given intraperitoneally (i.p.) in the treatment of cancer. These are both naturally derived lymphokines, such as IL-2 or interferons, which can stimulate immune responsiveness. In addition, BRM compounds of synthetic origin, such as synthetic polyanions,[51,52] which are too toxic for intravenous (IV) administration, although they possess good therapeutic index for anticancer activity when given i.p. to mouse tumor models, can now be given in peritoneal dialysis fluid for the treatment of AIDS and cancer.[52,53]

Large molecular weight substances given i.p. behave very differently than when you give the same material intravenously.[51,52] If we are going to succeed clinically, using BRMs or cytokines, we have to be able to take advantage of the omentum with its monocytic "milky bodies" and its lymphatic arterial portal access. The omentum and the peritoneal cavity produce peritoneal exudate cells that have potent anti-tumor host defense activity and we have to see if the omentum as a monocyte- and lymphocyte-producing system can be utilized as a generating system for antigen processing to serve as a site for systemic immunization.

The peritoneal space can be used to generate exudate cells derived from the omentum by direct stimulation using intraperitoneal dialysis fluid placement to produce an artificial ascites. Lymphocytes or monocytes accumulated in the peritoneal space can migrate locally or systemically. We must use the intraperitoneal space to enhance immune responsiveness for stimulation of both nonspecific and specific host resistance. This is feasible because of Tenckhoff catheters attached to portacaths developed for peritoneal dialysis for the treatment of renal failure. We will use subcutaneous ports to avoid the major threat of peritonitis, so we can reach the omentum in the abdomen for the intraperitoneal treatment or immune effector cell generation for vaccine production.[51,52]

In regard to the above, we must determine if we can take advantage of the omentum for vaccine development instead of administering our vaccines subcutaneously or intramuscularly. We must learn to use the peritoneal space to impinge directly on the omentum's immune response capability.

The growing popularity of peritoneal dialysis with osmotic icodextrin in the treatment of renal insufficiency has made the intraperitoneal space a safe place for chemotherapy, immunotherapy, and vaccine adminstration.[53] The intraperitoneal space provides access to 80% of lymph nodes, and to the action of peritoneal effector cells. The intraperitoneal route provides direct contact with omental milky spots, as well as the thymus and the spleen involved in immune processing. In support of the value of the peritoneal space, intraperitoneal icodextrin with dextrin sulfate has resulted in the disappearance of HIV viral titers in chemotherapy-resistant AIDS patients.[53]

We must also examine if placement of the omental transposition to a regional site can assist in localized immune processing. In that regard, the vascular omentum can support tumor growth, as well as disrupt the blood-brain barrier[54] to enhance intracerebral chemotherapy.

NEUROTRANSMITTER, NEURAL REGENERATION, AND CYTOKINE NEUROTROPHIC ACTION

In 1987, Goldsmith et al.[55] and then McIntosh and Goldsmith[56] described the presence of dopamine and epinephrine produced by the omentum.

There was also evidence that the omentum produced acetylcholine as well.

In more recent work, Krist et al.[57] have found dopaminergic innervation of the milky spots of the human omentum.

de la Torre and Goldsmith[58-61] have shown that omental transposition can produce neural bridging following complete spinal cord transection in the cat. With omental stimulation, neural growth occurs through a defect utilizing a collagen stint.[58-61] The success of this procedure in a clinical case of almost complete spinal cord transection has been described by Goldsmith et al. in this text.[61] Thus, the action of the omental transposition on the cord not only relates to its action in decreasing edema and inflammation post-injury,[62] but also stimulates neural regeneration.

In regard to the omental production of neurotransmitters, we know that if we administer dopaminergic agents to mice, we delay aging and maintain functional motor effectiveness. The omentum theoretically could be useful trophically for maintenance of the substantia nigra, i.e., the basal ganglia, which deteriorate as a critical feature related to Parkinson's disease.[63]

With aging, we lose controlling neuroendocrine functional roles that are important. Among the key neurotransmitters that quantitatively decline are both dopamine and acetylcholine. In addition, we lose the capacity to generate catechols involved in postural vascular or cardiac responses.[63] For this reason, I repeat what I suggested in 1988[5]: "...that we await those neurologists and neurosurgeons concerned with symptoms of Parkinson's and Alzheimer's disease who will have the clinical nerve to try the omental transposition for their treatment." With growing justification for the use of the omental transposition in stroke, as described in this text,[64-67] the extension of this to treatment of Parkinson's disease is warranted, particularly in view of Goldsmith's demonstration of the value of the omental transposition in the treatment of Alzheimer's disease (AD).[68]

In regard to AD, we have shown that the cognitive response to tacrine in AD is due to increased cerebral blood flow.[69] In our 1997 review of AD,[70] we relate its pathology to decreases in cerebrovascular blood flow, a position confirmed by Scheibel et al[71], who showed the primary microvascular pathology of this disease.

de la Torre and Goldsmith[72] have described the decline in blood flow to the distal stump below the surgical transection of the cord. Again, as we discussed in 1988,[5] we must ask if this distal circulatory decline is the reason why we have muscle spasm and loss of functional automaticity that are characteristic of even minimal cord injury. Is the distal decline in spinal cord circulatory capacity after injury critical to many of the chronic clinical problems of paraplegia? Does the omental transposition restore circulatory function distal to the injury and is this a factor in reversing clinical muscle spasm and providing functional return?

In support of the above, we have the observation as to the effect of the omental transposition on cerebral blood flow presented by Rosadini et al.[73] We also have the clinical observations of Abraham[74] and others, and Berger's[75] work in animal models, where we saw the actual histologic demonstration of penetration into the brain of new blood vessels stimulated by the placement of the omental transposition. Certainly, the omental transposition must be enhancing blood flow relevant to its placement on the neural surfaces of the brain and spinal cord. Relevant to stroke injury, it was clearly shown that the transposition stimulated CNS blood flow after the procedure.

What is also intriguing to omental CNS placement is the fact that despite the observation that the blood-brain barrier is breached by the omental transposition, patients do not how any changes in their behavior.[75] What is the purpose of the blood-brain barrier, or is it just a developmental circulatory barrier whose existence is important to drug entry but not related to post-prandial amino acid influences?

In addition to neurotransmitter, angiogenic, and neurotrophic action, adipose cells of the omentum of obese subjects release two to three times more IL-6 than those of subcutaneous tissue. The glucocorticoid dexamethasone suppressed IL-6 production,[76] as does dehydroepiandrosterone (DHEA), a native hormone that is the precursor to the sex steroids and that declines with age. Steroid inhibition of IL-6 is involved in control of inflammation and inhibition of tumor growth.

There is a marked difference between adrenogenic-induced lipolysis of the omentum vs. subcutaneous fat in obese vs. non-obese men. The cells of the omentum in the obese mobilize fat more readily. This relates to omental ß-androgenic receptors,[77] which suggests that the omentum can play both a heat induction and nutritional role governing local and systemic lipid metabolism.

ALTERNATIVE USES

The omentum has a long history of application to plastic or reconstructive procedures, either as a source of supplemental blood for tissue maintenance and/or as a source of fat or connective tissue for plastic reconstruction or structural support. A review of publications shows the range of the omentum's applicability to surgical reconstructive procedures.[5,34] To discuss this would require a separate detailed review. Suffice it to say, the omentum has been used to control infection in vascularized infected sites, to close esophageal fistulae, for enhancing recovery in radiation tissue necrosis, to restore brachial palsies, to aid in prosthetic replacement for reconstruction procedures, for closing rectal or vaginal fistulas, for scalp or cranial skin and bone repair, for upper and lower limb circulatory enhancement, for chest wall reconstruction, for the treatment of osteomyelitis or mediastinitis, to provide splenic vascular support, for the treatment of Buerger's disease, and for plastic facial reconstruction.

In regard to alternative uses, Goldsmith was among the first to use the omentum to enhance lymphatic drainage from occluded peripheral limbs, and to provide vascular support for arteriosclerotic occlusive peripheral vascular disease, a program that is coming back in vogue.[78]

DISCUSSION

Since 1988, when the first edition of Goldsmith's omental text first appeared,[34] there has been further confirmation of the value of the omental transposition[79] in the treatment of CNS disease involving spinal cord and brain injury. Apart from confirmation, what has been discovered is the role of the omentum in producing true functional regeneration of the transected cord in both animal models and the clinic. Most importantly is the demonstration of the value of the omental transposition in the treatment of AD,[68,70,80] which has been further confirmed in two more of Goldsmith's patients. In addition, the value of the omentum in recovery of late cerebral palsy has been shown, as has its possible value in lumbosacral spinal adhesive pathology (in this text).

The value of the omental transposition in spinal cord injury, and in stroke and cerebral palsy, is discussed in this text. The value of its application to Moyamoya disease has been confirmed,[67] and its use in the treatment of post-viral encephalitic injury and hydrocephalus represents a new use of clinical value.

Levander's work[80] in CNS fluid mobilization has moved from dog models to more definitive clinical success in the treatment of hydrocephalus and spina bifida, showing the value of the omentum as a "sucker" for the relief of CNS pressure and edema. Pertinent to this are the reports of Chinese neurosurgical interventions using the omental transposition in the treatment of acute spinal cord and brain injury where edema predominates.

Again, I would like to reiterate that the courageous among us should consider the application of the omental transposition for use in the treatment of refractory schizophrenia, the post-polio syndrome, multiple sclerosis, and amyotrophic lateral sclerosis. These present wide clinical therapeutic options as these diseases can be severely debilitating or lethal and the alternatives for effective treatment and the opportunity to study animal models are nonexistent.

Finally, it is tragic that the proven value of the omentum as an angiogenic stimulus has not developed clinical acceptance despite its proven value in the treatment of coronary disease, as was shown by Vineberg in the clinic and confirmed repeatedly in past animal models.

The role of the omentum in bone repair should be extended and one should investigate its potential value as a possible stimulus to bone marrow recovery in myelofibrosis and aplastic anemia, recognizing its ontogenic place in embryonic hematopoiesis.

I feel that the data in this text and in the literature clearly support the omentum as an adult source of cytokines or stem cells involved in immune, angiogenic, and neurotrophic responses. We particularly need to encourage our neurosurgical confreres to visit China and other centers where the clinical use of the omentum in CNS disease has been routinized.

For the new millennium, the work reported in this text by those involved in CNS applications for the omental transposition will eventually make the omentum and its trophic products a regular part of our armamentarium.

REFERENCES

1. Jirasek JE. *Atlas of Human Prenatal Morphogenesis.* Boston: Martin Nijhoff; 1983.
2. Lieberman-Meffert D, White H. *The Greater Omentum: Anatomy, Physiology, Pathology, Surgery with an Historical Survey.* New York: Springer-Verlag; 1983;1-369.
3. Dux K. Anatomy of the greater and lesser omentum in the mouse with some physiological implications. In: Goldsmith HS, ed. *The Omentum: Research and Clinical Applications.* New York: Springer Verlag; 1988;19-43.
4. Williams R. Angiogenesis and the greater omentum. In: Goldsmith HS, ed. *The Omentum: Research and Clinical Applications.* New York: Springer Verlag; 1988;45-61.
5. Regelson W. Summation: ideas presented and lessons learned. The omentum: a physiological generating system of basic physiology. The need for its application to myocardial vavscularization and other problems. In: Goldsmith HS, ed. *The Omentum: Research and Clinical Applications.* New York: Springer Verlag; 1988;229-240.
6. Vineberg AM, Pifarre R, Merce C. An operation designed to promote the growth of new coronary arteries using the detached omental graft: a preliminary report. *Can Med Assoc J.* 1962;81:1116.
7. Ausprunk DH, Nighton DR, Folkman J. Vascularization of normal and neoplastic tissues grafted to the chick choriollantois. *Am J Pathol.* 1975;79: 597-618.
8. Rosenthal SM. Microcirculation and lymphatics. *CRC Handbook of Physiology in Aging.* Boca Raton: CRC Press; 1981;155.
9. Yamura H, Matsuzawa T. Decrease in capillary growth during aging. *Exp Gerontol.* 1980;15:145.
10. Goldsmith HS, Catsimpoolas N. Increased vascular perfusion after administration of an omental lipid fraction. *Surg Gynecol Obstet.* 1986;162:579-583.
11. Goldsmith HS, Griffith AL, Kupferman A, Catsimpoolas N. Lipid angiogenic factor from omentum. *JAMA.* 1984;252:2034-2036.
12. Nishimura A. Omental transplantation for Buerger's disease. In: Goldsmith HS, ed. *The Omentum: Research and Clinical Applications.* New York: Springer Verlag; 1988;87-206.
13. Regelson W. Personal communication. Omental Conference, Surgical Research Inst., Moscow, 1990.
14. Catsimpoolas N, Evans J, Sinn RS. Increased vascular perfusion following adminstration of lipids. US Patent 4 769,362. 1988.
15. US patent 4,778,787. 1988. US patent 4,710,490. 1987.
16. Leeden RW, Wu G, Lu ZH, Kozireski-Chuback D, Fang Y. The role of GM1 and other gangliosides in neuronal differentiation. Overview and new finding. *Ann NY Acad Sci.* 1998;19:161-175.
17. Angio-Medical Corp. Evaluation of porcine omental extract (POE) in wound healing in normal volunteers. Study Report. New York;1990.
18. Nickoloff BJ. Histological evaluation of the effectiveess of formula 24 as a trichotrophic agent in androgenic alopecia. Report submitted to Angio-Medical Corp, New York; 1989. (Formula 25: Thinning Hair Supplement, 1990).
19. Catsimpoolas N. Lipids with plasmin inhibitory. US patent 4,673,667. 1987.
20. Takada T, Kamei YI, Iwata T, Yokoi T, Torii S. Effect of omental lipid fraction on enhancement of skin flap survival. *Ann Plast Surg.* 1998;41:70-77.
21. Levy Y, Miko I, Hauchk M, Mathesz K, Furka I, Orda A. Effect of omental angiogenic lipid factor on revascularization of autotransplanted spleen in dogs. *Eur Surg Res.* 1998;30:183-193.
22. O'Shaughnessy C. Surgical treatment of cardiac ischemia. *Lancet.* 1937;1:145-147.
23. Knock FE. Cardiomentopexy and implantation of multiple omental loops for revascularization of the heart. *Surg Forum.* 1958;9:230-232.
24. Knock FE, Sessions RW, Beattle EJ. Surgical procedures for myocardial revascularization *Arch Surg.* 1960;81:807-811.
25. Vineberg AM, Baichwal KS, Syers J. Treatment of acute myocardial infarction by epicardiectomy and free omental graft. *Surgery.* 1965;57:836-838.
26. Vineberg AM, Shanks J, Pifarre R, et al. Myocardial revascularization by omental graft without pedicle: experimental background and report of 25 cases followed 6 to 16 months. *J Thor Cardiovasc Surg.* 1965;49:103-129.
27. Vineberg AM. Revascularization by unilateral ventricular mammary artery implants and pericoronary omental grafts. Ten year follow-up. *Vas Surg.* 1973;137:565-578.
28. Vineberg AM. The problem of blocked aorto-coronary artery vein grafts. Report of three cases with successful treatment by intraventricular arterial implants and omental grafts. *J Thor Cardiovasc Surg.* 1973;66:428-438.

29. Vineberg AM. Revascularization via healthy myocardial arteriolar networks compared with that through diseased surface coronary arteries. *Israel J Med Sci.* 1975;11:250-263.

30. Vineberg AM. *Myocardial Revascularization by Arterial Ventricular Implants.* Littleton: PSG Pub. Co.; 1982.

31. Vineberg AM, Syed AK. Arterial vascular pathways from subclavian arteries to coronary arterioles created by free omental myocardial implants. *Can Med Assoc J.* 1967;19:399-401.

32. Vineberg AM, Lwin MM. Fostering a natural artery bypass for disseminated coronary artery disease by pericoronary omental strips. *Surg Gynecol Obstet.* 1973;137:565-578.

33. Goldsmith HS. Pedicled omentum versus free omental graft for myocardial revascularization. *Dis Chest.* 1968;54:27-40.

34. Goldsmith HS. The omentum: present status and future application. In: Goldsmith HS, ed. *The Omentum: Research and Clinical Applications.* New York: Springer Verlag; 1988:131-145.

35. Galadja Z, Miko I, Hallay J, Maros T, Peterffy A, Furka I. Why the internal mammary artery is an ideal graft for myocardial revascularization? (An experimental model with omentopexy). *Acta Chirugica, Hungarica.* 1997;36:92-94.

36. Siek GC, Marquis JK, Goldsmith HS. Experimental studies of omentum-derived neurotrophic factors. In: Goldsmith HS, ed. *The Omentum: Research and Clinical Applications.* New York: Springer Verlag; 1988:83-95.

37. Wyatt JR, Freed WJ. Progress in neurografting as a treatment for degenerative brain disease: the Parkinson's model. In: Regelson W, Sinex M, eds. *Intervention in the Aging Process.* Part B, New York: Alan R. Liss; 1983:203-212.

38. Hitchcock ER, Clough C, et al. Embryos and Parkinson's disease. *Lancet.* 1988;I:1274.

39. Ratajczak MZ, Jaskulski D, Poida W, et al. Omental lymphoid organ as a source of macrophage colony stimulating activity in the peritoneal cavity. *Clin Exp Immunol.* 1987;69:198-203.

40. McClure RH, Evens JE, Williams M, et al. Characterization of feline omental lipids. *Lipid.* 1987;4:229-235.

41. Guiring DP. *Collateral Circulation*, Philadelphia: Leland Febinger; 1949:33-38.

42. Sewell WH, Koth DR. A basic observation on the ability of newly formed capillaries to develop into collateral arteries. *Surg Forum.* 1958;9:227-229.

43. Speiser W, Anders E, Preissner KT, et al. Differences in coagulant and fibrinolytic activities of cultured human endothelial cells derived from omental tissue microvessels and umbilical veins. *Blood.* 1987;69:964-967.

44. Bull HA, Pittilo RM, Drury J, et al. Effects of autologous mesothelial cell seeding on prostacyclin production within Factron arterial prosthesis. *Br J Surg.* 1988;75:671-674.

45. Brunelli GA, Brunelli F, DiRosa F. Neurolized nerve padding in actinic lesions: omentum versus muscle use. An experimental study. *Microsurg.* 1988;9:177-180.

46. Liebermann-Meffert D. Historical images and ideas about the greater omentum. In: Goldsmith HS, ed. *The Omentum: Research and Clinical Applications.* New York: Springer Verlag; 1988:5-17.

47. Huber B, John A, Mohler D, et al. Time and dose-dependent profile of omental angiogenic factor on bone repair. In: Goldsmith HS, ed. *The Omentum: Research and Clinical Applications.* New York: Springer Verglag; 1988:97-108.

48. Nottebaert M, Lane JM, June A, et al. Omental angiogenic lipid fraction and bone repair, An experimental study in the rat. *J Orthop Res.* 1989;7:157-169.

49. Wurzler KK, DeWeese TL, Sebald W, Reddi AH. Radiation-induced impairment of bone healing can be overcome by recombinant human bone morphogenic protein-2. *J Craniofac Surg.* 1998;2:131-137.

50. Reddi AH. Role of morphogenic proteins in skeletal tissue engineering and regeneration. *Nat Biotechnol.* 1998;16:247-252.

51. Regelson W. Advances in intraperitoneal (intracavitary) administration of synthetic polymers for immunotherapy and chemotherapy. *J Bioactive Compatible Polymers.* 1986;1:84-107.

52. Regelson W, Shaunuk S. The systemic therapeutic value of the peritoneal space. Submitted for publication.

53. Shaunuk S, Thornton M, John S, et al. Reduction in the viral titer of administration of dextrin-2-sulphate in patients with AIDS. *AIDS.* 1998;12:399-409.

54. Berger MS, Weinstein PR, Goldsmith HS, Hattner R, Longa EZ, Perira B. Omental transposition to bypass the blood-brain barrier for delivery of chemotherapeutic agents to malignant brain tumors. Preclinical investigation. In: Goldsmith HS, ed. *The Omentum: Research and Clinical Applications.* New York: Springer Verlag; 1988:117-129.

55. Goldsmith HS, McIntosh T, Vezina RM, Colton T. Vasoactive neurochemicals identified in omentum: a preliminary report. *Brit J Neurosurg.* 1987;1:359-364.

56. McIntosh TK, Goldsmith HS. Vasoactive neurochemicals in the omentum. Implications for CNS injury. In: Goldsmith HS, ed. *The Omentum: Research and Clinical Applications.* New York: Springer Verlag; 1988:75-95.

57. Krist LF, Estermans IL, Steinbusch HW, Cuseta MA, Meyer S. Beelen, RH. An ultrastructural study of dopamine-immunoreactive nerve fibers in milky spots of the human greater omentum. *Neurosci Lett.* 1994;28:143-146.

58. de la Torre JC, Goldsmith HS. Supraspinal fiber and apparent synaptic remodeling across transected-reconstructed feline spinal cord. *Acta Neurochir.* (Wien). 1992;114:118-127.

59. de la Torre JC, Goldsmith HS. Collagen-omental graft in experimental cord transection. *Acta Neurochir.* 1990;102:152-163.

60. Goldsmith HS, Brandt M, Waltz T. Near total transection of human spinal cord. Functional return following omentum-collagen bridge reconstruction. In: Goldsmith HS, ed. *Omentum Application to Brain and Spinal Cord.* Wilton: Forefront Publishing; 1999:76-92.

61. Goldsmith HS, de la Torre JC. Effect of the omentum on axonal regeneration following complete spinal cord transection. In: Goldsmith HS, ed. *Omentum Application to Brain and Spinal Cord.* Wilton: Forefront Publishing; 1999:61-75.

62. Yoshito S, Nagashima C. Experimental study on effects of omental transposition in cats with spinal cord injury. In: Goldsmith HS, ed. *Omentum Application to Brain and Spinal Cord.* Wilton: Forefront Publishing; 1999:44-60.

63. Regelson W. Biomarkers in aging. In: Regelson W, Sinex M, eds. *Intervention in the Aging Process. Part A: Quantitation, Epidemiology and Clinical Research.* New York: Alan R. Liss; 1983:2-98.

64. Mrowka R, Hendryk S. LatkaD. Omental transposition to the ischemic brain—a critical review of 60 patients. In: Goldsmith HS, ed. *Omentum Application to Brain and Spinal Cord.* Wilton: Forefront Publishing; 1999:143-151.

65. May CH, Vogel S. Omental transplantation in patients with severe visual disturbances due to ischemia. In: Goldsmith HS, ed. *Omentum Application to Brain and Spinal Cord.* Wilton: Forefront Publishing; 1999:198-213.

66. Wu W, Xu S, Liu M, Hua X, Jiang F. Omental transposition following arachnoid excision to treat post-cerebral anoxia (cerebral palsy). In: Goldsmith HS, ed. *Omentum Application to Brain and Spinal Cord.* Wilton: Forefront Publishing; 1999:161-168.

67. Karasawa J, Touho H. Application of omental transplantation to Moyamoya disease. 109-129.

68. Goldsmith HS. Omental transposition to the brain for Alzheimer's disease. In: Goldsmith HS, ed. *Omentum Application to Brain and Spinal Cord.* Wilton: Forefront Publishing; 1999:184-197.

69. Harkins SW, Taylor JR, Mattay V, Regelson W. Tacrine treatment in Alzheimer's disease enhances cerebral blood flow and mental status and decreases caregiver suffering. Cerebrovascular pathology in Alzheimer's disease. *Ann NY Acad Sci.* 1997;826:472-474.

70. Regelson W, Harkins SW. "Amyloid is not a tombstone." A summation: the primary role for cerebrovascular and CSF dynamics in AD. *Ann NY Acad Sci.* 1997;826:348-374.

71. Scheibel AG, Doung T, Tomiyasu U. Microvascular changes in Alzheimer's disease. In: Sheibel AB, Weschler AF, Brazier MAB, eds. *The Biological Substrates of Alzheimer's disease.* New York: Academic Press; 1996:177-192.

72. de la Torre JG, Goldsmith HS. Can transected spinal cord axons be bribed into regeneration. In: Goldsmith HS, ed. *The Omentum: Research and Clinical Applications.* New York: Springer Verlag; 1988:63-73.

73. Rosadini G, Cossu M, Goldsmith HS, et al. A CBF follow-up study in stroke patients after omentum transposition to the brain. In: Goldsmith HS, ed. *The Omentum: Research and Clinical Applications.* New York: Springer Verlag; 1988:109-115.

74. Abraham J. Omental transposition to the brain: experimental and human application. In: Goldsmith HS, ed. *The Omentum: Research and Clinical Applications.* New York: Springer Verlag; 1988:147-157.

75. Berger MS, Weinstein PR, Goldsmith HS, Hattinger R. Longa EZ, Perira B. Omental transposition to bypass the blood-brain barrier for delivery of chemotherapeutic agents to malignant brain tumors. Preclinical investigation. In: Goldsmith HS, ed. *The Omentum: Research and Clinical Applications.* New York: Springer Verlag; 1988:117-129.

76. Fried SK, Bunkin DA, Greenberg AS. Omental and subcutaneous adipose tissues of obese subjects release interleukin-6: depot difference and regulation by glucocorticoid. *J Clin Endocrinol Metab.* 1998;83:847-850.

77. Hoffstedt J, Arner P, Hellers G, Lonnqvist F. Variation in adrenergic regulation of lipolysis between omental and subcutaneous adipocytes from obese and non-obese men. *J Lipid Res.* 1997;38:795-804.

78. Bhargava JS, Makker A, Bhargava K, Shaunik AV, Sharda A, Kumar PS. Pedicle-omental transfer for ischaemic limbs—a 5-year experience. *J Indian Med Assoc.* 1997;95:100-102.

79. Baskov A, Shevelev IN, Iarikov DE, Iundin VI, Kolpachkov VA, Sokolova AA. The results of omentomyelopexy in the late period of traumatic spinal cord disease. *Zh Vopr Neirokhir Im N N Burdenko.* 1998;2:9-17.

80. Goldsmith HS. Application of the omentum to the brain and spinal cord. In: Goldsmith HS, ed. *Omentum Application to Brain and Spinal Cord*. Wilton: Forefront Publishing; 1999:25-43.
81. Levandar B. Lumbo-omental shunt and its CSF absorption capacity: experimental and clinical studies. In: Goldsmith HS, ed. *Omentum Application to Brain and Spinal Cord*. Wilton: Forefront Publishing; 1999:93-100.

CHAPTER 1

HISTORICAL IMAGES AND IDEAS ABOUT THE GREATER OMENTUM

DOROTHEA LIEBERMANN-MEFFERT

The following report summarizes earlier searches for "the nature of the greater omentum" as it was seen through the centuries. This paper shows not only previous misinterpretations, errors, and speculations, but also the endeavors and highlights in the discovery of this useful organ in modern surgery that has for so long been disregarded.[1,2]

THE VARIOUS TERMS USED FOR THE STRUCTURE

The first historical account of the visceral tissue apron in the abdomen was found in 800 BC *(Figure 1.1)* in the Greek literature: in Homer's *Odyssey* it is reported that the giant Tityos was eternally punished for crime by vultures that *"plunged deeply into his DERTRON to feed an eagle on his liver."*

A search through medical and non-medical writings revealed various expressions pertaining to the omentum throughout history. The terms used were related to cultural centers and to political superiority *(Figure 1.1)*, but all clearly allude to the structure or position of the organ *(Table 1.1)*.

While many vernacular terms were abandoned in the course of time, cultural diversities continued with the designation of the structure. Today, the structure is called *omentum* in the English, *epiploon* in the French, *Netz* in the German, and *rete* in the Italian medical literature.

The speculative hypothesis of the German physician F. Rebmann in 1753, that the Latin term *"omentum"* was deduced from *"omen,"* became so attractive that it was still used in 1963 in the remarkable work on the function of the omentum by the British surgeon F.C. Walker. The Romans, however, used the flight of birds for their prophecy, and there is no proof that they used the intestines.[1]

ANATOMY OF THE OMENTUM IN THE LIGHT OF HISTORY

After the first short note found on the anatomy of the omentum around 450 BC in the Hippocratic writings, the Greek philosopher and physician Aristotle (384-322 BC) mentioned the structure in more detail as being a *"fatty material present in all warm-blooded animals."* The Roman physician Pliny the Elder (23-79 AD) introduced into the medical literature the term omentum, formerly used by the poet Catullus, and described it as a *"fatty membrane covering stomach and intestines."*

The distinguished physician Claudius Galen (128-199 AD) of Asia Minor had schooling in logic, philosophy, mathematics, and, of course, medicine in all the famous institutions of ancient Greece, and at the University of Alexandria in Egypt. He later became the personal physician of the Emperor Marcus Aurelius in Rome, and due to his reputation and skill, he was the uncontested authority of medicine for the next 14 centuries.[1]

Apart from writing philosophical essays, Galen's particular interest was anatomy. Like all his contemporaries, he admired Hippocrates and regarded the ancient doctrines as unimpeachable. He added no new concepts to anatomy but he gave the most accurate description of the omentum in classical times. Autopsy of human corpses was still impossible because of the taboos of religion and society. Galen had to content himself with the study of animal cadavers. Many of Galen's anatomical errors obtained from the animal model and transferred to man were not corrected until the end of the Middle Ages.[1]

Throughout the Middle Ages, anatomical knowledge stagnated with medicine being strictly controlled by the church; medicine remained dogmatic and philosophical rather

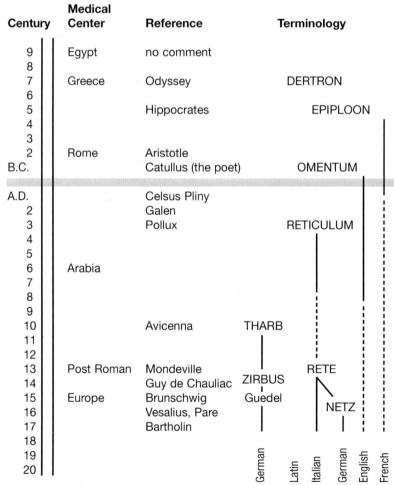

Figure 1.1 Terms used for the greater omentum since ancient times.

Table 1.1 Commonly used historical and modern terms in medical literature, and their meanings

Term	Language	Root	Meaning	Character
Dertron	Greek	Derma	Skin	Membrane
	Greek	Dero	To fly	Membrane
Epiploon	Greek	Eplma	Sole of the root	Cover
	Greek	Plein	Floating, drifting on	Cover
Omentum	Latin	Operimentum	Cover (of intestines)	Cover
	Latin	Opimus	Fat	Fat
	Latin	Ovimentum	Induo=1 clothe or	Cover
Rete	Latin	Reticulum	Net (of a fisherman)	Membrane
Mappa ventris	Latin	Mappa	Napkin (of the abd.)	Cover
Cupeus	Latin	Clipeus	Shield	Cover
Zirbus	German	Tharb	Fat	Fat
Coefe	French	Coiffe	Lace bonnet	Membrane
Crepine	French	——	Sieve or riddle	Membrane
Coul	French	——	Hair-net	Membrane
Guedel	German	——	Sac	Sac
Gidel	German	——	Sac	Sac
Mirach	German	——	Greasy hood of meat	Cover
Netz	German	——	Net of a fisherman	Membrane

than scientific. Anatomical knowledge progressed very slowly *(Table 1.2)*. Systematic anatomical studies on the human did not start until the 18th century.

The ignorance about the omentum is reflected in fanciful pictures in surgical books of the late Middle Ages. The first and most accurate illustration of the omentum was not made by an anatomist or surgeon but by the Italian artist and painter Leonardo da Vinci (1452-1519) in 1504. It is a lifelike drawing with copious notes by a man who procured ample human dissection material. However, this beautiful natural drawing of the omentum influenced neither medical knowledge nor medical concepts at that time because da Vinci´s illustration (which is preserved in the library of Windsor Castle) was not published until 200 years after the artist's death.

In 1543, the renowned Belgian anatomist Andreas Vesalius (1514-1564) published the first somewhat accurate medical illustrations of the human greater omentum *(Figures 1.2A and 1.2B)*. As a result of firsthand knowledge gained from dissection of human corpses, Vesalius now was able to criticize the Galenic prejudices and doctrines. By doing so, he marked the beginning of modern anatomy.

Shortly later, Adrian van den Spieghel (1548-1621) gave a comprehensive description of the topography of the omentum and its vessels *(Figure 1.3)*, which were also documented in 1656 in the delightful artwork by Daniel Bucretius in Julius Casserius Placentini's anatomical tables *(Figure 1.4)*. By 1789, the wax cabinet of the Josephinum at Vienna displayed a splendid lifelike model showing the omentum *in situ (Figure 1.5)*. The precise and varying pattern of the vessels was demonstrated through consecutive vascular injections in man *(Figure 1.6)* not before the middle of the 20th century by Liebermann-Meffert.[1] This pattern proved to be instrumental for the surgical use and the lengthening techniques of the omentum.

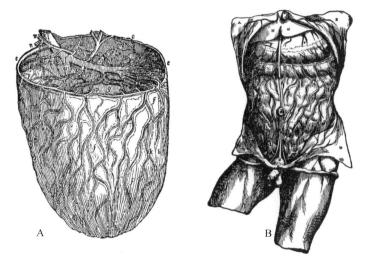

A   B

Figure 1.2A and 1.2B Ideas showing the vessels in the greater omentum by Andreas Vesalius. A = omental sac, B = topographical position of the omentum. In: De humani corporis fabrica, Basel, 1543.

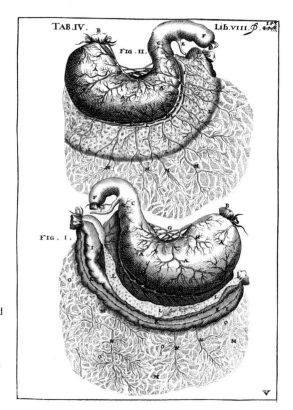

Figure 1.3 Illustration of the greater omentum attached to the stomach and transverse colon showing its vascularization by Adrian van den Spieghel. In: De Omento. De humani corporis fabrica. Libr. X, Frankfurt/Main, 1632.

Table 1.2 Knowledge of omental anatomy from classical to recent times. Poor knowledge of omental anatomy progressed slowly from classical times to the 19th century

Year	Author	Claim
200	Aristotle	Warm fatty material, attachment to stomach
50	Pliny	Membrane
200	Galen	Peritoneal purse, delicate membrane, arteries, veins
1000	Avicenna	Peritoneal purse, delicate membrane, arteries, veins
1267	Theodoric	Peritoneal purse, delicate membrane, arteries, veins
1300	Mondino Da Luzzi	Attachment to diaphragm, stomach, spleen, colon
1500	Leonardo Da Vinci	Life-like picture
1543	Vesalius	'Bird catcher's sac', two layers, tributaries to the portal vein, glands excreting liquid individual fat amount, first accurate picture of anatomy
1632	Van Den Spieghel	Comprehensive description, vessel, no glands
1659	Wharton, Bartholin	Lymph vessels
1687	Malpighi	Adipose ducts or vessels
1702	Ruysch	Vascularity (by wax injection) confirms Spieghel, membranes have no perforations, no true net
1732	Winslow	Reflections, opening into the omentum
1874	Ranvier	Taches laiteuses (milky spots)

THE LONG WAY TO DISCOVER FUNCTION

The highly respected and famous medical school of Alexandria at Egypt taught during ancient times that the omentum had no special functions. This nihilistic attitude was adopted by the Greek anatomist and surgeon Erasistratus (ca. 300-250 BC), and probably represented the overall view of this epoch. The concept entered future anatomical and surgical textbooks, and persisted up to modern times.

Over the years, various obscure and mysterious functions have been attributed to the greater omentum *(Table 1.2)*.

The physician Galen (128-199 AD) believed that the main function of the omentum was to warm the intestines. He gained this impression as a consequence of an injury endured by a Roman gladiator. This man claimed that he "suffered greatly from cold for the rest of his life after an abdominal stab injury and an omental resection." Several other erroneous ideas of omental function were not only preserved and passed on to the Middle Ages, but new errors and fanciful philosophies were also added, even by respected medical authorities *(Table 1.2 and 1.3)*.

The scientific discovery of true omental function finally began in the first decades of the 19th century when protective properties were observed after application to inflamed surfaces. The French anatomist Louis Ranvier (1835-1922) discovered special tiny ovoid structures throughout the membranous parts of the omentum, which he called "taches laiteuses" (milky spots) because of their white color. Much later they were recognized as specialized immunocompetent lymphoreticular organs.[3-7]

The British surgeon Rutherford Morison in 1906 called the omentum *"the policeman of the abdomen,"* which indicated that the omentum is a protective organ, demonstrating adhesive and cohesive properties to traumatized and

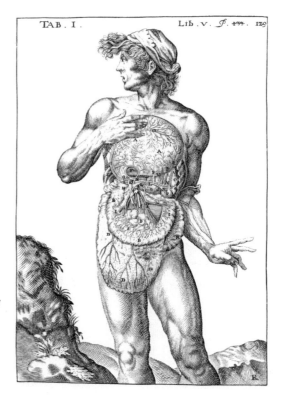

Figure 1.4 The Omentum by Julius Casserius Placentini. Anatomische Tafeln mit denselben, welche Daniel Bucretius hinzugetan. Götzen, Frankfurt/Main, 1654.

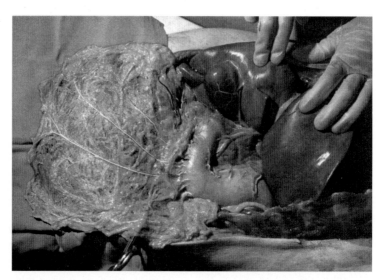

Figure 1.5 The greater omentum in natural position in man. Anatomical waxwork. Collection Josephinum, Vienna 1789 (courtesy of the photographer R. Nedorost, Vienna).

Table 1.3 Claims for omental function from classical to the turn of our century. Speculations about the functions of the omentum were mostly erroneous until they were followed by experiments since the late 19th century.[18]

Year	Author	Claim
450	Hippocrates	Prevents conception in obese by pressing upon and occluding the uterus
200	Aristotle	Inflow of ingested fat after compression of the gravid uterus upon stomach into omentum; from there it ascends to the breast and turns into milk
200	Galen	Warmth of fat accelerates digestion, fat content lubricates peritoneum
1300	Mondeville	Fat storage, heat exchanger Heat compensatory for hairless human skin
1619	Ab Acqua Pendente	Receptacle for waste products of stomach, liver and spleen
1620	Riolan	Ruler of the whole abdomen
1659	Wharton	Fat transport via omental lymph vessels to distant body regions
1660	Bartholin	
1743	Boerhaave	
1747	Haller	
1666	Vesling	Production of pus and serous fluid
1687	Malpighi	Fat transport via adipose omental ducts
1727	Petit	Lubricant production to smooth peristalsis
1747	Culmus	Nourishes the body, adds fat to the bile
1840	Robert	Ability to enclose foreign bodies.
1903	Renzi	
1874	Ranvier	Protection against infection
1898	Roger	
1903	Renzi	
1906	Morison	
1882	Maffucci	Peritoneal absorption
1895	Muscatello	
1899	Milian	Active migration
1903	Heger	
1910	Boljarski	Revascularization

inflamed surfaces.[1,2] Soon after, omental functional abilities such as phagocytosis and foreign body reactions were shown experimentally *(Table 1.3)*. This knowledge and the spread of scientific research at that time paved the way for the modern understanding of the value of the omentum.

However, not until decades later, in the 1970s, was the omentum recognized as an *"immune-competent organ"* in the abdomen by the immunologists Herbert Fischer[3] in Germany and Kazimierz Dux[4] in Poland. They, and later the Japanese surgeons Shimotsuma et al[5,6] and Beelen from the Netherlands,[7] related this function to the cellular contents in the milky spots and the specific structures of the organ *(Figure 1.7)*. Additionally, hemostatic properties and angiogenic substances,[8-10]

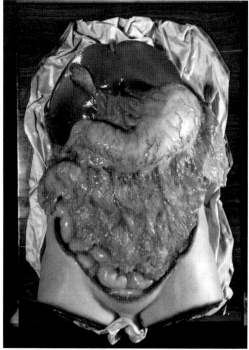

Figure 1.6 Arterial distribution in the human omentum. Intra-aortal injection specimen. Liebermann-Meffert, 1979.

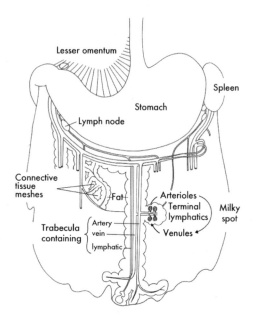

Figure 1.7 Main tissue texture and constituents of the omentum (drawing by Liebermann-Meffert, 1979).

neurotransmitters,[11] and dopamine-immunoreactive nerve fibers have been established to be present in the omental tissue.

THE ROLE OF THE OMENTUM IN SURGERY OVER THE CENTURIES

The Hippocratic writings compiled in Greece around 450 BC contain a number of references to the omentum and particularly to case reports of abdominal injuries in which the omentum became extruded and gangrenous. Subsequently, famous surgeons such as the Greek physician Paul of Aegina (625-690 AD) gave detailed accounts of the treatment of abdominal wounds involving the omentum, but added nothing new to the classical techniques and concepts. Surgical knowledge, however, passed to the Arabian world where it was further developed during the Dark Ages and protected from the persecution of the Christian church in Europe.

During the Middle Ages, no important information was added to Galen's doctrine. Nothing was found in the surgical textbooks of Albucasis (936-1013) who taught in Spain, nor in the Italian writings of Roger (Frugardi) of Salerno (ca. 1150), Bruno di Laburgo (1252), William of Saliceto (1210-1276), or Guido Lanfranchi of Milan (1250-1315) who laid the foundation of French surgery. No new concepts or surgical techniques were presented in the textbooks of the famous French surgeon Pierre Franco (1500-1561), whom William Harvey referred to as his teacher. Hieronymus Brunschwig (1450-1530) and Johannes Scultetus (1595-1645), the outstanding German surgeons, nicely illustrated the traditional technique for treating omental prolapse.[1]

Following this period, there were excellent accounts of strangulated omental hernias in the lectures of the French surgeon Guillaume Dupuytren (1777-1835),[1] which were published between 1830 and 1834. These are of interest since in 1832 the death rate from herniotomy and reduction of the omental contents was very high and remained at 22% even at the end of the 19th century.

NEW IDEAS AND CONCEPTS OF USING THE OMENTUM IN SURGERY

The catching idea of using the omental properties for protection *(Figure 1.8)* was popularized in 1826 by the observation of the French military physician Jobert de Lamballe (1799-1867), later court surgeon to Napoleon III. Lamballe reported his surgical experience accumulated during the civil wars in a publication that showed the readiness of the omentum to form adhesions with the injured bowel.[1] This, as he said, saved many soldiers from peritonitis, a death-threatening event in those days.

Abdominal operations were undertaken only as a last resort until 1867 when Lister introduced antiseptic techniques, and satisfactory general anesthesia became available. Following this, initial use of the greater omentum to protect wounds in surgery was presumably made by the renowned Swiss-American surgeon Nicholas Senn (1844-1909), who was known for his special interest in abdominal surgery.[12] By 1888, Senn recommended free omental grafts to protect unsafe suture lines at bowel anastomoses. In time, the value of the omentum was used to treat gastroduodenal perforation and hepatic injury, and in bladder surgery. Pioneers and their main working subjects are cited in *Figure 1.8*.

By 1937, the American surgeon Walter Walters[13] used the omentum to treat vesicovaginal fistula. In the same year, the

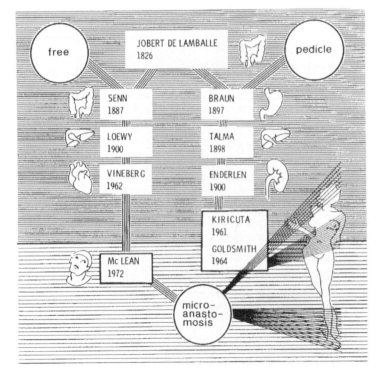

Figure 1.8 Development of three techniques of reconstructive surgery using the omentum at pedicle, microanastomosis, and free graft.[1]

British surgeon O'Shaughnessy[14] published his experience with the omentum in the treatment of cardiac ischemia in the *Lancet*. He used the omental potential for revascularization, a feature which was established by Paunz in 1929 in Germany.

The German surgeon Knazozovicky was the first to exteriorize the omentum from the abdominal cavity in 1926 in order to perform an arthroplasty. However, distant organs could not be reached satisfactorily at that time. It remained for the American surgeon J.E. Cannaday to master this problem in 1948 by lengthening the omentum on a vascular pedicle.[15]

The beneficial role of the greater omentum was well realized by the Romanian surgeon oncologist Ion Kiricuta (1918-1988),[2] who by the 1950s gave a fresh impetus to the application of the omentum for surgical problems. Among these were the treatment of bladder defects after irradiation (1961) and chest wall defects after surgery and irradiation for breast cancer (1963). Kiricuta, by his tremendous continuous pioneering work and publications, was instrumental in promoting the use of the greater omentum in modern surgery.[2]

A comparable marathon of extensive work on various fields of treating diseases with the omentum was done by the North American surgeon Harry S. Goldsmith in 1968.[1,2] He finally became well known for his enthusiastic struggles and enormous attempts to bypass the blood-brain barrier, to treat stroke, paraplegia, and Parkinson's disease. He and his coworkers also performed many basic physiological studies that demonstrated vasoactive neurochemicals,[8,9] neurotransmitters, and growth factors within the omental tissue, as well as omentum-derived angiogenic and neurotrophic factors.[8,9]

In China, Wu Wei Lei and his colleagues treated motor impairment resulting from viral encephalitis successfully by transposition of the pedicled omentum to the brain. Also, the German neurosurgeons Vogel and May started the treatment of Parkinson's disease by omental transposition. In Japan, Moyamoya has been treated with success since the first report of Miyamoto et al in the late 1980s.

The development of microvascular and laparoscopic surgery has opened up areas of new promise.[16-24] The American vascular surgeons McLean and Buncke (1972) were first to transfer the detached omentum to the scalp using microvascular anastomoses. There have since been many reports of this technique for a variety of conditions, including the transfer to the lower extremities by Harii and Ohmori (1973) in Japan, and to the brain by the Swiss neurosurgeons Yasargil *et al* (1974) in Zurich. After the first reports on the successful repair of large skull, face, and neck defects by Banzet and Le Quang in France (1976), Arnold of the Mayo Clinic (1976), and Erol and Spira (1980) in the United States, the greater omentum gained increasing interest worldwide in plastic and reconstructive surgery and in vascular surgery.

REFERENCES

1. Liebermann-Meffert D, White H, eds. *The Greater Omentum Anatomy, Physiology, Pathology, Surgery, With an Historical Survey*. Berlin, Heidelberg, New York: Springer; 1983:1-369.
2. Kiricuta I. Use of the omentum in plastic surgery. Cluj, Roumania: Ed. Medicala; 1980:1-290.
3. Fischer H, Ax W, Freund-Molbert E, et al. Studies on phagocytic cells of the omentum. In: Furth R, ed. Mononuclear phagocytes in immunity, infection and pathology. Oxford: Blackwell; 1975:528-547.
4. Dux K. Anatomy of the greater and lesser omentum in the mouse with some physiological implications. In: Goldsmith HS, ed. *The Omentum. Research and clinical applications*. New York: Springer; 1990:19-43.
5. Shimotsuma M, Kawata M, Hagiwara A, Takahashi T. Milky spots in the human greater omentum. Macroscopic and histological identification. *Acta Anat.* 1989;36:211-216.

6. Shimotsuma M, Takahashi I, Kawata M, Dux K. Cellular subsets of the milky spots in the human greater omentum. *Cell tissue Res.* 1991;264:599-601.

7. Beelen RHJ. The greater omentum. Physiology and immunological concepts. *Neth J Surg.* 1991;43:145-150.

8. Cartier R, Brunette I, Hashimoto K, et al. Angiogenic factor: a possible mechanism for neovascularization produced by omental pedicles. *J Thor Cardiovasc Surg.* 1990;99:264-268.

9. Goldsmith HS, Griffith AL, Kupfermann A, et al. Liquid angiogenic factor from omentum. *JAMA.* 1984;252:2034-2036.

10. Goldsmith HS, McIntosh T, Vezina RM, et al. Vasoactive neurochemicals identified in omentum: a preliminary report. *Brit J Neurosurg.* 1987;1:359-364.

11. Krist LFG, Eestermans IL, Steinbusch HWM, et al. An ultrastructural study of dopamine-immunoreactive nerve fibers in milky spots of the human greater omentum. *Neurosci Lett.* 1994;168:143-146.

12. Senn N. An experimental contribution to intestinal surgery with special reference to the treatment of intestinal obstruction. *Ann Surg.* 1889;7:84-89.

13. Walters W. An omental flap in transperitoneal repair of recurring vesicovaginal fistulas. *Surg Gynecol Obstet.* 1937;64:74-75.

14. O'Shaughnessy L. Surgical treatment of cardiac ischemia. *Lancet.* 1937;1:185-194.

15. Cannaday JE. Some use of undetached omentum in surgery. *Am J Surg.* 1948;76:502-505.

16. Liebermann-Meffert D, Siewert JR. The role of the greater omentum in intrathoracic transposition. *Neth J Surg.* 1991;43:154-160.

17. Logmans A, van Lent M, van Geel AN, et al. The pedicled omentoplasty, a simple and effective surgical technique to acquire a safe pelvic radiation field, theoretical and practical aspects. *Radiother Oncol.* 1994;33:269-271.

18. Williams RJLL, White H. Transposition of the greater omentum in the prevention and treatment of radiation injury. *Neth J Surg.* 1991;43:161-166.

19. Hultman CS, Carlson GW, Losken A, et al. Utility of the omentum in the reconstruction of complex extraperitoneal wounds and defects. *Ann Surg.* 2002;235:782-795.

20. Reade CC, Meadows WM Jr, Bower CE, et al. Laparoscopic omental harvest for flap coverage in complex mediastinitis. *Am Surg.* 2003;69:1072-1076.

21. Samson MJ, van Ooijen B, Wiggers T. Management of extended radionecrosis in the pelvic area with repeated surgical débridement and omental transposition. *Eur J Surg. Oncol.* 1994;20:571-575.

22. Shilov BL, Milanov NO, Liebermann-Meffert D. Biological activity of tissue flaps in the treatment of complicated irradiation wounds. *Eur J Plast Surg.* 1995;18:46-49.

23. Shrager JB, Wain JC, Wright CD, et al. Omentum is highly effective in the management of complex cardiothoracic problems. *J Thorac Cardiovasc Surg.* 2003;125:526-532.

24. Liebermann-Meffert D. Chirurgie des groben Netzes. In: Siewert JR, Rothmund M, Schumpelick V, eds. *Praxis der Viszeralchirurgie,* 2. Aufl., Kap.42, Heidelberg: Springer; 2006:745-751.

HISTORICAL SOURCES

Liebermann-Meffert D, White H, eds. *The Greater Omentum Anatomy, Physiology, Pathology, Surgery, With an Historical Survey.* Berlin, Heidelberg, New York: Springer; 1983:1-369.

Talbott JH. A biographical history of medicine. Experts and essays on the men and their work. New York, London: Grune and Stratton; 1970:1-1211.

Toellner D. *Illustrierte Geschichte der Medizin.* Salzburg: Andreas & Andreas; 1986. 6 volumes.

Chapter 2

FACTORS IN THE OMENTUM THAT ENDOW IT WITH HEALING POWER

NATALIA O. LITBARG AND ASHOK K. SINGH

INTRODUCTION

The unique healing power of the omentum was long realized by surgeons who observed that the omentum sensed injured sites in the peritoneal cavity and spontaneously extended itself to fuse with the injured area. Fusion of the omentum to the injured site improved its healing and prevented infections. Subsequently, the omentum was used to repair injured extraperitoneal organs such as the heart, brain, spinal cord, and limbs, either by using it as a detached piece of tissue (free omental graft) that could be sutured to an injured organ or by lengthening it in a manner that preserved its blood vessels and subsequently attaching it to the injured organ (called omentopexy or omental transposition).[1-4] The omentum is being applied in many more creative ways now that the underlying biological factors are better understood. Below, we review the studies of these special properties of omentum and their application for tissue repair and regeneration.

OMENTUM IS A HIGHLY PLASTIC TISSUE THAT RAPIDLY UNDERGOES CELLULAR CHANGES BY INJURY (ACTIVATION)

Similar to its response to injury, the omentum also reacts to foreign bodies placed in the abdominal cavity, such as in peritoneal dialysis patients when an intraperitoneal catheter is placed for dialysis access, or when surgical instruments or supplies are inadvertently left in the abdominal cavity by surgeons.[5,6] On sensing a foreign body, the omentum rapidly spreads to encapsulate it as if to protect the internal organs from direct contact with it. This phenomenon, called activation of the omentum, was used as an experimental model to study cellular and vascular changes that take place after the omentum encounters a foreign body.[7]

As the omentum gets activated by injury or by a foreign body, it changes its cellular character. While the native omentum consists of 95% fat cells and 5% nonfat cells, an activated omentum consists of 70% nonfat cells and 30% fat cells, suggesting that it is the nonfat cell compartment in the omentum (tissue commonly known as milky spots) that undergoes expansion in response to injury.[7] The extent of tissue expansion that takes place during activation is dictated by the size of the foreign body. In rats, one could expand the omentum mass 20 to 50-fold by injecting either polydextran or polyacrylamide particle slurry (particle size approximately 120 μM). Interestingly, the omentum handled each particle individually by growing a new tissue

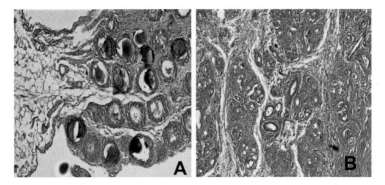

Figure 2.1 Response of the omentum upon encountering a foreign body. **A:** One week after injecting polyacrylamide gel slurry (particle size approx. 120 uM) in the peritoneal cavity; the non-fat component of the omentum (milky spots) expanded to surround each particle individually with new tissue. **B:** One week after a solid polyvinyl rod was attached to the stomach wall, the omentum expanded to surround the foreign body. Similar to **A,** the non-fat milky spot of the omentum expanded to surround the foreign body, but in contrast to **A,** the tissue that was formed was more compact.[7]

around each particle as a result of an active cell proliferation (*Figure 2.1A*). On the other hand, when a larger foreign body such as solid polypropylene rod was sutured to the stomach wall, the omentum grew to surround the rod as a continuous pocket of tissue (*Figure 2.1B*).

In addition to the capacity of omentum to surround foreign bodies of varied shape and size, it can also be extended, stretched, and folded to create a tissue pouch, or dissected to create a long pedicle with uninterrupted vascular supply for grafting at distal anatomical regions.[1-5]

OMENTUM FORMS VASCULAR ANASTOMOSES WITH IMPLANTED OR INJURED TISSUE

In studies on the application of the omental pedicle to repair an ischemic heart, Vineberg angiographically demonstrated formation of vascular anastomoses between the omental graft and the adjacent great vessels.[8] For the same reason, it has become a standard practice to rescue splenic function (when total splenectomy is necessary because of traumatic or ischemic damage) by implanting small pieces of spleen into the omentum.[9] The implanted spleen fragments remain viable due to anastomoses of splenic vessels with those of the omentum.[10] Similarly, application of the omentum to the injured heart as an adjunct to stem cell therapy improved blood perfusion to the heart.[11]

In current practice of pancreatic islet transplantation in humans to treat type 1 diabetes, harvested islets are injected into the portal vein for hepatic implantation. However, there is a high failure rate with this technique due to poor vascularization of the transplanted islets. Therefore, multiple islet injections (pooled from multiple donors) are often required to make the diabetic patient insulin-free.[12] In recent studies on large animals, omentum was tested as an alternate implantation site for donor pancreatic islets. In these studies, animals remained normoglycemic for a longer time, suggesting that pancreatic islets were better vascularized in the omentum.[13,14]

The natural predilection of the omentum to

invade a material placed in it with an extensive network of blood vessels has been used to grow embryonic organs to maturity and prime engineered tissue for transplantation (discussed below).

OMENTUM PRODUCES ANGIOGENIC FACTORS AND A MYRIAD OF OTHER GROWTH FACTORS

Because omentum is efficient in forming blood vessels, it must produce angiogenic factors. What are these factors? Goldsmith's group and others isolated an angiogenic factor from the lipid fraction of omentum.[15] When injected systemically, this factor increased vascularity around a severed femoral artery.[16] Later, several independent groups reported improved vascularization of autotransplanted splenic chips,[17] improved bone repair,[18] and healing of skin flaps[19] after systemic injection of the omentum-derived lipid angiogenic factor. One awaits further purification and molecular characterization of this lipid-soluble angiogenic factor from the omentum.

Vascular endothelial growth factor (VEGF) is one of the most powerful angiogenic factors. Omental extracts contain high concentrations of VEGF.[7,20] Of the several adult organs studied, the omentum was found to contain the highest concentration of VEGF (approximately 10- to 100-fold higher than other organs).[20,21] Omental VEGF production increases to even higher levels by a foreign body activation.[7] Consistent with this, cells cultured from the activated omentum were also found to produce high levels of VEGF in culture.[21,22] This well-studied angiogenic factor is water soluble and thus presumed to be different from the earlier reported lipid-derived angiogenic factor.[15]

In addition to the lipid-soluble angiogenic factor and VEGF, omentum also secretes several other growth factors. One of the technical problems of demonstrating growth factors in tissues is that these factors are secreted and therefore eluded by immunohistochemical techniques. One must extract the tissue and perform growth-factor–specific immunoassays. These assays unfortunately are not readily available, especially for animal species commonly used for experimental work (such as for the rat). Our group showed indirectly that omental extracts contain many types of growth factors equivalent to those present in fetal bovine serum, a mixture of natural growth factors used as an essential additive to the growth media for culturing cells.[7] By comparing cell growth in media containing omental extracts versus in media containing fetal bovine serum, we found that the omental extract was equal or superior in potency in supporting the cell growth of several mammalian cell lines tested.[7]

OMENTUM POSSESSES EFFICIENT LYMPHATICS

While blood vessels are important for oxygen and nutrient delivery to the organ, lymphatic vessels are important for maintaining tissue homeostasis by draining excess fluid, cellular debris, infectious agents, and particles accumulated in the interstitial space. These vessels also transport proteins from inflamed tissues to lymph nodes for antigen presentation and facilitation of an appropriate immunological response. Lymphatic vessels are present in most organs. One distinguishing feature of the lymphatic vessels is that they are open at the peripheral tissue end in contrast to the un-open continuous network of blood capillaries. Distribution of lymphatic vessels in omenta of humans and animals has been studied and described in detail by the anatomist Dr. Simer in the 1930s.[23,24] There is ample indirect evidence from the surgical and veterinary literature, wherein the omental pedicle has been used as a hose to efficiently drain edema from tissues, that the omental lymphatics are capable of anastomosing with the lymphatics of the injured organ upon contact as do the omental blood vessels.[25-28]

OMENTUM HAS ANTI-INFLAMMATORY PROPERTIES

Among the non-adipose cells in the milky spots of the omentum, there are progenitor cells, white blood cells, and stromal cells.[7,29] A few studies have suggested that milky spots may be sites of hematopoiesis independent from the bone marrow.[29] Macrophages are visible at all levels of maturation in the milky spots and can readily enter or leave milky spots. They can be activated by an intraperitoneal injection of carbon particles or bacteria. After activation, their ability to phagocytose particles increases.[29] Also, capillaries in the milky spots of omentum are uniquely adapted for transmigration of white blood cells and rapid fluid absorption under inflammatory conditions. Such adaptation includes 1) fenestrated capillary endothelium (similar to the endothelium of the kidney glomerular capillaries—therefore, these capillaries are also known as "omental glomeruli") *(Figure 2.2)*; 2) mesothelium with intercellular pores; and 3) discontinuous basal

lamina in the submesothelial connective tissue.[29] This unique combination of macrophages capable of activation, proliferation, and easy transfer from milky spots into peritoneal cavity with the special "interrupted" structure of capillaries renders the omentum with a robust infection-scavenging property.

Antibacterial and anti-inflammatory properties of omentum were elegantly demonstrated in a series of experiments in dogs in which an aortic graft was placed in the abdomen followed by injection of fecal material into the graft area to deliberately introduce infection. In dogs in which the grafts were not wrapped by the pedicled omentum, the survival rate was 20%, while in dogs in which the grafts were wrapped with the pedicled omentum, the survival rate was 70% to 80%.[30] These findings were followed by other reports in the veterinary and human surgical literature on the effective use of the omentum for resolution of infections in different body organs.[31-34] The specific proteins, chemokines, or cytokines responsible for the antibiotic activity of omentum have not yet been characterized and therefore remain a fertile area of future research.

In addition to its antibacterial properties, there is indirect experimental evidence

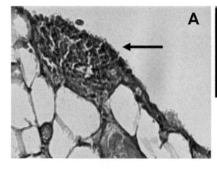 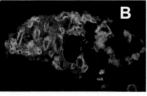

Figure 2.2 Microanatomy of an omental milky spot. **A**: Arrow shows a milky spot representing an island of tightly packed cells surrounded by adipose cells (empty spaces). **B**: Immune-staining of the milky spot with anti-collagen IV antibody showing the fine blood vessels in the milky spot similar to those in a kidney glomerulus.

suggesting that omentum also exhibits immunosuppressive properties. Keyser et al[35] compared the immunosuppressive properties of mesenchymal stem cells derived from the bone marrow, omentum, and muscle by mixed lymphocyte reactions. In this common test for T cell activation, either generic mitogen (concanavalin A, a lectin) or allogeneic T cells were used as inducers of T cell activation. Mitogen-induced T cell activation, as well as allogeneic T cell activation, was inhibited in the presence of mesenchymal stem cells from all sources. However, allogeneic T cell activation was mostly inhibited in the presence of mesenchymal stem cells from omentum. These data demonstrated that omentum-derived mesenchymal stem cells exhibit immunosuppressive effects that may be more potent than those of the mesenchymal stem cells from other sources. That the omentum provides an immune-privileged (or immunosuppressive) environment was also noted by Rogers et al., who performed xenogeneic and allogeneic embryonic pancreatic and kidney transplants into adult omenta.[36,37] They observed that both xenogeneic and allogeneic allografts could be protected by low doses of immunosuppressive medication when transplanted into the omentum.

OMENTUM CONTAINS STEM CELLS

Several reports demonstrate that omentum contains a population of cells with mesenchymal stem cell properties. Cells expressing markers of the mesenchymal stem cells were identified in intact omentum.[38,39] Cells isolated from intact omentum exhibited mesenchymal stem cell behavior,[21,35,40-42] ability for hematopoiesis,[43,44] and capacity to transdifferentiate into hepatocytes in culture.[45] Endothelial cells isolated from omentum were used for lining of vascular grafts, indicating the presence of endothelial progenitor cells in the

omentum.[46]

The cell populations present in the omentum that expanded in response to foreign body activation were studied in more detail by our group.[7,21] We showed that milky spots of the omentum normally contained cells positive for stem cell markers. These cells proliferated when omentum was activated by an inert foreign body (polyacrylamide particles). In the activated omentum, the cells immediately surrounding the polyacrylamide particles expressed markers of adult stem cells (WT1, SDF-1α, CXCR4) and of pluripotent embryonic stem cells (Nanog, Oct-4, SSEA-1).[7] When cells isolated from activated omentum were cultured, they attached to the culture dish and could be propagated for more than 10 passages. Through the passages, these cultured omental cells retained the expression of the stem cell markers and secreted high levels of VEGF.[21] These findings were recently confirmed by Gomez-Gil et al.,[42] who isolated cells from omental adhesions induced by placing a polypropylene mesh in the parietal peritoneum of rabbits. The cells cultured from the omental adhesions showed a proliferation rate that was significantly higher than the proliferation rate of cells from unactivated omentum. Also, cells from omental adhesions exhibited epithelial-to-mesenchymal transition in culture and expressed embryonic stem cell markers showing that omentum activated by a foreign body induces proliferation of its stem cell populations.

APPLICATIONS OF OMENTUM IN TISSUE ENGINEERING

Omentum is a favorable site for growing embryonic tissues

In the past 10 years, several reports have appeared showing that embryonic kidney and pancreas precursors implanted into omental pouch continued to develop and reach structural maturity. Kidney tissue grown by this approach contained adult kidney structures but remained functionally deficient, forming an ultrafiltrate that is concentrated to only 10% compared to that achieved by a normal kidney.[37,47] Similarly, embryonic pancreas implanted into omentum developed to maturity, secreted insulin in response to ambient glucose, and reversed hyperglycemia of diabetes. However, a glucose tolerance test was not performed to confirm full functional capacity of this pancreatic tissue.[36] Interestingly, the blood vessels that developed in the implanted organs were of host origin, thus likely derived from the omentum.[48]

In another set of experiments, omentum was used as a site to grow embryonic kidney precursors seeded with human mesenchymal stem cells. In these experiments, human mesenchymal cells were shown to incorporate into developed kidney structures. Using the lacZ transgenic animals, the authors showed that the vasculature of the obtained neo-kidney originated from the host omentum.[49] Moreover, the implanted hybrid organoid produced human erythropoietin, indicating that human mesenchymal cells not only incorporated into embryonic renal parenchyma, but also differentiated into functioning kidney cells.[50] Another group obtained a hybrid pig tooth and bone by implanting the bone-dentin embryonic tissue complex into the omentum.[51] Using omentum as an implantation site, intestinal tissue has also been successfully grown from embryonic small intestine[52-54] and colon.[55]

Omentum as a site to cellularize, vascularize, and functionalize bioengineered tissues for subsequent transplantation

Engineering a functional tissue from cultured cells seeded onto synthetic or biological scaffolds for subsequent transplantation is being developed as an alternative to organ transplantation. Such experiments encountered rapid loss of the graft, largely due to lack of proper vascularization of the bioengineered tissues. Omentum as a pre-transplantation site for vascularizing engineered tissue was tested by several groups. Autologous canine oral epithelial cells and rib chondrocytes seeded on a porous biodegradable scaffold and implanted into the omentum proliferated to form multi-cell layered structures rich in blood vessels, whereas scaffolds cultured *in vitro* showed only isolated cell growth over scaffolds and a lack of blood vessels.[56] Attempts have also been made to engineer liver by seeding cultured hepatocytes on similar three-dimensional (3-D) scaffolds. The 3-D construct was then implanted at different sites in the body. It was found that, of the several sites tested, the omentum provided the best site for graft vascularization and hepatocyte proliferation.[57] Additional reports have recently appeared in the literature describing maturation of other bioengineered tissue constructs by implanting them into the omentum. These include cardiac patch (for ventricular wall repair),[58] intestine,[59] ureter, [60] bladder,[61,62] esophagus,[63] and trachea.[64] In all cases, omentum provided appropriate structural support and vascularization of the transplanted tissue, and the omentum-matured tissue constructs showed appropriate physiological responses in a few cases.[58,61,63]

The mechanism of omental contribution to the maturation of implanted tissues awaits further investigation. At this time, one can only speculate that among the omental factors favoring tissue maturation must be its plasticity, capacity to elaborate angiogenic and other growth factors, and permissive immunological environment, and an expandable population of stem cells.

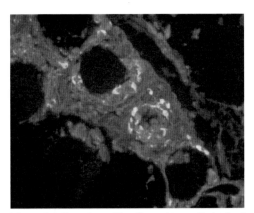

Figure 2.3 Detection of insulin-positive cells (stained green by immunohistochemical staining) in the activated omentum (activated by polyacrylamide) of rats autotransplanted with fragments of diabetic pancreas. The empty spaces were occupied by polyacrylamide particles. Many of the cells immediately surrounding the polyacrylamide particles were insulin-positive. Tissue was counterstained with ethidium bromide to highlight cell nuclei (red).[65]

ACTIVATED OMENTUM CAN REGENERATE ADULT ORGANS *IN VIVO*

β-cells of pancreas

Singh and his group[65] hypothesized that, in its activated state, the omentum could present a stimulating environment rich in growth factors and stem cells for adult β-cell progenitors, normally present in the pancreatic ducts, to differentiate and grow to mature insulin-producing β-cells. Fragments of pancreas from rat with streptozotocin-induced diabetes (pancreas with absent β-cells) were autotransplanted into the activated omentum. After several weeks, new insulin-secreting cells had appeared in the omentum (*Figure 2.3*). Extracts of the omentum containing pancreatic fragments showed measurable amounts of insulin consistent with the number of insulin-positive cells seen by immune staining. Those diabetic rats containing higher amounts of insulin in the omentum became normoglycemic. When pancreatic fragments

were transplanted into native (unactivated) omentum (control animals), measurable insulin in the omentum was negligible and insulin-positive cells were not seen. The control animals remained hyperglycemic, showing that the activated omentum was responsible for regenerating insulin-producing β-cells, presumably from the progenitor cells present in the diabetic pancreas.

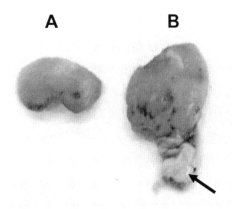

Figure 2.4 Regenerating rat liver using activated omentum. The maneuver included making a small V-shaped wound in the rat liver (A) and activating the omentum by injecting polyacrylamide gel slurry intraperitoneally. After 2 weeks, the liver mass grew to 50% more than the mass of the original liver (B). Arrow in B shows the omental attachment at the point of injury.[66]

Liver

Using a different maneuver of allowing the foreign body activated omentum to fuse with a deliberately created surgical injury to the liver, Singh et al[66] showed that liver could be expanded to 150% of its original mass, a remarkable finding considering that other commonly applied methods of inducing regeneration in the liver, such as massive

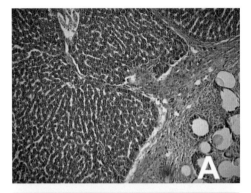

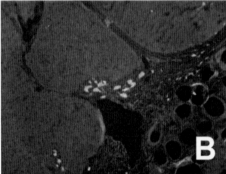

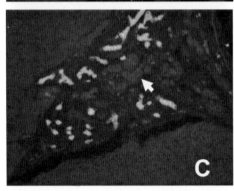

Figure 2.5 Border tissue between the injured liver and activated omentum. A: Trichrome staining of the tissue showing the omentum (with polyacrylamide gel particles) attached to the liver 1 week after injury. B: The section in A immune-stained with cytokeratin 19 (liver-specific stem cell marker normally present in liver bile ducts), showing bile ducts of the liver extending extrahepatically in the border tissue (stained green). C: Larger view of the immune-stained border tissue showing small islands of liver tissue formed in the border tissue (white arrow).[66]

hepatectomy, only restore the liver to its original mass (*Figure 2.4*). Examination of the tissue formed between the activated omentum and the liver showed that biliary ducts, normally containing oval cells (known to be liver-specific stem cells), had expanded to give rise to the new liver tissue (*Figure 2.5*). Further, the expression of several genes (measured by RT-PCR) associated with 1) embryonic activity (Nanog, Oct-4), 2) liver embryonic differentiation (WT1, WNT4, HNF-6), and 3) fetal liver synthetic activity (α-fetoprotein; AFP) were significantly elevated (7- to 20-fold) in the tissue formed between the injured liver and activated omentum, indicating that developmental events were induced in this tissue liver.

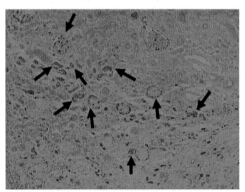

Figure 2.6 Examination of tissue formed by fusion of the kidney parenchyma with activated omentum at the point of injury for WT1 (Wilms' tumor antigen-1, a common marker of kidney regeneration by immune-staining (reaction product is brown). In this tissue were present structures resembling embryonic bodies, commonly seen in a developing kidney (comma, S-shaped bodies, crown-shaped structures, young glomeruli, etc.), suggestive of kidney regeneration.[67]

Kidney

In their preliminary studies, Litbarg et al[67] attempted to induce kidney tissue regeneration in rats using activated omentum. They surgically wounded rat kidneys and allowed activated omentum to fuse with the wound. The tissue formed between the normal kidney parenchyma and activated omentum showed high number of cells expressing WT1, an early marker of nephrogenesis, and structures resembling embryoid bodies, commonly seen in a developing kidney (comma, S-shaped bodies) (*Figure 2.6*). Several developmental nuclear factors (WNT4, Nanog, Oct-4 and WT1) were upregulated up to10- to 20-fold in the zone of kidney-omentum fusion as measured by RT-PCR. Based on these findings, they hypothesized that adult mammalian nephrogenesis, previously never observed, can be induced by the interaction between the surgically injured kidney and omentum.

REFERENCES

1. Goldsmith HS. *The Omentum. Application to Brain and Spinal Cord.* Wilton, CT: Forefront Publishing; 2000.
2. Liebermann-Meffert D. The greater omentum. Anatomy, embryology, and surgical applications. *Surg Clin North Am.* 2000;80:275-293.
3. Vernik J, Singh AK. Omentum: power to heal and regenerate. (editorial). *Intl J Artif Organs.* 2007;30:95-99.
4. Collins D, Hogan AM, O'Shea D, Winter DC. The omentum: Anatomical, metabolic, and surgical aspects. *J Gastrointest Surg.* 2009;13:1138-1146.
5. Goh YH. Omental folding: A novel laparoscopic technique for salvaging peritoneal dialysis catheters. *Perit Dial Intl.* 2008;28:626-631.
6. Rodrigues D, Perez N, Hammer PM, Weber JD. Case report: laparoscopic removal of a retained intra-abdominal ribbon malleable retractor after 14 years. *J Laparoendosc Adv Surg Tech.* 2006;16:369-371.
7. Litbarg, N, Gudehithlu KP, Sethupathi P, Arruda JAL, Dunea, G, Singh AK. Activated omentum becomes rich in factors that promote healing and regeneration. *Cell Tiss Res.* 2007;328:487-497.
8. Vineberg AM, Shanks J, Pifarre R, Criollos R, Kato Y, Baichwal KSJ. Myocardial revascularization by omental graft without pedicle: Experimental background and report on 25 cases followed 6 to 16 months. *Thoracic Cardiovasc Surg.* 1965;49:103-129.
9. Marques RG, Petroianu A, Coelho JM, Portela MC. Regeneration of splenic auto transplants. *Ann Hematol*; 81: 622-626, 2002.
10. Malagó R, Reis NS, Araújo MR, Andreollo NA. Late histological aspects of spleen autologous transplantation in rats. *Acta Cirúrgica Brasileira.* 2008;23:274-281.
11. Kanamori T, Watanabe G, Yasuda T, Nagamine H, Kamiya H, Koshida Y. Hybrid surgical angiogenesis: Omentopexy can enhance myocardial angiogenesis induced by cell therapy. *Ann Thorac Surg.* 2006;81:160-167.
12. Gaglia JL, Shapiro AM, Weir GC. Islet transplantation: progress and challenge (review). *Arch Med Res.* 2005;36:273-280.
13. Hefty TR, Kuhr CS, Chong KT, Guinee DG. Omental roll-up: a technique for islet engraftment in a large animal model. *J Surg Res.* 2009 (In press).
14. Bermana DM, O'Neil JJ, Coffeya LCK, et al. Long-term survival of nonhuman primate islets implanted in an omental pouch on a biodegradable scaffold. *A J Transplant.* 2009;9:91-104.
15. Goldsmith HS, Griffith AL, Kupferman A, Catsimpoolas N. Lipid angiogenic factor from omentum. *JAMA.* 1984;252:2034-2036.
16. Goldsmith HS, Griffith AL, Catsimpoolas N. Increased vascular perfusion after administration of an omental lipid fraction. *Surg Gynecol Obstet.* 1986;162:579-583.
17. Levy Y, Miko I, Hauck M, Mathesz K, Furka I, Orda R. Effect of omental angiogenic lipid factor on revascularization of autotransplanted spleen in dogs. *Eur Surg Res.* 1998;30:138-143.
18. Nottebaert M, Lane JM, Juhn A, et al. Omental angiogenic lipid fraction and bone repair. An experimental study in the rat. *J Orthop Res.* 1989;7:157-169.
19. Takada T, Kamei YI, Iwata T, Yokoi T, Torii S. Effect of omental lipid fraction on enhancement of skin flap survival. *Ann Plast Surg.* 1998;41:70-77.
20. Zhang QX, Magovern CJ, Mack CA, Budenbender KT, Ko W, Rosengart TK. Vascular endothelial growth factor is the major angiogenic factor in omentum: mechanism of the omentum-mediated angiogenesis. *J Surg Res.* 1997;67:147-154.
21. Singh AK, Patel J, Litbarg NO, et al. Stromal cells cultured from omentum express pluripotent markers, produce high amounts of VEGF, and engraft to injured sites. *Cell Tissue Res.* 2008;332: 81-88.
22. Sako A, Kitayama J, Yamaguchi H, et al. Vascular endothelial growth factor synthesis by human omental mesothelial cells is augmented by fibroblast growth factor-2: Possible role of mesothelial cell on the development of peritoneal metastasis. *J Surg Res.* 2003;115:113-120.

23. Simer P. On the morphology of the omentum with especial reference to its lymphatics. *Am J Anat.* 1934;54:203-228.

24. Simer PH. Omental lymphatics in man. *Anat Rec.* 1935;63:253-262.

25. Campbell BG. Omentalization of a nonresectable uterine stump abscess in a dog. *J Am Vet Med Assoc.* 2004;224:1799-1803, 1788.

26. White RA, Williams JM. Intracapsular prostatic omentalization: a new technique for management of prostatic abscesses in dogs. *Vet Surg.* 1995;24:390-395.

27. Yasuura K, Okamoto H, Morita S, et al. Results of omental flap transposition for deep sternal wound infection after cardiovascular surgery. *Ann Surg.* 1998;227: 455-459.

28. Abalmasov KG, Yegorov YS, Abramov YA, Chatterjee SS, Uvarov DL, Neiman VA. Evaluation of the greater omentum in the treatment of experimental lymphedema. *Lymphology.* 1994;27:129-136.

29. Platell C, Cooper D, Papadimitriou JM, Hall JC. The omentum. *World J Gastroenterol.* 2000;6:169-176.

30. Goldsmith HS, de los Santos R, Beattie EJ Jr. Experimental protection of vascular prosthesis by omentum. *Arch Surg.* 1968;97:872-878..

31. Goldsmith HS. The treatment of postsurgical lymphedema. *Surg Clin North Am.* 1969;49:407-412.

32. Kuwabara Y, Sato A, MD, Mitani M, et al. Use of omentum for mediastinal tracheostomy after total laryngoesophagectomy. *Ann Thorac Surg.* 2001;71:409-413.

33. Johnson MD, Mann FA. Treatment for pancreatic abscesses via omentalization with abdominal closure versus open peritoneal drainage in dogs: 15 cases (1994-2004). *J Am Vet Med Assoc.* 2006;228:397-402.

34. Carlson GW, Thourani VH, Codner MA, Grist WJ. Free gastro-omental flap reconstruction of the complex, irradiated pharyngeal wound. *Head Neck.* 1997;19: 68-71.

35. Keyser KA, Beagles KE, Kiem HP. Comparison of mesenchymal stem cells from different tissues to suppress T-cell activation. *Cell Transplant.* 2007;16:555-562.

36. Rogers SA, Liapis H, Hammerman MR. Normalization of glucose post-transplantation of pig pancreatic anlagen into non-immunosuppressed diabetic rats depends on obtaining anlagen prior to embryonic day 35. *Transplant Immunol.* 2005;14:67-75.

37. Rogers SA, Liapis H, Hammerman MR. Transplantation of metanephroi across the major histocompatibility complex in rats. *Am J Physiol.* 2001;280:R132-R136.

38. Sakurai S, Hishima T, Takazawa Y, et al. Gastrointestinal stromal tumors and KIT-positive mesenchymal cells in the omentum. *Pathol International.* 2001;51:524-531.

39. Todoroki T, Sano T, Sakurai S, et al. Primary omental gastrointestinal stromal tumor (GIST). *World J Surg Oncol.* 2007;12:66.

40. Van Harmelen V, Rohrig K, Hauner H. Comparison of proliferation and differentiation capacity of human adipocyte precursor cells from the omental and subcutaneous adipose tissue depot of obese subjects. *Metabolism.* 2004;53:632-637.

41. Tchkonia T, Giorgadze N, Pirtskhalava T, et al. Fat depot–specific characteristics are retained in strains derived from single human preadipocytes. *Diabetes.* 2006;55:2571-2578.

42. Gomez-Gil V, Pascual G, Garcia-Honduvilla N, Rodriguez M, Bujan J, Bellon JM. Characterizing omental adhesions by culturing cells isolated from a novel in vivo adhesion model. *Wound Repair Regen.* 2009;17:51-61.

43. Pinho M de F, Hurtado SP, El-Cheikh MC, Borojevic R. Hematopoietic progenitors in the adult mouse omentum: permanent production of B lymphocytes and monocytes. *Cell Tissue Res.* 2005;319:91-102.

44. Rangel-Moreno J, Moyron-Quiroz JE, Carragher DM, et al. Omental milky spots develop in the absence of lymphoid tissue-inducer cells and support B and T cell responses to peritoneal antigens. *Immunity.* 2009;30:731-743.

45. Liu Z, Shi ZY, Zhou HX, Wu MH, She ZJ, Li YN. A study on the transdifferentiation of adipose mesenchymal stem cells into hepatocytes. *Zhonghua Gan Zang Bing Za Zhi.* 2007;15:601-604.

46. Salacinski HJ, Punshon G, Krijgsman B, Hamilton G, Seifalian AM. A hybrid compliant vascular graft seeded with microvascular endothelial cells extracted from human omentum. *Artificial Organs.* 2001;25:974-982.

47. Rogers SA, Lowell JA, Hammerman NA, Hammerman MR. Transplantation of developing metanephroi into adult rats. *Kidney International.* 1998;54:27-37.

48. Hammerman MR. Renal organogenesis from transplanted metanephric primordia. *J Am Soc Nephrol.* 2004;15:1126-1132.

49. Yokoo T, Fukui A, Ohashi T, et al. Xenobiotic kidney organogenesis from human mesenchymal stem cells using a growing rodent embryo. *J Am Soc Nephrol.* 2006;17:1026-1034.

50. Yokoo T, Fukui A, Matsumoto K, et al. Generation of a transplantable erythropoietin-producer derived from human mesenchymal stem cells. *Transplantion.* 2008;85:1654-1658.

51. Young CS, Abukawa H, Asrican R, et al. Tissue-engineered hybrid tooth and bone. *Tissue Eng.* 2005;11:1599-1610.

52. Kim SS, Kaihara S, Benvenuto MS, et al. Effects of anastomosis of tissue-engineered neointestine to native small bowel. *J Surg Res.* 1999;87:6-13.

53. Rocha FG, Sundback CA, Krebs NJ, et al. The effect of sustained delivery of vascular endothelial growth factor on angiogenesis in tissue-engineered intestine. *Biomaterials.* 2008;29:2884-2890.

54. Agopian VG, Chen DC, Avansino JR, Stelzner M. Intestinal stem cell organoid transplantation generates neomucosa in dogs. *J Gastrointestinal Surg.* 2009;13:971-982.

55. Grikscheit TC, Ochoa ER, Ramsanahie A, et al. Tissue-engineered large intestine resembles native colon with appropriate in vitro physiology and architecture. *Ann Surg.* 2003;238:35-41.

56. Suh S, Kim J, Shin J, Kil K, Kim K, Kim H, Kim J. Use of omentum as an in vivo cell culture system in tissue engineering. *Am Soc Aritif Int Organs J (ASAIO J).* 2004;50:464-467.

57. Lee H, Cusick RA, Utsunomiya H, Ma PX, Langer R, Vacanti JP. Effect of implantation site on hepatocytes heterotopically transplanted on biodegradable polymer scaffolds. *Tissue Engin.* 2003;9:1227-1232.

58. Dvir T, Kedem A, Ruvinov E, et al. Prevascularization of cardiac patch on the omentum improves its therapeutic outcome. *Proc Natl Acad Sci, USA.* 2009;106:14990-14995.

59. Chen DC, Avansino JR, Agopian VG, et al. Comparison of polyester scaffolds for bioengineered intestinal mucosa. *Cell Tiss Organs.* 2006;184:154-165.

60. Baumert H, Mansouri D, Fromont G, et al. Terminal urothelium differentiation of engineered neoureter after in vivo maturation in the "omental bioreactor". *Euro Urol.* 2007;52:1492-1498.

61. Hattori K, Joraku A, Miyagawa T, Kawai K, Oyasu R, Akaza H. Bladder reconstruction using a collagen patch prefabricated within the omentum. *Int J Urol.* 2006;13:529-537.

62. Baumert H, Simon P, Hekmati M, et al. Development of a seeded scaffold in the great omentum: Feasibility of an in vivo bioreactor for bladder tissue engineering. *Euro Urol.* 2007;52:884-892.

63. Nakase Y, Nakamura T, Kin S, et al. Intrathoracic esophageal replacement by in situ tissue-engineered esophagus. *J Thorac Cardiovasc Surg.* 2008;136:850-859.

64. Kim J, Suh SW, Shin JY, Kim JH, Choi YS, Kim H. Replacement of a tracheal defect with a tissue-engineered prosthesis: early results from animal experiments. *J Thor Cardiovasc Surg.* 2004;128:124-129.

65. Singh AK, Gudehithlu KP, Litbarg NO, Sethupathi P, Arruda JAL, Dunea G. Transplanting fragments of diabetic pancreas into activated omentum gives rise to new insulin producing cells. *Biochem Biophys Res Comm.* 2007;355:258-262.

66. Singh AK, Pancholi N, Patel J, et al. Omentum facilitates liver regeneration. *World J Gastroenterol.* 2009;15:1057-1064.

67. Litbarg NO, Pancholi N, Vujicic S, et al. Activated omentum induces nephrogenesis in the wounded adult rat kidney. *J Am Soc Nephrol.* 2008;19:116A. Abstract.

Chapter 3

APPLICATION OF THE OMENTUM TO THE BRAIN AND SPINAL CORD

HARRY S. GOLDSMITH

INTRODUCTION

The omentum has for decades been known to have important biological characteristics. Surgeons have been particularly impressed by the ability of the omentum to seal intestinal suture lines and wall off inflammatory processes within the peritoneal cavity, such as in appendicitis. Recently, there has been increasing interest in immunologic, angiogenic, and neurochemical agents that have been reported to be present in omental tissue. It is these known and as yet unknown biological substances in omental tissue that may prove a major importance in the future treatment of a host of serious neurological conditions.

BIOLOGICAL PROPERTIES OF THE OMENTUM

Edema absorption

It has been demonstrated that the omentum has an enormous capacity to absorb edema fluid.[1] In order to appreciate this absorptive ability of the omentum, simply place an intact piece of an animal's omentum into a beaker filled with dye (India ink) and saline. Within 30 seconds the dye can be observed in omental lyphatics[2] (*Figure 3.1*). A more practical

experimental study has shown that the omentum can absorb one third of the entire cerebrospinal fluid reservoir when it is placed in the subarachnoid space of an animal.[3] This ability of the omentum to absorb vasogenic edema from the central nervous system (CNS) has obvious clinical potential in conditions where edema fluid removal would be beneficial, as in an acute spinal cord injury.

When an injury to the spinal cord occurs, the force impacting on the spinal cord is delivered either directly or indirectly. From the moment of injury, a cascade of pathobiological events begins to develop within the cord with rapid development of post-injury vasogenic edema, which can become a major factor leading to irreversible cord damage. Shortly after the injury, edema fluid begins to leak through the endothelial lining of damaged blood vessels, mainly the capillaries located in the central gray matter of the cord, with subsequent propagation of the extravasated fluid toward the peripheral white matter. Edema fluid that develops within the injured spinal cord is rich in plasma protein, which has a high osmotic pressure that attracts an increasing amount of edema fluid. As the edema volume increases, it causes the spinal cord to expand within the non-yielding confines of its dura mater covering and the surrounding bony vertebral canal. This cord swelling causes the veins that

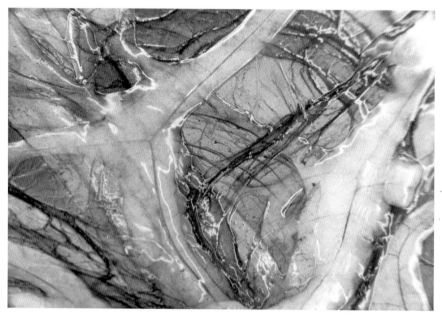

Figure 3.1 (See color section.) Omental lymphatics absorb dye within 30 seconds after immersion in India ink solution.

drain the area of the injury to become compressed thereby elevating venous pressure, which further enhances the capillary extravasation of the edema fluid. The edema-swollen spinal cord, which is being compressed in a confined space, results in an associated interstitial fluid pressure elevation. This increased pressure now begins to exert a progressive compressive effect upon the capillaries located within and adjacent to the site of the spinal cord injury. Fluid mechanics attempt to lower the increased spinal cord interstitial pressure by displacing some of the edema fluid up and down the cord.[4] However, this longitudinal fluid movement cannot compensate for the increasing vasogenic edema that develops within the cord at the injury site. If the spinal cord tissue pressure becomes excessive in the area of the cord injury, capillary perfusion pressure in that area may ultimately be diminished to the point of total vascular cessation. This phenomena leads to irreversible neurologic damage if capillary

circulation is not restored within 4 to 6 hours after injury.

Over the years, decompression laminectomy and, on occasion, myelotomy has been performed in an attempt to lower the elevated spinal cord interstitial pressure caused by the vasogenic edema that develops within an injured spinal cord. However, the uncertainty of clinical improvement that followed these surgical procedures failed to justify their routine performance. It now appears that the simple lowering of a high interstitial tissue pressure within a traumatized spinal cord is important but it is not the only factor that must be addressed in the attempt to prevent permanent cord damage. Another factor that appears necessary to address is the absorption of the vasogenic edema fluid that accumulates at the site of the cord injury, a consideration that may prove of major importance in the future treatment of spinal cord injuries, a subject that will be subsequently discussed.

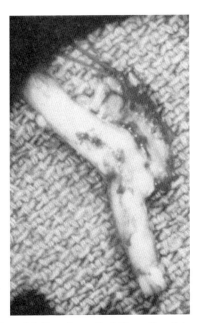

Figure 3.2 (See color section.) Circumferential scar formation has developed several weeks following a standard 400 g cm⁻¹ injury to cat spinal cord. Note dense scar at point of impact with persistent fluid accumulation in area where still-edematous spinal cord has herniated into laminectomy site.

Fibrotic inhibition

It has been observed that spinal cord swelling caused by vasogenic edema persists in the animal and man for weeks after injury by which time a severe fibrotic reaction can develop at the site of trauma[5] (*Figure 3.2*). The reason for the poor neurological results that so frequently persist after a spinal cord injury may well be due largely to the production of this scar tissue. This idea began when it was first noted that improvement occurred in the treatment of experimental spinal cord trauma when the vasogenic edema that accumulates within and around the spinal cord was absorbed by the omentum.[2] This observation raised the question as to whether the decreased edema

fluid that resulted from its absorption by the omentum was the major reason for the decreased scar formation found at the injury site. The spinal cord itself was not felt to be responsible for the edema fluid absorption since there is an absence of a lymphatic system in the CNS.

Surgical procedures on the spinal cord, such as decompression laminectomy and myelotomy, can lower spinal cord interstitial tissue pressure but these operations have no effect on edema. One hypothesis to explain why laying the omentum on the spinal cord leads to minimal scar formation is that a dynamic equilibrium develops at the site of the cord injury between the production of vasogenic edema within the cord and its absorption by the overlying omentum. The fibrotic reaction produced at the site of spinal cord injury is believed to be initiated by the fibrinogen in the plasma-derived vasogenic edema fluid; the fibrinogen being activated to fibrin (scar) by the presence of free blood or petechial hemorrhages in the injured area.[6] When vasogenic edema fluid is absorbed by the omentum, the fibrinogen in the edema fluid would be proportionately decreased, thereby lessening the opportunity for scar development (*Figure 3.3*). Conversely, if a significant volume of vasogenic edema fluid is not absorbed at the injury site, scar formation would more readily develop (*Figure 3.4*). When scar is developing, it would be expected to compress spinal cord capillaries resulting in the progressive ischemia of injured but still viable axons in the area of injury, a situation not conducive to subsequent functional improvement. This suggested hypothesis as to how the omentum can help in a spinal cord injury highlights the importance of limiting the development of scar formation at the site of cord injury so that adequate blood flow can be maintained to injured neurons that survived the force of the spinal cord impact. Maintaining adequate blood flow to prevent progressive ischemia to injured but still repairable neurons

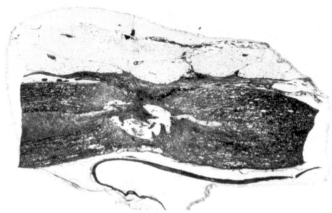

Figure 3.3 Cat spinal cord 30 days after standard spinal cord injury (400 g cm⁻¹). Note omental placement on area of injury with only minimal development of fibrosis. Cat could walk and had positive SEPs (H&E, x12).

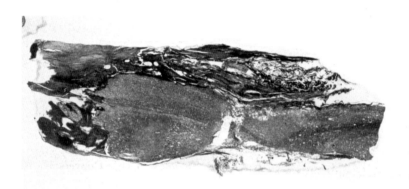

Figure 3.4 Cat spinal cord 30 days after standard spinal cord injury (400 g cm⁻¹). Note extensive scar formation at point of injury. Animal was paralyzed with negative SEPs (H&E, x12).

may prove crucial if neurological improvement is to occur after a spinal cord injury. The omentum can apparently fulfill the requirements for limiting scar formation at a spinal cord injury site by absorbing edema fluid and by increasing vascular perfusion at that location.[7] There is also the unexplored possibility that the omentum, which is replete with a host of biological substances, may contain collagenolytic agents within its tissues that directly impede scar formation.

Blood supply

It was first shown by Vineberg that the omentum can produce vascular channels that grow into surrounding tissues. His classic experiment demonstrated that an isolated piece of omentum placed in the anterior chamber of an animal's eye results in the development of blood vessels between the omentum and the iris within 72 hours[8] (*Figure 3.5*).

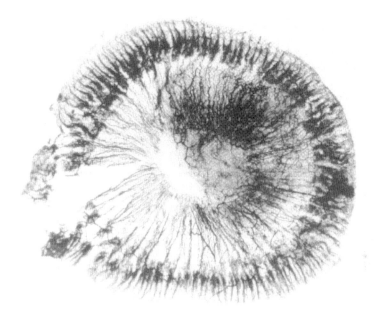

Figure 3.5 First historical slide showing piece of omentum in anterior chamber of rabbit eye. Note robust vascularization within 72 hours between omentum and iris. (Personal gift of the late Dr. Arthur M. Vineberg.)

Starting in the late 1960s, interest in my laboratory began to focus on learning whether omental transposition to the brain and spinal cord could result in the formation of new blood vessels that penetrate the interface that separates the omentum from the underlying CNS tissue. Proof of the development of blood vessels at this omental-cerebral interface was unequivocally confirmed using fluorescein and India ink as dye markers.[9] This confirmation was accomplished by injecting these dye markers into a small catheter that had been inserted within the peritoneal cavity into an omental artery that supplied the elongated omental pedicle that had been previously transposed to the surface of the brain. In order to eliminate any possibility that the injected dye markers might have arrived at the brain through vascular channels other than through omental blood vessels, the head of the dead animal was transected at the neck so that the animal's brain was completely separated from its body except for preservation of the omentum pedicle, which remained intact and connected within the peritoneal cavity. This experimental model ensured that any dye marker found in the brain following its injection into an intra-abdominal artery that supplied the omental pedicle had to have passed through blood vessels at the omental-cerebral interface since complete severance of the animal's head from its body allowed no other vascular route into the brain except through the omental pedicle. Post-mortem studies showed the depths of both cerebral hemispheres. Comparable studies performed on the spinal cord confirmed that injected dye markers travel through vascular connections that develop at the omental-spinal cord interface with the markers being seen within capillaries located on the spinal cord surface (*Figure 3.6A*) and in capillaries deeply positioned in the cord[10] (*Figure 3.6B*)

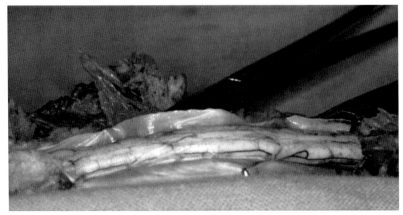

A

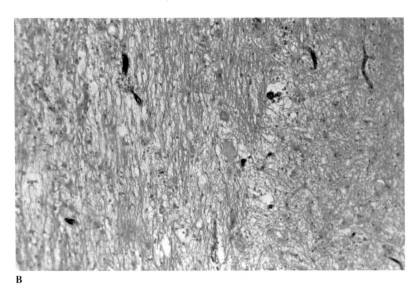

B

Figure 3.6 (See color section.) Omental-spinal cord segment of cat removed *en bloc.* Dye markers injected into an omental artery are apparent **A:** on spinal cord surface and **B:** in deeply located spinal cord capillaries.

After demonstrating that vascular channels did develop between the omentum and underlying CNS tissue (*Figure 3.7*), it was subsequently shown that the pedicled omentum could supply sufficient blood flow through these new vascular channels to prevent cerebral infarction in the dog[11] and the monkey[12] even in the presence of middle cerebral artery (MCA) ligation, as long as the omentum was placed on the brain days to weeks prior to the MCA occlusion. This protection by the omentum against the development of a cerebral infarction indicated that an extensive collateral circulation had formed from the omentum to the brain during the period prior to MCA ligation, which meant that the collateral

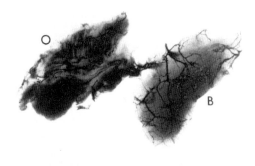

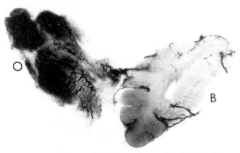

Figure 3.7 Omental (O) and cerebral (B) tissue connected at omental-cerebral interface by blood vessels filled with India ink injected into omental pedicle. Transparency accomplished using methyl salicylate.

circulation had to have developed in the presence of a non-ischemic brain, i.e., there was no need for supplemental cerebral blood flow and, therefore, there was probably an extra cerebral factor causing the collateral circulation to occur. This observation became the basis for the search for an omental angiogenic factor in our laboratory, which took years to discover.[13] The ability of the omentum to develop an extensive collateral circulation to the brain has also been demonstrated to occur in the spinal cord.[10]

Blood-brain barrier penetration

It is now known that omental blood vessels grow directly and deeply into underlying brain (*Figure 3.8*) and spinal cord tissue. When omental transposition to the human brain was first performed in the late 1970s, a theoretical question arose as to whether disruption of the blood-brain barrier (BBB) by penetration of omental blood vessels into the brain might result in detrimental long-term neurological consequences resulting from the continuing entrance into the brain of various neurologically toxic substances present in the systemic circulation. This has not occurred and a large number of patients throughout the world have had their omentum lying on their brain for over a decade with no indication of subjective or objective neurological consequences.[14] In fact, the omentum's ability to allow the introduction of various substances into brain parenchyma, which previously could not penetrate the BBB because of large molecular size or water solubility factors, may now open new areas of clinical investigation and therapy (see Chapter 14).

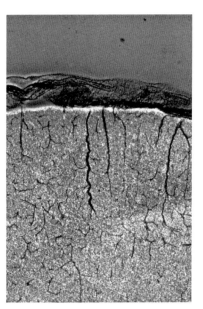

Figure 3.8 (See color section.) Omentum placed on brain shows blood vessels filled with India ink penetrating directly into underlying brain tissue. The blood–brain barrier is broken.

CLINICAL APPLICATION (BRAIN)

It was first reported in 1973 that it is possible to transpose the pedicled omentum to an animal's brain, which results in the delivery of an additional source of blood to that organ.[9] This experiment was the basis for first performing omental transposition (OT) in man in 1978.[15] A request was made at that time of the hospital administrative authorities that the first omental procedures be approved for patients suffering from transient ischemic attacks (TIAs). However, permission for this was not given based on the belief that OT should not be done in the hope of preventing a possible stroke that might never occur in the future. Omental transposition to the brain was therefore first performed on patients who had already suffered a cerebral infarct. (It is still the belief of the author that one of the best indications for the operation is a patient with frequent TIAs.)

The rationale for performing OT in post-stroke patients was based on the concept that there are penumbral cells surrounding cerebral infarcts that remain viable or else they would be part of the infarct. These cells are likely to be depressed, both neurophysiologically and neuroelectrically. It was believed

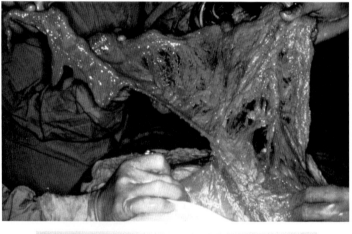

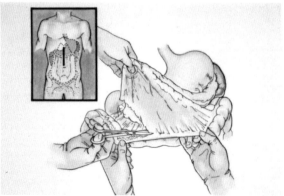

Figure 3.9 First major surgical maneuver is to remove the omentum from the transverse colon. This dissection is relatively avascular.

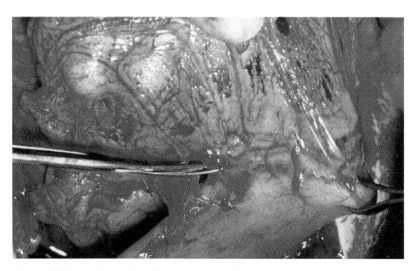

Figure 3.10 (See color section.) Second major surgical maneuver is to remove the omentum from proximal portion of the greater curvature of the stomach. This is tedious because of the numerous small blood vessels connecting the stomach to the omental apron.

that increasing cerebral blood flow (CBF) and neurochemicals to these depressed penumbral cells by way of the omentum might lead to increased biological activity of these cells as reflected by increased dendritic growth, greater synaptic activity, and new nervous pathways that ultimately could result in increased neurological benefit.

Based on the above concept, a small number of patients who had sustained a cerebral infarction months to years earlier underwent omental transposition to their brain. The technical steps in transposing the omentum to the brain has been reported in detail in earlier publications.[16,17] In summary, the first maneuver in the operation is to remove the omentum from the transverse colon (*Figure 3.9*). This is a relatively avascular procedure but one must be gentle since even the handling of the omentum can lead to spontaneous hematoma development, which can expand very rapidly within the omentum.

After the omentum is separated from the colon, it is then removed from the proximal portion of the greater curvature of the stomach, leaving the gastroepiploic vessels within the omental apron. This part of the operation is tedious since there are many small vessels between the greater curvature of the stomach and the gastroepiploic arcade within the omentum that must be individually divided and ligated (*Figure 3.10*). At this point, a decision is required as to whether to divide the left or the right gastroepiploic vessels. I almost always divide the left-sided vessels since the right-sided vessels are larger. (Frequently, no definite left gastroepiploic vessels will be found as one moves proximally up the greater curvature of the stomach.) Following this, the omentum is surgically tailored in a manner so as to obtain its greatest length with the arterial supply to the omental pedicle being maintained primarily along its periphery (*Figure 3.11*). After the omentum has been lengthened sufficiently so that it can reach the top of the head without tension, several transverse skin incisions are made along the chest with an additional incision (transverse or longitudinal, depending on the width of the omentum) made along the medial edge of the sternocleidomastoid muscle on the side of the neck below the cerebral hemisphere that is to be revascularized. A

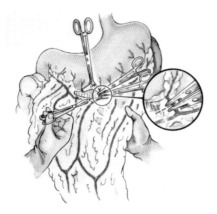

Figure 3.11 Common technique used to surgically tailor the omentum to gain extensive length of the structure with preservation of a major omental artery and vein.

subcutaneous tunnel is then developed, connecting the incisions along the chest and neck through which the omentum is placed. At this stage, the omentum consists of an elongated pedicle that rests in a subcutaneous tunnel on the chest wall and along the anterolateral neck (*Figure 3.12*). The omentum is then brought out from behind the ear and placed directly on the brain, which has been exposed by a craniotomy followed by the opening of the dura mater and excision of pieces of the arachnoid membrane. The scalp flap for the craniotomy must be undermined back from the ear so that the omentum can be brought up to the brain without pressure from the scalp being exerted on the underlying omentum.

After the omentum is laid on the brain, several interrupted sutures are placed between the omentum and the edges of the surrounding dura. The cranial defect is closed by replacing the bone, which has its edges rongeured at the location where the omental pedicle crosses over the intact skull prior to entering the rongeured craniotomy opening to the brain. Tailoring the bone in this manner prevents direct pressure from being exerted on the

omental pedicle by the overlying bone flap.

The initial operative steps in performing OT to the injured spinal cord are comparable to those used with OT to the brain. The abdominal cavity is entered and the omentum is freed from the transverse colon and from a major portion of the greater curvature of the stomach. The omentum is subsequently tailored to gain the omental length that is required for spinal cord application. If a cervical cord injury is to be treated, the omental pedicle is brought to the cervical laminectomy site through a subcutaneous tunnel developed along the chest wall, over the shoulder, and then down to the spinal cord that has had the overlying dura scar tissue and arachnoid membrane removed. The omentum is laid parallel to and directly upon the spinal cord and secured carefully by suturing the omentum to the cut edges of the dura. This is a very important step in the operation since, if done incorrectly, the omentum can subsequently lose its adherence to the spinal cord. Sutures are closely placed in a running fashion between the omentum and the dura which minimizes the possibility of a cerebrospinal fluid (CSF) leak and its subsequent collection. The overlying muscle and fascial layers are then carefully approximated.

When the spinal cord injury to be treated is in the thoracolumbar region, the omentum is brought through a subcutaneous tunnel developed around the flank to the back where it is placed directly on the spinal cord at the appropriate laminectomy site. As more operative experience is gained, improved surgical approaches may be developed that are superior to the standard posterior laminectomy approach. An anterolateral surgical approach deserves evaluation.

Regardless of the surgical approach, what must be stressed to the patient is the importance of intensive postoperative physiotherapy if the procedure is to be effective.

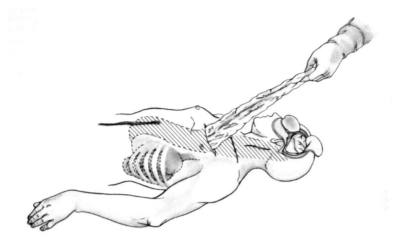

Figure 3.12 (See color section.) Omentum is brought up through a subcutaneous tunnel to the exposed brain.

EXPERIMENTAL AND CLINICAL DATA (BRAIN)

There have been numerous papers published over the past decade that have demonstrated the physiological effects that can occur after the omentum is placed on the brain of an experimental animal. An example is the finding that when OT to the rabbit brain is performed prior to MCA ligation, blood-flow studies using inhaled hydrogen clearance techniques showed only a slight decrease in cerebral blood flow.[18]

Another example of the physiological effectiveness of the omentum was seen in a study in which MCA occlusion in control animals resulted in a marked decrease in somatosensory evoked potential (SEP) amplitude immediately following ligation of the MCA, with a fall to zero level within one half hour.[19] Along with this decrease in neuroelectrical activity was a marked and parallel drop in CBF. In contrast to this were experimental animals who had OT to their brain prior to MCA ligation. These animals with OT showed preservation of their neuroelectrical activity after MCA ligation, as measured by positive SEPs in association with only a mild drop in CBF.

Additional experimental studies have shown that OT to the brain markedly reduced the lowering of cortical levels of biogenic amines that routinely occurs after MCA occlusion.[20] It has also been shown that OT can maintain protein synthesis in the brain to a significant degree[21] and can prevent the formation of brain edema and sodium-potassium flux.[22]

Many human studies have been reported from numerous institutions that have shown that placing the omentum on an ischemic brain can result in neurological improvement in patients treated for the sequelae of a long-standing stroke.[23-25] The clinical improvement that occurred following OT to a stroke victim's brain was obviously independent of any effect on the cerebral infarct itself. The neurological improvement that did occur was most likely caused by the omentum's ability to increase the CBF to the penumbral cells that surround a cerebral infarct, causing the subsequent development of increased physiological and/or bioelectrical activity. The reported omental-derived angiogenic factors,[13,26] neuro-transmitters,[27,28] and neurotrophic substances[29] are also presumed to play an important role following OT to the ischemic brain.

THE FUTURE (BRAIN)

The most common use for the omentum in the presence of brain pathology has been in the treatment of cerebral ischemia. Literally thousands of post-stroke patients have been treated in China by OT and undoubtedly many TIA patients have also been treated successfully in this manner.[30] As described earlier (see Chapter 15), there has been initial information that the omentum may play some future role in the treatment of Alzheimer's disease (AD). The rationale for using the omentum for this condition is to augment acetylcholine (ACh) activity and to increase cerebral blood flow, phenomena known to be depressed in AD. These deficiencies can be rectified by the omentum since it has been shown to increase CBF[31] in addition to having high levels of angiogenic factors[13,26] and neurotransmitters, including choline acetyltransferase (CHAT), the marker for ACh activity.[28]

Based on the above findings for the first time, a patient with AD underwent OT to his brain for this tragic neurodegenerative disease. The patient subsequently showed improvement in his mental status.[32] Of interest and possibly of major importance were the neuropathological findings that were found when the patient was ultimately autopsied 2½ years after OT. On microscopic examination of his brain, the conventional criteria for a definite diagnosis of AD were clearly met in terms of increased density of neocortical senile plaques and neurofibrillary tangles. Moderate cerebrovascular amyloid deposition was also present. Of major interest was the finding in the neocortex beneath the omentum of numerous hypertrophic astrocytes that contained fine

granules of Prussian blue-positive cytoplasmic hemosiderin, a finding not seen in AD patients. Where these unexpected intracellular hemosiderin deposits were observed, significantly fewer senile plaques were seen in the cerebral cortex at the crests of gyri beneath the omentum compared to those present in contiguous depths of the sulci. No comparable gradient of neurofibrillary tangles was observed in these areas and multiple examinations of other cortical regions of both cerebral hemispheres failed to reveal either hemosiderin inclusions or a similar density gradient of senile plaques outside of the area of the omental transposition.[33]

It is unknown at this time whether the neurologic and neuropathologic changes that occurred subsequent to OT resulted from trophic effects of the omentum on local blood flow, microglial activity, or anti-inflammatory action, or by mechanisms that still remain unknown. Control studies on the use of the omentum in the treatment of AD seems warranted and conceivably might lead to mechanisms for reducing senile plaque burden that could lead to a beneficial effort in AD patients, especially in the early stages of the disease.

There are other therapeutic avenues that remain to be explored in the years ahead relating to OT to the CNS. The huge number of patients who have suffered the sequelae of a severe brain injury is a good example. At the First International Congress of Omentum in 1995, Zheng and associates reported 11 patients with hemiplegia and/or aphasia resulting from brain contusion and laceration who were treated by omental transposition to the injured cerebral hemisphere. They reported excellent results in five patients, good in four patients, and fair in two patients, with no postoperative complications.[30] Another paper delivered at this congress by Shao et al entitled "Intracranial pedicled omentum transplantation for grave sequelae of cerebral trauma" also reported favorable results in three patients using this technique.

Another area with potential clinical significance with the use of the omentum is in the treatment of patients with cerebral palsy (CP). An overwhelming number of patients who have this condition do so as a result of a birth injury that causes varying degrees of cerebral anoxia. Assuming that an increased blood flow to the brain could increase oxygen to the structure, omental placement to the brain of CP patients might prove beneficial. Professor Wu has been successful in treating patients suffering from the neurological sequelae of encephalitis (see Chapter 12). He has recently treated more than 125 CP patients with OT and the postoperative results have been encouraging.[34] His long term follow-up results are awaited.

SPINAL CORD: EXPERIMENTAL AND CLINICAL DATA

Since omental transposition was first reported in 1985 on humans with spinal cord injuries,[35] interest continues to increase in evaluating the experimental and clinical effects of the operation.

Based on the biological properties of the omentum, which include absorption of edema and augmentation of blood flow and limiting production of scar development, I believe future clinical studies may show that the optimal way to manage an acute spinal cord injury is to treat the condition as a surgical emergency using the combined effects of decompressive laminectomy, dura mater opening, vertebral column stabilization, and OT to the spinal cord.[36] This belief that the rapid treatment of an injured spinal cord deserves clinical investigation is based on a series of cats who were subjected to a 400 g cm^{-1} injury to their spinal cord using the standard weight-drop technique of Allen. Motor and neuroelectrical somatosensory evoked potential (SEP) evaluations were made 30 days after injury following which the animals were sacrificed. It

was learned from these studies that when the omentum was applied to the spinal cord within 3 hours of injury, there was a statistically significant neurologic and neuroelectrical improvement in these animals compared to controls. However, when there was a 6- to 8-hour delay before omental application to the injured spinal cord, no improvement over control animals was observed[2] (*Figure 3.13*). (*P* values ranged from 0.005 to 0.05 using the Mann-Whitney Test.)

The aforementioned experiments supported the hypothesis that OT to the spinal cord within hours of experimental injury was a major factor in the return of motor and neuroelectrical activity, but transposing the omentum to the spinal cord within 3 hours of injury imposes severe time restrictions in terms of surgical practicality. In order to see if the time limit for the operation could be extended with the same success, additional experiments were undertaken in which OT in conjunction with a variety of pharmacological agents were evaluated for this purpose. Dexamethasone, methylprednisolone, and banamine were studied for their effectiveness but these drugs did not extend the 3-hour time period that OT could be successfully applied after spinal cord injury. However, when dimethyl sulfoxide (DMSO) was used along with OT, a statistically significant difference in preventing paralysis was seen compared to control animals (*Figure 3.14*). Different concentrations of DMSO were infused intravenously 1 hour after trauma, followed by OT 6 hours after injury. It was found that a 40% concentration of DMSO (2 g k^{-1}) was the amount that was most effective in extending the time that the intact omentum could be transposed to the injured spinal cord with an associated improvement in motor and neuroelectrical activity.[37] Since only a single injection of DMSO was given 1 hour after injury, the question that should be asked is whether

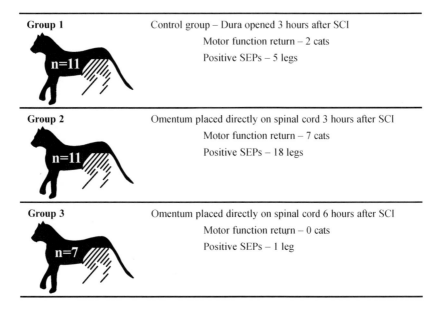

Group 1   Control group – Dura opened 3 hours after SCI
n=11   Motor function return – 2 cats
Positive SEPs – 5 legs

Group 2   Omentum placed directly on spinal cord 3 hours after SCI
n=11   Motor function return – 7 cats
Positive SEPs – 18 legs

Group 3   Omentum placed directly on spinal cord 6 hours after SCI
n=7   Motor function return – 0 cats
Positive SEPs – 1 leg

Figure 3.13 Data showing effect of omentum on a spinal cord injury in relation to time of omental placement.

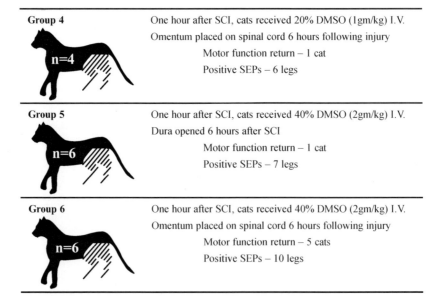

Group 4   One hour after SCI, cats received 20% DMSO (1gm/kg) I.V.
n=4   Omentum placed on spinal cord 6 hours following injury
Motor function return – 1 cat
Positive SEPs – 6 legs

Group 5   One hour after SCI, cats received 40% DMSO (2gm/kg) I.V.
n=6   Dura opened 6 hours after SCI
Motor function return – 1 cat
Positive SEPs – 7 legs

Group 6   One hour after SCI, cats received 40% DMSO (2gm/kg) I.V.
n=6   Omentum placed on spinal cord 6 hours following injury
Motor function return – 5 cats
Positive SEPs – 10 legs

Figure 3.14 Data showing effect of omental transposition on injured cord in association with DMSO administration.

additional DMSO administration, either at more frequent intervals after injury or by continuous intravenous infusion, might allow OT to be effective far longer than 3 hours after injury. The surgical-pharmacological combination of DMSO and OT to the injured spinal cord deserves further investigation.

The goal that has been sought for decades is to develop a method for re-establishing axonal continuity after spinal cord transection that could lead to the return of motor function. Experimental studies using an omental-collagen bridging technique following

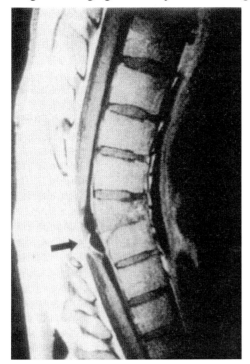

Figure 3.15 Arrow points to what was originally described radiologically as a total anatomical spinal cord transection.

complete spinal cord transection has been reported to be successful in developing axonal outgrowth and coordinated walking in cats.[38,39] The studies showed that surgically reconstructed spinal cords develop dense supraspinal fiber outgrowth across the collagen

matrix bridge supplied by an omental blood source and that these fibers apparently made neo-synaptic contacts with appropriate distal spinal cord target tissue. Of major importance is the report of the early results of a patient who had a long-standing near total transection defect in her spinal cord that extended for 1.6 inches in length, with only 5% to 10% of the posterior cord remaining intact *(Figure 3.15)*. The defect was filled 3½ years after her cord injury with collagen which was then covered with omentum. The patient has achieved continuing and progressive improvement in motor function at 2 years after surgery (see Chapter 6). The future role for the omentum in experimentation and clinical application appears extensive.

REFERENCES

1. Goldsmith HS, de los Santos R, Beattie EJ. The relief of chronic lymphedema by omental transposition. *Ann Surg.* 1967;166:573-585.
2. Goldsmith HS, Steward E, Duckett S. Early application of pedicled omentum to the acutely traumatized spinal cord. *Paraplegia.* 1985;23:100-112.
3. Levander B, Zwetnow NW. Bulk flow of CSF through a lumbo-omental pedicled graft in the dog. *Acta Neurochir.* 1978;41:147-155.
4. Nemecek ST, Peter R, Suba P, Rozsival V, Melka O. Longitudinal extension of edema in experimental spinal cord injury. *Acta Neurochir.* 1977;37:7-16.
5. Goodkin R, Campbell JB. Sequential pathologic changes in spinal cord injury. *Surg Forum.* 1969;20:430-432.
6. Ryan GB, Grobety J, Majno G. Postoperative peritoneal adhesions. *Am J Path.* 1971;65:117-148.
7. de la Torres JC, Goldsmith HS. Increased blood flow augments CNS axon regeneration. In: Goldstein AL, ed. *Biomedical Advances in Aging,* New York: Plenum Press; 1990:447-484.
8. Vineberg A, Shanks J, Pifarre R, et al. Combined internal mammary artery implantation and free omental graft operation: a highly effective revascularization procedure. *Can Med Assoc J.* 1964;90:717-722.
9. Goldsmith HS, Chen WF, Duckett S. Brain vascularization by intact omentum. *Arch Surg.* 1973;106:695-698.

10. Goldsmith HS, Ducklett S, Chen WF. Spinal cord vascularization by intact omentum. *Am J Surg.* 1975;129:262-265.

11. Goldsmith HS, Duckett S. Chen WF. Prevention of cerebral infarction in dog by intact omentum. *Am J Surg.* 1975;130:317-326.

12. Goldsmith HS, Duckett S, Chen WF. Prevention of cerebral infarction in monkey by omental transposition to the brain. *Stroke.* 1978;9:224-229.

13. Goldsmith HS, Griffith AL, Kupferman A, Catsimpoolas N. Lipid angiogenic factor from omentum. *JAMA.* 1984;252:2034-2036.

14. Goldsmith HS, Sax DS. Omental transposition for cerebral infarction: a thirteen year follow-up study. In press.

15. Goldsmith HS, Saunders RL, Reeves AG, Allen CP, Milne J. Omental transposition to the brain of stroke patients. *Stroke.* 1979;10:471-472.

16. Alday ES, Goldsmith HS. Surgical techniques for omental lengthening based on arterial anatomy. *Surg Gynecol Obstet.* 1972;135:103-107.

17. Goldsmith HS. Omental transposition to the brain and spinal cord. *Surg Rounds.* 1986;9:22-33.

18. DeRiu PL, Falzoi A, Papavero L, Rocca A, Viale GL. Local cerebral blood after middle cerebral artery occlusion in rabbits following transposition of omentum to the brain. *J Microsurg.* 1980;1:321-324.

19. DeRiu PL, Rocca A, Falzoi A, Carai M, Papavero L. Physiological function after middle cerebral artery occlusion in rabbits with neovascularization of the brain by transposed omentum. *Neurosurgery.* 1980;7:57-60.

20. Pau A, Viale ES, Turtas S. Effect of omental transposition to the brain on the cortical content of norepinephrine, dopamine, 5-hydroxytryptamine and 5-hydroxy-indoleacetic acid in experimental cerebral ischemia. *Acta Neurochir.* 1982;66:159-164.

21. Cucca GS, Papavero L, Pau A, Viale ES, Turtas S, Viale GL. Effect of omental transposition to the brain on protein synthesis in experimental cerebral ischemia. *Acta Neurochir.* 1980;51:253-259.

22. Pau A, Viale ES, Turtas S, Viale GL. Cerebral water and electrolytes in experimental cerebral ischemia following omental transposition to the brain. *Acta Neurochir.* 1980;54:213-218.

23. Goldsmith HS. Brain and spinal cord revascularization by omental transposition. *Neurol Res.* 1994;16:159-162.

24. Zhu ZC, Wu WL, Mo YZ. Omental transposition to the brain for cerebrovascular occlusive disease. *Chung Hua Wai Ko Tsa Chih.* 1982;20:11-13.

25. Wang CC, Chao YT, Jung DA. Omental transposition and revascularization. In: Bignami A, Bloom FE, Bolis CG, Adeloyle A, eds. *Central Nervous System Plasticity and Repair.* New York: Raven Press; 1985:159-163.

26. Zhang QX, Magovern CJ, Mack CA, Budenbender KT, Ko W, Rosengart TK. Vascular endothelial growth factor is the major angiogenic factor in omentum: mechanism of the omentum-mediated angiogenesis. *J Surg Res.* 1997;67:147-154.

27. Goldsmith HS, McIntosh T, Vezena RM, Colton T. Vasoactive neurochemicals identified in omentum. *Br J Neurosurg.* 1987;1:359-364.

28. Goldsmith HS, Marquis JK, Seik G. Choline acetyltransferase activity in omental tissue *Br J Neurosurg.* 1987;1:463-466.

29. Seik GC, Marquis JK, Goldsmith HS. Experimental studies of omentum derived neurotrophic factors. In: Goldsmith HS, ed. *The Omentum—Research and Clinical Applications.* New York: Springer-Verlag 1990:83-95.

30. Goldsmith HS. The First International Congress of Omentum in CNS. *Surg Neurol.* 1996;45:87-90.

31. Goldsmith HS, Cosso M, Pau A, et al. Regional cerebral blood flow after omental transposition to the ischemic brain in man: a five year follow-up study. *Acta Neurochir.* 1990;106:145-152.

32. Goldsmith HS. Omental transposition for Alzheimer's disease. *Neurol Res.* 1996;18:103-108.

33. Relkin NR, Edgar MA, Gouras GK, Gandy SE, Goldsmith HS. Decreased senile plaque density in Alzheimer neocortex adjacent to an omental transposition. *Neurol Res.* 1996;18:291-294.

34. Professor Wu Wei Lei. Personal communication.

35. Goldsmith HS, Neil-Dwyer G, Barsoum L. Omental transposition to the chronically injured human spinal cord. *Paraplegia.* 1986;24:173-174.

36. Goldsmith HS. Acute spinal cord injuries: a search for functional improvement. In press.

37. Goldsmith HS. The omentum: present status and future applications. In: Goldsmith HS, ed. *The Omentum— Research and Clinical Applications,* New York: Springer-Verlag; 1990:131-145.

38. de la Torre JC, Goldsmith HS. Collagen-omental graft in experimental spinal cord transection. *Acta Neurochir.* 1990;102:152-163.

39. Goldsmith HS, de la Torre JC, Axonal regeneration after spinal cord transection and reconstruction. *Brain Res.* 1992;589:217-224.

CHAPTER 4

EXPERIMENTAL STUDY ON EFFECTS OF OMENTAL TRANSPOSITION IN CATS WITH SPINAL CORD INJURY

YOSHIHITO SHIMADA AND CHICAO NAGASHIMA

INTRODUCTION

Human spinal cord injury experimentation has recently been addressed by several new approaches. One of these involves the use of omentum transposition to the injured spinal cord using vascular anastomoses as proposed by Nagashima.[1,2] The basis for this approach is to treat spinal cord ischemia caused by trauma by preventing or decreasing secondary spinal cord damage. The theory for this is that the omentum, when placed on an injured spinal cord, will absorb vasogenic edema fluid in the area of cord injury. As will be discussed, increased edema absorption improved spinal cord circulation.

The omentum is known to have a variety of neurobiological activities that have been evaluated experimentally[1,3-10] and clinically.[2,11-18] In China, there have been more than 3,000 patients with spinal cord injury who have been treated with an omental pedicle flap placed on their cord, with improvement being reported in motor function, sensory awareness, sphincter activity, autonomic nervous, and sexual recovery.[18] Nagashima has reported the successful use of omental transplantation using a free omental graft with vascular anastomoses,[1,2] as opposed to an omental pedicle.

Goldsmith was the first to show experimentally the favorable biological effects of omental transplantation to the spinal cord.[5,9,10,19] He postulated that one of the main characteristics of the omentum is its ability to absorb edema fluid. Goldsmith considered this function allowed a "dynamic equilibrium" to develop between the formation of vasogenic edema fluid caused by a spinal cord injury and the ability of the omentum to absorb the fluid produced by the injury. Absorption of edema fluid following spinal cord injury (SCI) has been theorized to reduce spinal cord interstitial tissue pressure, which increases capillary perfusion pressure. Additionally, absorbing edema fluid results in a lessening of fluid accumulation at the site of SCI.

There are pathological events that occur in the spinal cord following trauma. Specifically, these are edema, hemorrhage, and necrosis. These post-injury changes create a cavity, which Kao has reported is critical to our understanding of spinal cord degeneration and subsequent cord healing.[20-22] This work was the basis for deciding to study in detail the formation of a spinal cord cavity following injury and the progress of its resolution.

A reproducible spinal cord injury model was used based on a modified Allen weight-drop method.[23,24] This experimental technique resulted in comparable spinal cord injury cavities that were carefully measured using an image Digital Analyzer (MG-002, Muto Co., Japan) that allowed for the evaluation of the healing process of an injured spinal cord. This technique was used in all the animals in the study so that spinal cord cavity characteristics following injury could be carefully evaluated pathohistologically and neurophysiologically.

MATERIALS AND METHODS

Twenty-three adult cats (weight range 3.0-4.0 kg) were used in this experiment. After the animals were anesthetized, they were subject to a laminectomy that extended from T12 to L3. Allen's original weight-drop method was carried out to create the spinal cord injury. However, dropping a 2.9-g weight from a height of 17 cm directly onto the posterior surface of the spinal cord proved unsuccessful in creating a reproducible cord injury. Allen's weight-drop technique was then modified to that proposed by Sasaki, in which a 2x8x1 mm, 5-mg weight made of a balsa wood plate was used. The plate was placed on the dura-over the surface of the spinal cord and a 5.8g weight was dropped on the plate from a height of 17 cm, which created a 100 g cm^{-1} injury that was successful in creating reproducible spinal cord injuries.

The 23 cats in the study were divided into two groups. Twelve cats had their omentum placed directly on their injured spinal cord by mobilizing the omentum on a long pedicle, after which it was brought to the spinal cord for placement. These surgical manipulations were done under the microscope according to the techniques of Goldsmith[19] and Masumori.[6,25]

The control group in this study was comprised of 11 cats whose spinal cord was injured in an identical manner as the experimental group. The control animals, however, did not have their spinal cord covered with omentum, but with a layer of dental cement.

India ink perfusion techniques and histological studies

An India ink perfusion study was performed.[25] At 1, 2, 3, and 4 weeks after SCI, both control and omental transposition cats underwent a laparotomy under anesthesia at which time their celiac artery was cannulated with a #5 French catheter. The spleen was then removed, the common hepatic artery ligated, and branches from the celiac artery coagulated. At this point, the thoracic cavities were opened and 10 mL 1% xylocaine was injected directly into the heart. Thirty milliliters of India ink were drop infused under 150 cm H_2O pressure through the catheter that had been previously placed in the celiac artery. Following this infusion, the spinal cords of the cats were removed from T10 to L3 in an *en bloc* manner, which included spinal bone elements and meninges. These specimens were fixed and processed in an alcohol dehydration series, after which they were embedded in paraffin. Serial sections were made and stained with hematoxylin and eosin (H&E) and Kluver Barrera (KB), after which the slides were studied under a light microscope. Other immunohistochemical stains were used on some specimens when it was felt appropriate.

Spinal cord cavity analysis

The spinal cord cavities that developed within the cord following injury were carefully analyzed to measure the areas of the cavity. This was done by taking the H&E stained sections and photographing them at 30-times magnification. By this technique, the spinal cord cavities caused by the SCI could be precisely measured. The largest area of the cavity was determined microscopically by evaluating serial sections of the cord and, if the margins of a particular cavity were unclear, adjacent serial sections were measured. Statistical determinations of these measurements were performed using a student *t*-test.

Somatosensory evoked potentials

Somatosensory evoked potential (SEP) recordings were recorded using an MEB 5100 Neuropack 2 (Nihon Kohden Corp.). Stimulating electrodes were placed on the sciatic nerve, which had been exposed at the dorsal area of the thigh with the recording electrodes inserted epidurally 1 cm rostral from T13. After stimulating the sciatic nerves, the SEPs were recorded. These recordings were taken immediately before and after SCI, and weekly thereafter until the animal's death. The recording electrodes were kept in their inserted position during the cat's survival period.

FINDINGS

As previously mentioned at the beginning of the study, a 2.9-g weight was dropped from a 17 cm height (50 g cm-¹) according to Allen's original weight-drop method. However, this method did not always create a spinal cord injury cavity. In order to rectify this situation, the weight dropped on the spinal cord was increased to 7.9 g from a height of 17 cm (150 g cm-¹ injury). This caused spinal cord cavitation in the cats but they all died within one week after injury. At this point, 5.8 g was used for the weight drop (100-g/cm injury). This technique allowed all the animals to survive but the size of the spinal cord injury cavities differed in each animal. A final experimental modification was developed that produced a reproducible cavity and survival in all the cats by dropping a 5.8-g weight on a "balsa plate" overlying the spinal cord, which created a 100-g/cm injury. Two to three days after their spinal cord, injury, the cats began to walk dragging their hind limbs, with no differences noted in the abnormal walking patterns of the control and the omental-collagen cats.

Macroscopic examination

The injured spinal cords of all the animals were removed *en bloc* at different times following injury. At 1 week post-injury, the spinal cords were swollen to 1½ times the size of a normal cord but by 3 to 4 weeks after trauma, the size of the spinal cords had returned to normal with no macroscopic changes being noted.

Microscopic examination

Figures 4.1 and 4.2 demonstrate by light microscopy the findings at 1 and 4 weeks after injury in the spinal cords of control and omental cats. Both groups at 1 week showed hemorrhagic and necrotic changes most notably at the posterior horn and at the funiculus with extension into the lateral funiculus, the changes being asymmetrical. Hemorrhagic necrosis was noted in the cord tissue surrounding the injury-caused cavity. The areas with hemorrhagic necrosis also had many small vacuoles and when these findings were most pronounced, cavity formation had already begun. In association with this was demyelination, which was most notable around the posterior horn and the posterior and anterior funiculi: with these pathological changes radiating in a central to peripheral direction.

In comparing the control and omental groups, the proliferation of connective tissue with lymphocyte infiltration was noted in the control group adjacent to the "dental cement," which had been laid directly on the cord after its injury. However, in the cats who had the omentum laid on their injured spinal cord, a fibrous coat (FC)[19] had developed that was 2 to 4 µm in width and extended to the edges of the dura, which had previously been incised over the injured spinal cord. Both groups of cats displayed almost comparable degrees of hemorrhagic necrosis, with this finding being observed mainly around the posterior horn and funiculi. It was also noted that the cavity caused by the weight-drop injury to the cord appeared to be more lucent at the margin of the cavity in the omental cats as compared to the control animals. The margins of the cavity seen in the omental cats was partially formed by glial processes by the end of the first   week following injury, indicating that the healing process had already begun.

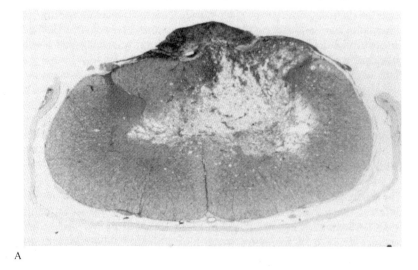

A

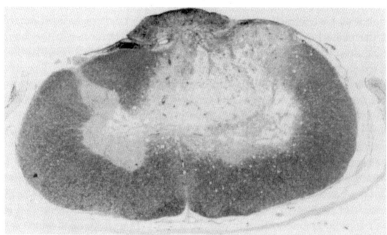

B

Figure 4.1 Light micrographs of the spinal cord 1 week after trauma (x20). Control group stained with **A:** H&E, **B:** KB. Omental transposition group stained with **C:** H&E, **D:** KB. In **C, D,** the omentum (O) and fibrous coat (FC) is seen overlying the spinal cord. Force of the weight dropping on the midposterior dural-enveloped spinal cord produced hemorrhagic necrosis in the areas of the posterior columns, posterior and anterior horns, and gray commisure in both groups. Size and extent of the injured areas are almost the same in both groups, more clearly shown in KB stains in **B** and **D.**

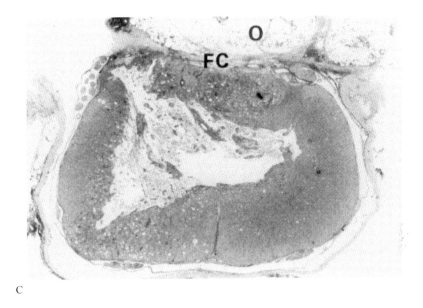

C

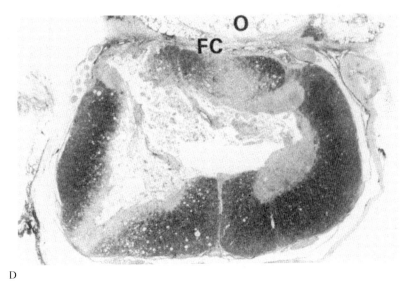

D

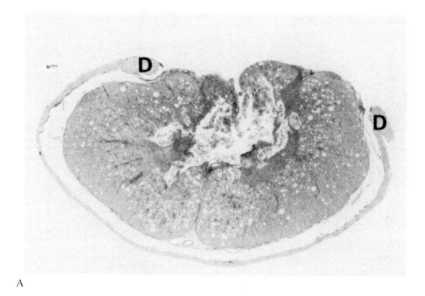

A

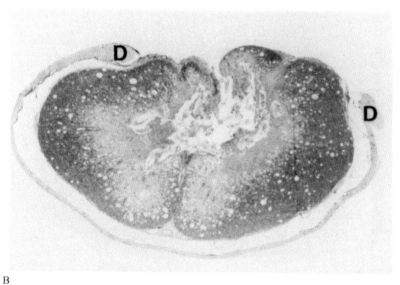

B

Figure 4.2 Light micrographs of the spinal cord at 4 weeks after trauma (x20). Control group stained with **A:** H&E, **B:** KB. Omental transposition group stained with **C:** H&E, **D:** KB. In **C, D,** transposed omentum is seen above the fibrous coat (FC) connecting both dural edges. Underneath the FC is seen fine structures resembling the arachnoid, the   subarachnoid space and pia with probable re-establishment of the CSF pathway. In **A, B,** dural edges (D) are kept opened, the spinal cord is slightly protruded with probable obstruction of CSF circulation due to leptomeningeal adhesions. There is persistent hemorrhagic necrosis and numerous, scattered, small and large vacuoles throughout the injured cord (**A** and **B**) controls. In **C, D,** omentum hemorrhagic necrosis is not observed. Note central polygonal cavity lined by ependymal cell layer and glial fibrils, with preservation of surrounding spinal cord parenchyma.

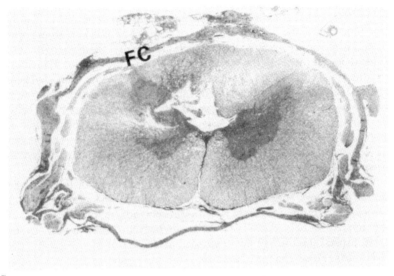

C

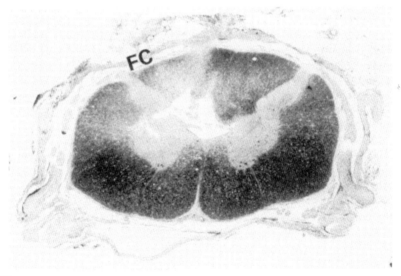

D

The spinal cord injury cavities in both groups decreased in size by this time but in the control animals, an increase in ischemic injury was more histologically evident. By a month after injury, these changes were evident in the area of the posterior horn and the anterior funiculus, locations that received the brunt of the weight-drop injury. These changes included multilobular tissue-lacking spaces in which there were many small amorphous tissue fragments intermingled with red blood cells. Surrounding these fragments were white blood cell accumulations in association with lymphocytes. Additionally, many vacuoles were present in the white matter with spongy degeneration and severe demyelination occurring in a central to peripheral direction.

When the dura mater had been opened over the site of the SCI, the spinal cord was found to be bulging out from the dural edges in association with the arachnoid, which was found adherent to the surface of the injured spinal cord. These changes lead to what appear to be cerebrospinal fluid (CSF) flow blockage at the site of SCI (*Figures 4.2A and 4.2B*). These changes, however, were not found in the cats whose injured cord had been covered with

omentum, which was still intact with the underlying FC that was continuous with the incised dural edges. The FC was a thin mesenchymal covering that was loosely attached to the pia mater and resembled arachnoid membrane. This physical arrangement suggested that it was possible for CSF to flow around the area of the SCI.

Within the spinal cord of these omental-treated cats was the absence of hemorrhagic necrosis. However, a polygonal irregular-shaped cavity was present in the center of the cord but it was markedly smaller than the cavity seen in control cats. In the white mater surrounding the cavity, no spongy degeneration was observed in either group of cats but demyelination was noted in both groups in the area of the posterolateral funiculus, with the process being much less in the omental cats as compared to the control animals (*Figures 4.2C and 4.2D*).

Cross-sectional areas of the injury-induced spinal cord cavities in all the cats in this study (*Table 4.1*) were carefully measured by evaluation serial histological sections by an image digital analyzer (*Figure 4.3*). The mean value of the cross-sectional areas of all cavities

Table 4.1 Maximum cross-sectional areas (μm^2) of the cavities obtained from serial histological slides of 23 cats' spinal cords measured by Image Digital Analyzer

Week(s) Post-trauma	Control group (n =11)				Omental transposition group (n =12)			
	1	2	3	4	1	2	3	4
μm^2	2723.33	7420.88	1042.38	2307.85	4553.67	6733.71	1858.66	520.02
	2943.65	377.00	2899.40	951.72	1823.48	1201.68	840.70	372.23
	5050.03			1075.03	7432.37			739.01
				758.03				423.33
								108.90
Means	3572.33	5398.94	1970.89	1279.90	4603.17	3967.69	1349.68	432.69
SD	1284.45	2859.45	1313.11	695.52	2804.77	3911.73	719.80	299.15

* Image Digital Analyzer: MG-002, Muto Co., Ltd.

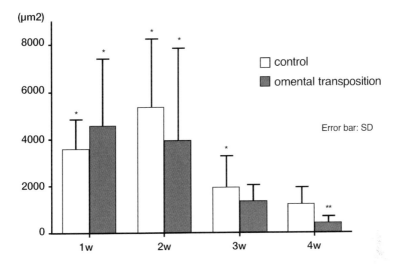

Figure 4.3 Bar graph illustrating mean changes in size of cavities between control and omental transposition groups at 1, 2, 3, and 4 weeks after injury. *$P<0.05$ compared to 4 weeks post-trauma of each group. **$P<0.05$ compared to   4 weeks post-trauma of control group

showed a tendency for the cavities to reduce in size. Cavities were smaller 2 weeks following injury compared to 1 week but at 4 weeks, both groups had significantly smaller cavities than those that were present at 1 and 2 weeks ($P<0.05$). However, 4 weeks after surgery, the animals with omental covering their SCI had statistically significant reduction in their spinal cord cavity size as compared to the control cats ($P<0.05$).

Immunohistochemistry: macrophages and glia cells

Histological examination of the omental-treated cats at 1 week following SCI showed that hemosiderin was being phagocytized by macrophages.[26] The macrophages were seen adjacent to the FC and pial vessels, and along vessels penetrating into the injured spinal cord (*Figure 4.4*). The macrophages were believed to be related to tissue repair. Situated around endothelial tissue within the injured spinal cord were round-shaped, chromatin-rich cells that

had accumulated and formed the so-called perithelial cell-proliferation pattern. At first, these cells were believed to be microglia but various staining techniques did not confirm this. Additionally, gemistocytic astrocytes were observed. Of major interest is that these histologic findings were found only in the omental-treated cats; they were not found in the control cats.

India ink perfusion

By the first and second week after SCI in the cats treated with omental placement, newly formed sinusoidal vessels were clearly evident in the pial membrane and in the spinal cord itself. By week three, India ink particles were seen in large numbers in the sinusoidal vessels of the FC (*Figure 4.5*). By the fourth week, the India ink particles were seen along vessels that had penetrated into the spinal cord. The finding of India ink particles that were evident in the omental transposition cats was not observed in control cats.

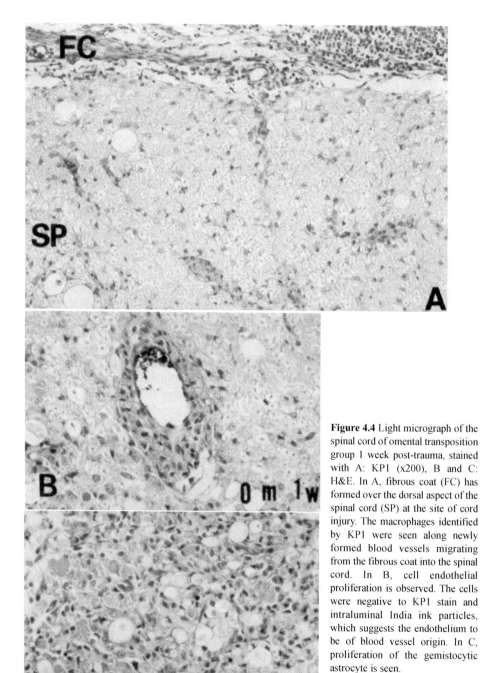

Figure 4.4 Light micrograph of the spinal cord of omental transposition group 1 week post-trauma, stained with A: KP1 (x200), B and C: H&E. In A, fibrous coat (FC) has formed over the dorsal aspect of the spinal cord (SP) at the site of cord injury. The macrophages identified by KP1 were seen along newly formed blood vessels migrating from the fibrous coat into the spinal cord. In B, cell endothelial proliferation is observed. The cells were negative to KP1 stain and intraluminal India ink particles, which suggests the endothelium to be of blood vessel origin. In C, proliferation of the gemistocytic astrocyte is seen.

Neurophysiological findings: SEPs

Somatosensory evoked potentials taken in all cats prior to SCI showed normal wave patterns consisting of biphasic and triphasic components. These patterns disappeared immediately after injury. This loss of reproducible wave patterns persisted over the next several weeks but by the third and fourth postoperative week, a normal wave pattern with a smaller amplitude became apparent in the omental transposition cats. This wave pattern was seen in three of five experimental cats (*Figure 4.6*). But the wave pattern remained flat in the control animals.

DISCUSSION

We have found that placing omental pedicle on a spinal cord injured by a modified Allen technique successfully reduced the development of hemorrhagic necrosis and cavity formation, a situation not seen in control animals. This is believed to be due to self-defense mechanisms inherent in omental tissue and its ability to absorb fluid. In addition, the presence of angiogenic factors,[9,27] neurotransmitters,[28,29] and nerve growth factors[30] in omental tissue may also play a role.

Of interest was the finding that macrophages migrated to the spinal cord from the newly formed and overlying fibrous coat, which was located directly below the omentum. Also of interest were "omental milky spots" and the more recent "omentum-associated lymphoid tissue" reported by Shimotsuma, which is an accumulation of lymphatic cells and macrophages. These macrophages apparently phagocytise the injured spinal cord in which there is decreased blood flow, hypoxia, and lactic acid accumulation, which results in tissue swelling, necrosis, and cavitation.[18] Of major importance is that these macrophages, which originate in the omentum and migrate to the injured cord, occurred only in the cats with omental placement. They were not found to be present in control animals. Perithelial cell proliferation was present adjacent to the macrophages (*Figure 4.4B*), which was believed to be caused by microglia, but the cell of origin remains unknown. Also associated with the macrophages were clusters of gemistocytic astrocytes (*Figure 4.4C*), which are believed to be related to microglia[31,32] that are involved in dendritic elongation and neuronal activity.

The macrophage proliferation and migration from the omentum is believed to be of major importance in the repair of an injured spinal cord.

Goldsmith first reported the presence of an FC on the surface of a spinal cord, which developed within 4 days following omental transposition.[10,19] Masumari further studied the effect of omental transposition on the normal spinal cord and found that neurtrophils and macrophages rapidly infiltrated at the omental spinal cord interface, with these cells decreasing and disappearing by 1 week.[6,25] By the second week, fibroblast proliferation had begun and the FC began to form from the dural edges. By 3 weeks after omental transposition, the FC had become rich with sinusoidal vessels, collagen, and elastic fibers that appeared to be comparable to dural tissue. In the authors' experience, however, it was found that placing the omentum on the injured cord caused considerable fibrous development within the first week and the early appearance of the FC thereafter (*Figures 4.1C and 4.1D*).

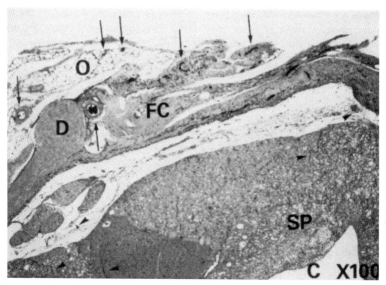

Figure 4.5 Light micrograph of spinal cord of omental transposition group 3 weeks after trauma, with India ink perfusion. SP: spinal cord and C: cavity. India ink particles are seen in small vessels of omentum, fibrous coat (vertical arrows), pial vessels, and in the intramedullary small vessels (arrow heads) (x100, H&E stain).

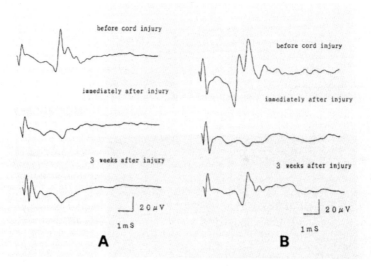

Figure 4.6 Pre- and post-injury somatosensory evoked potential waves in A: control, B: omental transposition group. Before injury, normal wave pattern consisting of successive positive, negative, positive waves were seen in A and B. This disappears immediately post-injury. Three weeks after injury, a more normal wave pattern can be detected in B.

In the healing of a wound, cytokines and cell growth factors are secreted from inflammatory cells, which leads to the proliferation of more cells and fibers.[33] The reason FC developed slowly in non-injured spinal cords with omental transposition but faster in injured cords suggests that mesenchymal cells originating from the omentum are stimulated by the injured cord and play a key role in forming the FC, which is considered important in the healing process of the injured cord. Increased blood flow might also play a key part in FC development since India ink particles were clearly seen in sinusoidal vessels of the FC at 4 weeks (following omental transposition to the injured spinal cord, whereas this observation was not present in cats with spinal cord injury and no omental coverage.

Somatosensory evoked potential recordings have proved useful in estimating spinal cord function.[34] All cats in this present study showed a flat wave pattern, which occurred immediately after spinal cord injury. This flat wave pattern persisted in the control animals but by 3 weeks after injury, three of the five cats with omental transposition showed reappearance of their SEP. Goldsmith reported the same SEP findings 30 days after injury in animals with omental transposition to their injured cord.[10] Demyelination was also noted to be less severe in their omental transposition cats as compared to control animals (*Figures 4.2B and 4.2D*).

CONCLUSION

The effects of omental transposition on injured spinal cords of cats were studied using a modified Allen weight-drop method.

- Cavity formation was noted histologically at 1 week after injury in both the omental transposition and control groups. As the weeks passed, the size of the cavity became progressively smaller. By 4 weeks after injury, the size of the cavity in the omental transposition cats was statistically less than that in the control animals.

- After injury, the severity and extent of demyelination around the injured cavity was far greater in control animals than in omental transposition cats.

- Hemorrhagic necrosis, which occurred following spinal cord injury, persisted in control animals but by 4 weeks had disappeared in omental transposition cats.

- By 1 week after injury a FC developed on the surface of the injured spinal cord of cats with omental transposition. The FC thickened by 3 weeks and by 1 month following trauma, the FC had become continuous with fusion to the incised dural edges, which had become rich in sinusoidal vessels. The arachnoid membrane was clearly evident beneath the FC in the omental transposition cats, a finding not present in control animals.

- India ink was observed in sinusoidal vessels of the FC by 3 weeks after SCI in omental transposition cats and by 4 weeks, the dye marker was present within the spinal cord. No India ink was observed in the control animals at any time in these locations.

- Somatosensory evoked potentials reverted to flat wave pattern immediately after SCI in all the cats. However, in the omental transposition group, there was reappearance of a normal wave pattern 3 to 4 weeks after injury. Somatosensory evoked potentials did not reappear in the control animals.

The above findings strongly suggest that omental transposition facilitates the healing of an injured spinal cord. This could be expected to be most effective in treating an acute spinal cord injury as quickly as possible following the injury.

REFERENCES

1. Nagashima C. Spinal cord regeneration and omental transplantation to the cord with microangioanastomosis. *Spine Spinal Cord.* 1991;4:879-886.
2. Nagashima C, Masumori Y, Shimada Y, Kubota S, Hori E, Heshiki J. Omentum transplantation to the cervical cord with microangioanastomosis. *Neurol Surg.* 1991;19:309-318.
3. Azzena GB, Campus G, Mameli D, et al. Omental transposition or transplantation to the brain and superficial temporal artery-middle cerebral artery anastomosis in preventing experimental cerebral ischemia. *Acta Neurochir.* 1983;68:63-83.
4. DeRiu PL, Rocca A, Falzoi A, Carai M. Papavero L. Physiological function after middle cerebral artery occlusion in rabbits with neovascularization of the brain by transplanted omentum. *Neurosurgery.* 1980;7:57-60.
5. Goldsmith HS, Chen WF, Duckett S. Brain vascularization by intact omentum. *Arch Surg.* 1973;106:695-698.
6. Masumori Y. Ultrastructural study of neovascular connections between the spinal cord and transposed omentum in the cat. *J Saitana Med School.* 1991;18:345-357.
7. Yasagil MG, Yonekawa Y, Denton I, Piroth D, Benes I. Experimental intracranial transplantation of autogenic omentum majus. *J Neurosurg.* 1974;39:345-357.
8. Yonekawa Y, Yasagil MG. Brain vascularization by transplanted omentum: a possible treatment of cerebral ischemia. *Neurosurgery.* 1977;13:25.
9. Goldsmith HS, Griffith A, Kupferman A, Catsimpoolas N. Lipid angiogenetic factor from omentum. *JAMA.* 1984;252:2034-2036.
10. Goldsmith HS, Steward E, Duckett S. Early application of pedicled omentum to the acutely traumatized spinal cord. *Paraplegia.* 1985;23:100-111.
11. Abraham J, Paterson A, Bthra M. Omento-myelo-synangiosis in the management of chronic traumatic paraplegia. *Paraplegia.* 1987;25:44-49.
12. Goldsmith HS, Saunders RL, Reeves AG, Allen CD, Milne J. Omental transposition to brain of stroke patients. *Stroke.* 1979;10:471-472.
13. Goldsmith HS, Neil-Dwyer G, Barsoum L. Omental transposition to the chronic injured human spinal cord. *Paraplegia.* 1986;24:173-174.
14. Herold S, Frackoviak RSJ, Neil-Dwyer G. Studies of cerebral blood flow and oxygen metabolism in patients with established cerebral infarcts undergoing omental transposition. *Stroke.* 1987;18:46-51.
15. Goldsmith HS, Cossu M, Pau A, et al. Regional cerebral blood flow after omental transposition to the ischemic brain in man: a five year study. *Acta Neurochir.* 1990;106:145-152.
16. Karasawa J, Kikuchi H, Kawamura J, Sakai T. Intracranial transplantation of the omentum for cerebrovascular moyamoya disease: a two year follow up study. *Surg Neurol.* 1980;14:444-449.
17. Sayama I, Kukazawa H, Yasui N, Suzuki A. Child with moyamoya disease after bypass surgery. *Neurol Med Chir.* 1982;25:857-859.
18. Zhou T. The actual state of omental transposition for spinal cord injury in China. *Spine Spinal Cord.* 1992;5:127-130.
19. Goldsmith HS, Duckett S, Chen WF. Spinal cord vascularization by intact omentum. *Am J Surg.* 1975;129:262-265.
20. Kao CC, Chang LW. The mechanism of spinal cord cavitation following spinal cord transection. Part 1: a correlated histochemical study. *J Neurosurg.* 1977;46:197-209.
21. Kao CC, Chang LW, Bloodworth JMB. The mechanism of spinal cord cavitation following spinal cord transection. Part 2: electron microscopic observations. *J Neurosurg.* 1977;46:745-756.
22. Kao CC, Chang LW, Bloodworth JMB. The mechanism of spinal cord cavitation following spinal cord transection. Part 3: delayed grafting with and without spinal cord reconstruction. *J Neurosurg.* 1977;46:757-766.
23. Allen AR. Surgery of experimental lesion of spinal cord equivalent to crush injury of fracture dislocation of spinal column: preliminary report. *JAMA.* 1911;57:878-880.
24. Allen AR. Remarks on the hisotpathological changes in the spinal cord due to impact. An experimental study. *J Nerve Ment Dis.* 1914;41:141-147.
25. Masumori Y, Nagashima C, Nakamura H. Experimental omento-myelo-synangiosis. *Surg Neurol.* 1992;38:411-417.
26. Pulford KAF, Rigney EM, Micklem KJ, et al. KPI: a new monoclonal antibody that detects a monocyte/macrophages associated antigen in routinely processed tissue sections. *J Clin Pathol.* 1989;42:412-421.
27. Toshio I. Purification and characterization of endothelial cell growth factor from the bovine greater omentum. *J Sapporo Med.* 1989;58:59-70.
28. Goldsmith HS, McIntosh T, Vesina R, Colton T. Vasoactive neurochemicals identified in omentum. *Br J Neurosurg.* 1987;1:359-364.

29. Goldsmith HS, Marwuis JK, Siek G. Choline acetyl transferase activity in omental tissue. *Br J Neurosurg.* 1987;1:463-466.

30. Siek G, Maquis JK, Goldsmith HS. Experimental studies of omentum-derived neurotrophic factors. In: Goldsmith HS, ed. *The Omentum—Research and Clinical Applications,* New York: Springer-Verlag; 1990:109-116.

31. Matsumoto Y. Immune defense mechanism in the central nervous system: role of microglia and astrocytes. *Brain Nerve.* 1992;44:881-892.

32. Nakajima K, Kohsaka S. Rat microglia secrete plasminogen that is a potent stimulator for neuronal growth and function. *Exper Med.* 1993;11:139-145.

33. Clark RA. Cutaneous tissue repair: basic biological considerations. *J Am Acad Dermatol.* 1985;13:701-725.

34. Kubota S, Nagashima C, Ohmori S. Segmental spinal somatosensory evoked potentials in cervical myelopathies due to spondylosis, ossification of the posterior longitudinal ligament and developmental cervical stenosis. *Neuro-orthopedics.* 1988;5:25-35.

CHAPTER 5

EFFECT OF THE OMENTUM ON AXONAL REGENERATION FOLLOWING COMPLETE SPINAL CORD TRANSECTION

HARRY S. GOLDSMITH AND JACK DE LA TORRE

INTRODUCTION

When the mammalian spinal cord is completely divided, total paraplegia results due to a variety of factors, some of which can negatively influence axonal regeneration. Even though physical and chemical events occur in the cord that impede successful regeneration of divided central spinal cord axons, there has been increasing evidence that transected mammalian axons have the capacity to regrow and develop new connections with nerve tissue distal to the transection site. Such axons appear to display orderly neuroelectrical activity[1,2] and apparent functional return.[3]

Ramon y Cajal has often been misquoted as saying that successful central nervous system (CNS) regeneration was impossible when in fact, he claimed that functional regeneration could be accomplished if the chemical and physical obstacles to central neuritic outgrowth were identified and corrected.[4] It now appears that Cajal was correct in his reasoning.

A major observation that has been made following spinal cord injury (SCI) is the decreased blood flow that occurs at the site of injury.[5,6] The reduced microcirculation that results from SCI may be a major factor in contributing to the absence of effective regrowth of neural processes, since the trophic and metabolic substrates needed for neuritic repair are pathologically depressed. It has

therefore been theorized that a normalized blood supply to an area of SCI might be a crucial effect on the regenerative rate and/or the density of divided axons. Based on this concept, it was postulated and subsequently shown that placing an intact omental pedicle on a normal or injured spinal cord could revascularize underlying spinal cord tissue.[7-9] Also of experimental interest was the demonstration that a completely transected spinal cord could have the defect (gap) resulting from the cord transection reconstructed by a collagen matrix. The collagen matrix that connected the divided proximal and distal spinal cord segments led to morphological, neuroelectric, and apparent functional improvement in the animal model.[1,2]

MATERIALS AND METHODS

In order to evaluate the effect of the omentum on spinal cord blood flow (SCBF) following cord transection and whether an improved SCBF could influence the density or rate of axonal regeneration, cats were chosen for the animal model.[10] The reason this species of animal was used was the relative reliability of examining the neurophysiological and morphological end points in a feline model, whose functional improvement could be tested by analysis of the cat's well-known gait pattern.

Twelve conditioned female cats were given 20,000 U kg^{-1} of long-acting penicillin-streptomycin intravenously and fasted for 12 hours. Following the administration of a methoxyflurane-oxygen mixture to anesthetize the animals, a posterior laminectomy was performed between T8 and T10. After the spinal cord with its dural covering was exposed, it was cooled for 10 minutes using an ice-saline slush mixture to harden the cord and promote vasoconstriction. Following the cord cooling, the dura was cut between T8 and T10 and a guide suture was placed under the cord to facilitate and verify spinal cord transection at T9. The spinal cord was completely transected at this level using a very fine-edged razor blade. Completeness of the spinal cord transection was verified by two observers using a surgical microscope set at high power. Total confidence that the spinal cord had been completely transected was proven by the ability to lift and remove the previously placed guide suture through the gap separating the divided spinal cord stumps.

The 3-mm gap at the spinal cord transection site was then flooded with ice-saline sludge for 15 minutes, which almost totally prevented axoplasmic extrusion from the cord stumps, a situation that normally occurs after spinal cord transection. The ice-saline sludge also accelerated hemostasis. At this point, the gap between the spinal cord stumps was gently dried with cotton pledgets.

Ten cats were randomly divided into 2 groups. Group I had the gap between the transected spinal cord filled with collagen, which was covered with an omental pedicle graft (COM). The cats in Group II had spinal cord transection only. Two additional cats without cord transection were used as nonsurgical intact controls.

The collagen used in Group I was sterile Type I 35 mg mL^{-1} (Collagen Corporation, Palo Alto, Calif). The material was taken directly from the refrigerator at a temperature of 4°C and

dispensed from a sterile syringe into the cord transection site until the interstump gap was totally filed with the semi-liquid collagen. The collagen was then allowed to polymerize for 45 to 60 minutes, after which time it had hardened into a gel that created a tight bond with the proximal and distal spinal cord interfaces at the transection site. Collagen is biocompatible and biodegradable.

In preparing the cats who were to have their omentum placed on the collagen at the cord transection site, a 4-cm left subcostal laparotomy incision was made, with the omentum subsequently being surgically lengthened into a long pedicle. This vascularized pedicle of omentum was then inserted in a subcutaneous tunnel that was developed at the abdominal incision, carried around the flank and then down to the spinal cord transection site at T9. The omentum was placed directly upon the surface of the collagen bridge that connected the transected proximal and spinal cord stumps. All incisions were closed in a routine layered fashion.[11]

The collagen used in the Group I (COM) cats had neuroactive agents mixed into the collagen before it hardened. The following materials were used: 4-aminopyridine (4-AP, 5 µg); laminin (LAM, 5 µg); glia maturation factor-B (GMF-B, 10 µg); lipid angiogenic factor (LAF, 5 mg); physiological saline (SAL, 5 mL); and the vehicle used for the above agents.

Cats were kept sedated for 36 hours after surgery to minimize vertebral movements and to allow for optimal fixation of the collagen to the proximal and distal spinal cord stumps. They received daily postoperative care, which included monitoring of vital signs, fluid intake-output recordings, and twice-daily bladder expression. Urine cultures were monitored weekly and physical status of the cats was recorded daily. There were no deaths or serious complications noted in any of the animals.

On postoperative day 75 following spinal cord transection, all cats had neurological evaluation with their gait movement recorded by video camera for analysis. On the following day (postoperative day 76), the animals underwent general anesthesia as previously performed with exposure of their spinal cord at the T10 to T11 level. In order to record SCBF, teflon-coated microelectrodes were inserted into the dorsal gray matter of the cord 1 cm distal to the collagen bridge and an Ag/AgCl reference electrode was placed in a subcutaneous pouch. Cats were exposed to 5% hydrogen gas and baseline SCBF was recorded using the initial slope technique.[12]

Following SCBF measurements and without disturbing the recording electrodes, the pedicled omentum overlying the collagen bridge was clamped above its point of contact with the collagen matrix and additional SCBF measurements were recorded. Following these determinations, a 2% aqueous solution of the retrograde axonal tracer Fluoro-Gold (5 µL) was injected bilaterally into the anterior-dorsal spinal cord columns 1.7 to 2.0 cm distal to the collagen bridge. Cats were allowed to recover and 14 days later (postoperative day 90) were deeply anesthetized and then killed by perfusing transcardially with 1 liter of heparinized saline followed by 2 liters of 4% paraformaldehyde in 0.1 M phosphate-buffered saline adjusted to a pH 7.4.

The brain and spinal cord were removed and cut coronally into 2- to 3-cm tissue blocks. The blocks were immersed in the perfusate for 6 hours at room temperature and then transferred to a 10% sucrose solution in 0.1 M phosphate-buffered saline and stored at 4°C for a minimum of 14 hours.

Sagittal cryostat sections from each brain and spinal cord block were taken and stained immunohistochemically using anti-serum against:

1. tyrosine hydroxylase (TH, 1:1000)
2. dopamine-B-hydroxylase (DBH, 1:1000)
3. phenylethanolamine n-methyltransferase (PNMT, 1:1000)
4. serotonin-like (5-HTL, 1:1000)
5. glial fibrillary acidic protein (GFAP, 1:400)

6. synaptophysin (SYN, 1:10)
7. neuropeptide Y (NPY, 1:2000)

Anti-serum for TH, DBH, PNMT, serotonin-like, GFAP, and NPY were obtained from Eugene Tech (Allendale, NJ); for synaptophysin from Boehringer (Montreal, Quebec); and for Fluoro-Gold from Fluorochrome Inc. (Englewood, Colo).

Serial sections from each block were taken for Fluoro-Gold, Nissl, and Palmgren silver impregnation stains. Sections were processed according to the peroxidase-antiperoxidase (PAP) and the fluorescein isothiocyanate (FITC) techniques using antibodies to the above enzymes.[12] When serial histologic sections were stained with TH, DBH, and PNMT, it was possible to identify by exclusion the presence of dopaminergic, noradrenergic, and adrenergic immunoreactive fibers. Serial sections were also double immunostained for TH or DBH using PAP, and for SYN using FITC. All sections were examined using a Zeiss epifluorescence microscope with a mercury vapor lamp as the light source. Fluoro-Gold was visualized using a BP 4045/8 exciter filter and a LP 418 barrier filter.

RESULTS

Motor preservation and activity

Neurological examination was carried out on postoperative days 75 and 90. The cats who had spinal cord transection only, with no collagen reconstruction, exhibited flaccid or spastic paraplegia of their hind limbs with associated thigh muscle atrophy, which was clearly apparent as early as 4 weeks after surgery. By contrast, cats with COM reconstruction showed only mild to absent thigh muscle atrophy at the time of their sacrifice.

Cats who had no reconstruction of their divided spinal cord (Group II) ambulated solely by way of their front legs with their hind limbs

Table 5.1 Mean SCBF* 76 days after spinal cord transection and reconstruction

Group	Omentum unligated	Omentum ligated	Omental % contribution to SCBF
4-AP	41 mL (±6)	16 mL (±3)	61%
LAM	38 mL (±1)	12 mL (±2)	68%
LAF	34 mL (±2)	18 mL (±1)	48%
GMF	46 mL (±4)	17 mL (±4)	63%
SAL	52 mL (±2)	24 mL (±3)	54%

*Mean spinal cord blood flow (SCBF) recorded 1 cm distal to collagen matrix bridge in cats with omentum collagen matrix (COM) treated with neuroactive agents or saline (SAL). SCBF ranged from 34-52 mL 100 g^{-1} tissue min^{-1} but are significantly reduced when omental pedicle blood supply to CM region is ligated. Values are mean ±SEM.
4-AP, 4-aminopyridine; LAM, laminin; LAF, lipid angiogenic factor; GMF, glia maturation factor; SAL, saline.
Normal cat dorsal gray SCBF = 49-54 mL. Cats with spinal cord transection and no spinal cord reconstruction (controls) SCBF = 11 mL (±3).

being dragged in the process. However, at 75 days after COM reconstruction of the spinal cord in Group I, one cat who had 4-aminopyridine placed in the collagen, and another with laminin, developed fore-hindlimb coordinated locomotion when supported by the tail. Slow motion videotape analysis of these cats indicated a near-normal gait pattern. We have not observed this type of locomotion during our experience over the years in a very large series of spinal cord transected cats. The coordinated locomotion in these 2 cats seen on postoperative day 75 became visibly impaired after 5 μL of Fluoro-Gold was injected below the collagen bridge for labeling purposes. It was felt that this decrease in coordinated locomotion was due to the neurotoxic nature of the Fluoro-Gold since the amount injected into the cord is sufficient to cause focal axotomy and limited tissue necrosis.

Spinal cord blood flow

Physical evidence of the omentum's contribution to the vascular supply adjacent to the spinal cord transection site was shown by a rich network of variable-sized blood vessels that traversed the collagen bridge, as was observed microsurgically following the removal of the cord.

The omental contribution to the SCBF was determined in each animal by measuring the blood flow before and after clamping the omental pedicle, which stopped the omental blood flow to the cord. Spinal cord blood flow measurements recorded 1 cm distal to the collagen bridge on day 76 after cord transection are shown in *Table 5.1*. Spinal cord blood flow in collagen-omental cats (Group I) ranged from 34 to 52 mL g-1 tissue min-1 and averaged 42 mL higher than the SCBF in transected cord only cats (Group II). When the omental pedicle was clamped to occlude its blood supply in the cats with cord reconstruction (Group I), SCBF was reduced 48% to 68%. These low SCBF volumes that resulted from omental blood flow occlusion were similar to flow measurements obtained in Group II cats (spinal cord transection only) whose SCBF averaged 11 mL 100 g^{-1} tissue min^{-1}.

Retrograde labeling

Fourteen days after SCBF recordings and Fluoro-Gold injection (postoperative day 90 after cord transection and the day of animal sacrifice), brain tissue processed for Fluoro-Gold accumulation showed the presence of this marker within the cytoplasm and the processes of neurons located in the pontomedullary region. Specifically, Fluoro-Gold was found in the cells and processes of the locus coeruleus, subcoeruleus, Kolliker-Fuse nucleus, and regions in the medulla, including the lateral reticular nucleus and an area lateral to the inferior olive (*Figure 5.1*). These nuclei are located in the brain stem and are known to contain noradrenergic cell bodies that project descending pathways to the spinal cord and make synaptic connections and adrenoceptive cells, including preganglionic sympathetic neurons and ventral/dorsal horn cells.[3] Fluoro-Gold was also observed within neurons known to send cholinergic fibers to the spinal cord. Cholinergic neurons accumulating Fluoro-Gold included scattered areas of the pontomesencephalic reticular formation, particularly gigantocellular neurons. No Fluoro-Gold particles were found in the raphe complex (spinal source of serotoninergic neurons) or in the rostral medulla C1 and C2 cell groups (spinal source of adrenergic neurons).

The injected Fluoro-Gold, which had been placed in the distal spinal cord below the collagen bridge, had followed a retrograde axonal pathway to the brain. Conversely and of major significance was the absence of injected Fluoro-Gold in the brain stem of any of the cats who had complete spinal cord transection without collagen reconstruction and omental application.

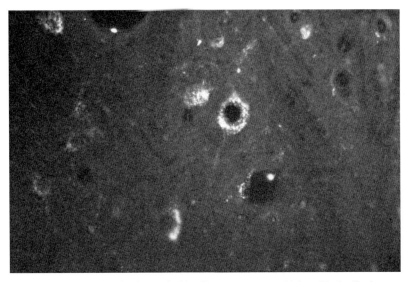

Figure 5.1 Kolliker-Fuse neurons in animal treated with collagen-omentum and injected in the distal stump with Fluoro-Gold. Note typical Fluoro-Gold granules accumulated in the cytoplasm, which extends into the neuronal process of one neuron (left side of picture). Other Kolliker-Fuse neurons (right and bottom of picture) show no uptake of the Fluoro-Gold tracer. X250.

Immunohistochemical staining

The brain and spinal cord were removed on postoperative day 90 and stained immunohisto-chemically using primary anti-sera that specifically recognize TH, DBH, PNMT, 5-HTL, GFAP, NPY, and SYN.

Histologic examination of the distal spinal cord below the cord transection site on an examiner's blind-to-treatment basis revealed the following consistent findings in all the cats with collagen-omentum reconstruction:

- Dense bundles of TH and DBH nerve fibers within and distal to the collagen bridge.
- Invasion of TH and DBH fibers into distal cord gray-white matter pathways.
- TH and DBH fiber sprouting for long anatomic distances distal to the collagen bridge.
- The appearance of large-size TH and DBH "terminal staining dots" on the somatic surface of adrenoceptive neurons (cells with catecholaminergic receptors).
- Large-size (SYN) (the marker for synaptogenesis) varicosities on the somatic surface of preganglionic sympathetic neurons located distal to the collagen bridge.
- Accumulation of Fluoro-Gold particles found in brainstem neurons.

Examination of the spinal cord at its junction with the proximal collagen bridge interface showed near-normal density of TH, DBH, PNMT, and 5-HT immunoreactive fibers in collagen-omental reconstructed cords, but a marked reduction of these fibers was noted in the same region in Group II cats who had spinal cord transection with no cord reconstruction. Immunofluorescent staining for GFAP showed little to no difference in the density of reactive astrocytes between the collagen-omentum reconstructive cats when compared to normal spinal cord tissue. In contrast, intense staining of GFAP fibers was observed in sections taken from spinal cord transected animals (Group II) at the proximal and distal junctions at the transection site. This suggests that astrocytosis was decreased or did not occur in collagen-omentum–treated cats, as opposed to animals with cord transection only.

Tyrosine hydroxylase is the enzyme that converts tyrosine to dOPA in the biosynthetic cascade that leads to the production of catecholamines and is present in dopamine, noradrenaline, and adrenaline-containing neurons. Dopamine-B-hydroxylase catalyzes the conversion of dopamine to noradrenaline and is present in noradrenergic and adrenaline-containing neurons. Phenylethanolamine n-methyltrans-ferase is the enzyme that converts noradrenaline to adrenaline and is present only in adrenaline-containing neurons.

Within the collagen bridge were dense bundles of TH and DBH fibers that were present in a ratio of 2:1 (*Figures 5.2A and 5.2B*). This same TH-DBH fiber density was observed at the distal cord-collagen bridge junction with these bundles invading gray and white matter regions where catecholaminergic tracts are normally found (*Figure 5.3*). By contrast, a lack of TH and DBH fibers was noted in the scar formation that developed between the proximal-distal cord stumps in the transection only cats. The scar in these Group I cats was located between the cord stumps and was composed of collagenous connective tissue derived mostly from proliferative fibroblasts, glial cells, and macrophages.

Distal to the collagen bridge in Group I cats were dopaminergic and noradrenergic "terminal staining dots" (characterized by large-size TH-DBH immunostaining varicosities), which were observed on the somatic surface of gray and white matter adrenoceptive neurons (*Figures 5.4A and 5.4B*). These terminal staining dots were

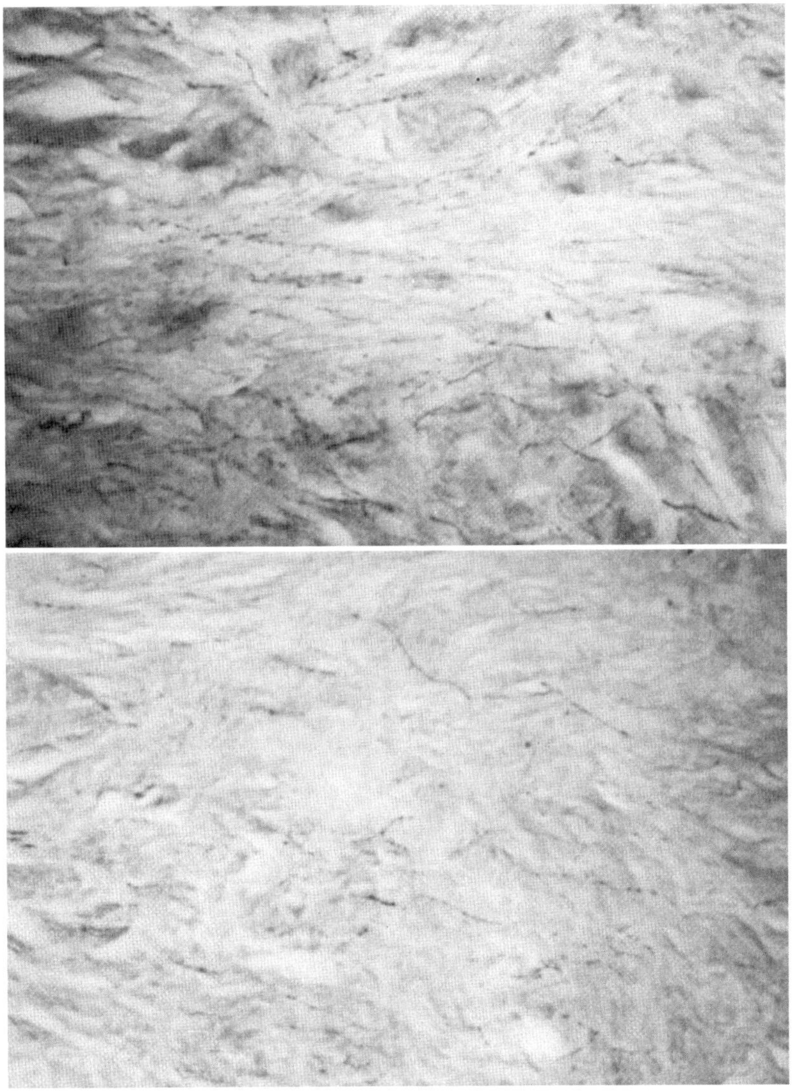

Figure 5.2 Sagittal serial sections of the spinal cord at the site of transection showing cell free collagen bridge in collagen-omentum treated animal. **A:** Numerous tyrosine hydroxylase immunopositive fibers containing dopamine and noradrenaline. **B:** Numerous dopamine-B-hydroxylase immunopositive fibers containing only noradrenaline, can be seen. Note approximate 2:1 density ratio of dopamine:noradrenaline in **A** compared to noradrenaline-containing fibers in **B**, suggesting a significant contribution of regenerating dopaminergic fibers after surgical treatment. Scale bar = 100 μm.

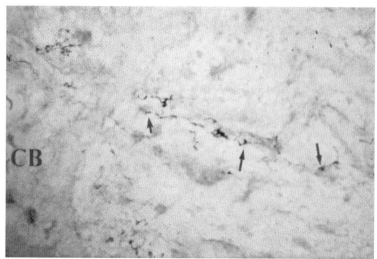

Figure 5.3 Large tyrosine-hydroxylase-immunoreactive for noradrenaline-dopamine varicosties exciting collagen bridge (CB). Some of these distal-to-lesion varicosities appear to be in contact with pre-ganglionic sympathetic neurons (arrows).

consistently noted on preganglionic sympathetic neurons and on their processes in the region of the intermediolateral nucleus (*Figures 5.5*). Dopaminergic terminal staining dots were also noted on lateral funiculus preganglionic sympathetic neurons in the white matter. A small number of gray matter dorsal and ventral horn neurons contained both dopaminergic and noradrenergic terminal staining dots.

Double immunostaining showed that SYN varicosities were often, but not always, found adjacent to the TH or DBH terminal staining dots when these dots were detected on the surface of adrenoceptic elements distal to the collagen bridge (*Figure 5.6*). Although SYN is normally present in spinal cord gray but not in white matter, collagen-reconstructive spinal cord tissue showed many large-size SYN varicosities often in contact with adrenoceptive neurons such as preganglionic sympathetic neurons in both gray and white matter. Other atypical SYN varicosities appeared densely distributed in the proximal and distal cord junctions at the collagen bridge. These atypical SYN varicosities extended 7 to 15 mm into the distal spinal cord stump where they eventually returned to their normal size and appearance. Large-size SYN varicosities are described here as atypical because they are punctuate in size and homogenous in appearance in normal spinal cord tissue.

Dopaminergic and noradrenergic distal fibers became progressively less abundant in relation to increasing distances from the collagen bridge in the collagen-omental cats. The maximum regenerating distal distance of dopaminergic/noradrenergic fibers in these cats was +90 mm, as measured from the proximal-cord–collagen bridge interface. How far these dopaminergic/noradrenergic fibers may have extended beyond 90 mm is uncertain since all spinal cords were cut approximately 10 cm below the cord transection site. Cats whose collagen bridge was treated with 4-aminopyridine (+90 mm) or with laminin (75 mm) showed the longest distal fiber outgrowth. Other treatments of the collagen material, which formed the spinal cord bridge, included glial maturation factor, lipid angiogenic factor, and saline. The distal fiber outgrowth length using these substances mixed

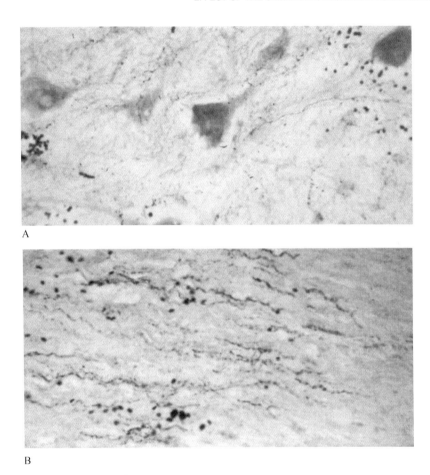

A

B

Figure 5.4 A: Sagittal section of normal (above lesion site) distribution of tyrosine-hydroxylase-immunoreactive varicosities in ventral horn region. Note the many fine-sized varicosities measuring about 0.8 μm in diameter, which appear to be in contact with several motor horn cells. Single dark spots at right of picture are peroxidase-positive artifacts. **B:** Large tyrosine-hydroxylase-immunoreactive fibers (measuring about 1.4 μm diameter) caudal to the lesion site in animal treated with collagen-omentum repair.

into the collagen averaged 56 mm. These distances may be underestimated since after spinal cord transection in mammals, axotomized fibers generally retract cranially for several millimeters.

DISCUSSION

Regeneration of CNS fibers is an endeavor that has been pursued by numerous investigators for many years. Even though the results have been known to be highly limited and generally nonfunctional, we showed in initial studies that a collagen reconstructed transected spinal cord with an omental graft can develop limited catecholaminergic outgrowth distal to the transection site.[1] These first experimental studies using a collagen bridge for a transected spinal cords showed that supraspinal catecholaminergic fibers crossed the bridge and continued distally for a maximum distance of 9.6 mm during a

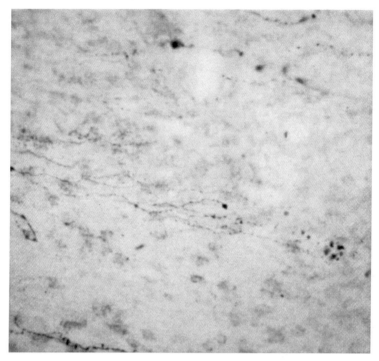

Figure 5.5 Sagittal section of typical (small-fine) and atypical (large-dark) tyrosine-hydroxylase-immunopositive fiber varicosities several millimeters caudal to the transection site in collagen-omentum–treated spinal cord. Note both fine and large varicosities, which meander and appear to contact numerous peripheral sympathetic neurons (dark-shaded cells) in the region around a number of spinal cells of the interomediolateral cell nucleus. X250.

12-week recovery period. In addition, spinal cord blood flow in the distal spinal cord tissue adjacent to the transection site was increased by a mean flow of 53% as compared to control cats. Also observed was the partial return of somatosensory evoked potentials when the electrical stimulus was applied below the lesion site. Cats with positive somatosensory evoked potentials also demonstrated short distance retrograde axonal transport of horseradish peroxidase in the proximal cord when the marker was injected distal to the collagen bridge.

However, these preliminary studies were done in the presence of a large gap (6 mm) between the spinal cord stumps after complete cord transection with no neurotrophic agents being added to the collagen bridge. In the study that has been described in depth in this chapter, a smaller gap was made between the transected spinal cord stumps (3 mm, made by approximating the cut dural edges at the transection site). This narrowing of the transection gap resulted in a considerable increase in this regeneration of supraspinal dopaminergic and noradrenergic fibers distal to the transection site.

Continuing work involving collagen bridging in association with an omental pedicle has been a logical progression of previous experiments in the attempt to clarify conditions concerning central regeneration after spinal

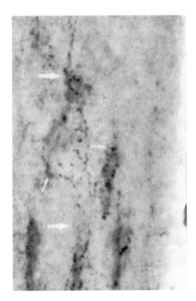 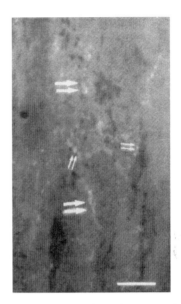

Figure 5.6 Double-immunostaining for **A:** tyrosine hydroxylase and **B:** the synaptic marker synaptophysin in distal stump of collagen-omentum–treated spinal cord. Note single arrows (A) pointing to immunopositive catecholaminergic fibers on the somatic surface of several neurons. Atypical medium-sized synaptophysin varicosities (double arrows, **B)** which are suggestive of new synaptic endings, appear in parallel location and distribution to the tyrosine-hydroxylase-immunopositive fibers seen in panel **A**. Scale bar = 100 μm.

cord transection. The primary goal has been to improve distal cord supraspinal regeneration; specifically, maximal distance outgrowth, axonal density, and appropriate target tissue reconnection caudal to the transection site.

The collagen-neuroprotective mixture used in association with an omental pedicle showed specific changes that were not observed in the control animals. The changes that have been demonstrated included:

- An increase of SCBF near the transection site. This SCBF increase was due to supplemental blood flow coming from the omentum, which increased the flow by a mean of 53% compared to the SCBF of control animals.
- Placement of the omentum on a collagen bridge connecting transected spinal cord stumps prevented hind-limb muscle atrophy. This was not observed in control animals.
- Well-coordinated hind-forelimb locomotion occurred in collagen-omental treated animals when the lower body was supported. This was observed at the time of the animals' sacrifice 3 months after surgery.[13] A longer postoperative survival period in association with an exercise program may, in the future, allow for coordinated locomotion without lower extremity support.
- It was found that an outgrowth of noradrenergic fibers crossed through the collagen bridge and continued to extend into the distal spinal cord. The growth rate of the regenerating fibers was approximately 1 mm per day, roughly the same growth rate that is seen in peripheral axonal regeneration.

- Animals who underwent collagen-omental reconstruction following spinal cord transection showed the synaptogenic marker, synaptophysin, to be present in preganglionic sympathetic neurons along with dopaminergic- and noradrenergic-containing varicosities distal to the collagen bridge. This indicates that axons grew through the collagen bridge and had synaptic activity within the distal spinal cord. However, direct evidence of synaptic connections can only be confirmed by an electron microscope study using double labeling of presynaptic aminergic vesicles (previously depleted by spinal cord transection), which would visually demonstrate a direct contact with postsynaptic target tissue.
- Fluoro-Gold deposition was found in the locus coeruleus and other pontine noradrenergic-containing neurons following retrograde labeling. This confirmed that this labeled marker, which was injected distal to the spinal cord transection, moved in a retrograde fashion up to the brain through the collagen bridge at the transection site. This finding was not seen in cats who did not undergo reconstruction of their transected spinal cord.

It appears that a surgically reconstructed spinal cord using collagen and omentum can result in the development of relatively dense supraspinal fiber outgrowth across a collagen bridge supported by increased blood flow from the omentum and by neurotrophic substances known to be in omental tissue. The effect of these experimental procedures awaits evaluation in treating humans with complete spinal cord transection.

REFERENCES

1. de la Torre JC, Goldsmith HS. Collagen-omental graft in experimental spinal cord transection. *Acta Neurochir.* 1990;102:152-163.
2. Goldsmith HS, de la Torre JC. Axonal regeneration after spina cord transection and revascularization. *Brain Res.* 1992;589:217-224.
3. de la Torre JC, Goldsmith HS. Coerulospinal fiber regeneration in transected feline spinal cord. *Brain Res Bull.* 1994;35:413-417.
4. Ramon y Cajal S. In: May R, ed. *Degeneration and Regeneration of the Nervous System.* New York: Hafner Publishing; 1959:749-750.
5. de la Torre JC. Spinal cord injury models. *Prog Neurobiol.* 1984;22:289-344.
6. Zhang Z, Guth L. Experimental spinal cord injury: Wallerian degeneration in the dorsal column is followed by revascularization, glial proliferation and nerve regeneration. *Exp Neurol.* 1997;147:157-171.
7. Goldsmith HS, Duckett S, Chen W. Spinal cord vascularization by intact omentum. *Am J Surg.* 1975;129:262-265.
8. Goldsmith HS, Steward E. Chen W. Duckett S. Application of the intact omentum on normal and injured spinal cord. In: Kao CC, Bunge RP, eds. *Spinal Cord Reconstruction.* New York: Raven Press; 1983:235-243.
9. de la Torre JC, Goldsmith HS. Increased blood flow enhances axon regeneration after spinal transection. *Neurosci Lett.* 1988;94:269-273.
10. de la Torre, Goldsmith HS. Supraspinal fiber outgrowth and apparent synaptic remodeling across transected-reconstructed feline spinal cord. *Acta Neurochir.* 1992;114:118-127.
11. Goldsmith HS. Omental transposition to the brain and spinal cord. *Surg Rounds.* June 1986:22-23.
12. Ingvar DH, Lassen N. Regional blood flow of the cerebral cortx determined by Krypton 85. *Acta Physiol Scand.* 1962;54:325-338.
13. Video of Coordinating Walking presented at the 31st Annual Scientific Meeting. International Medical Society of Paraplegia, Barcelona, Spain, September 16-19, 1992.

CHAPTER 6

NEAR-TOTAL TRANSECTION OF HUMAN SPINAL CORD: FUNCTIONAL RETURN FOLLOWING OMENTUM-COLLAGEN RECONSTRUCTION

HARRY S. GOLDSMITH, MATTHIAS BRANDT, AND THOMAS WALZ

INTRODUCTION

A major neuroscientific goal over the past decades has been to develop a method to re-establish axonal continuity after spinal cord transection that could lead to the return of motor function. Experimental studies using an omental-collagen bridging technique following complete spinal cord transection has been reported to be successful in developing axonal outgrowth and coordinated walking in cats.[1-5] The results of these initial studies are now supported by the patient reported in this paper who had a near-total spinal cord transection followed by omental-collagen reconstruction of her spinal cord more than 3 years after her injury and has exhibited return of motor activity. This is a preliminary report since her motor progress continues to evolve.

Past research

For over a quarter of a century, experimental studies have been conducted (in the laboratory of H.S. Goldsmith) to learn the result of transposing the pedicled omentum onto normal and injured spinal cords in animals and in man. Associated with these laboratory and clinical studies has been a specific search to learn the possible role of the omentum in axonal regeneration within the spinal cord.

The first publication involving omental transposition (OT) to the spinal cord was reported in 1975,[6] which clearly demonstrated that placing the omentum on a spinal cord led to the induction of omental blood vessels that traveled through the omental-spinal cord interface and penetrated directly into the spinal cord. Subsequent injection of dye markers through blood vessels that had developed at the omental-spinal cord interface showed the dye marker (India ink) in capillaries located on the spinal cord surface and in deeply positioned spinal cord capillaries.[6] Furthermore, when the spinal cord was completely transected, the omentum allowed blood vessels to grow in a longitudinal manner through the transection site,[7] a finding that was felt to be important if, at a later date, axons could be shown to grow in a comparable longitudinal manner across a spinal cord transection gap.

What was of further importance in the study of the omental-spinal cord vascularization process was that the omental blood vessels that penetrated the normal spinal cord did so within 72 hours (and possibly even sooner), the time period being later confirmed by others in 1978.[8] The rapidity of this revascularization activity was even more impressive when the omentum was placed directly on an acutely injured spinal cord.[9]

By 1986, it was felt that the blood vessels that grew from the omentum into the spinal cord and brain[10] were stimulated by a powerful omental angiogenic factor that was found to be glycolipid in character.[11,12] In addition to this angiogenic factor, it has been more recently shown that the highly angiogenic vascular endothelial growth factor (VEGF) is also present in omental tissue in high concentrations.[13] Our laboratory has also reported the presence of neurotransmitters[14,15] and nerve growth substances[16] in omental tissue. The combination of angiogenic and neurogenic agents acting either alone or together may account for the large number of patients who have had varying degrees of success following OT to their chronically injured spinal cord.[17] It is believed that if the omentum were applied directly onto the spinal cord shortly after injury, the beneficial effects of the surgical procedure might even prove greater.[18]

The question that has been asked in our laboratory over the years is whether OT might allow axonal regeneration to occur across a completely transected spinal cord, which could result in the return of distal motor function. This question was first addressed by us in cats who had a 5-mm piece of their spinal cord excised at the T9 level. In order to approximate the severed stumps of the divided cord without tension, a lumbar vertebrectomy was performed.[7] The proximal and distal vertebral bodies adjacent to the excised vertebral body were then solidly fixed by the insertion of stainless steel plates and screws. The next step in the reconstruction operation was to approximate, without any tension, the divided ends of the transected cord. This was accomplished by laser welding together the circular edges of the proximal and distal stumps of the transected cord using a CO_2 laser set at 1 to 2 watts of energy. The laser beam was carefully directed under microscopic control, with the heat energy of the laser beam known to penetrate only a modest 1.2 mm into the spinal cord, thus sparing the deeper-placed neuroanatomical tracts.

Following this fuse-welding laser process, which joined the ends of the divided spinal cord, a pedicled omental flap was wrapped around the transection site in order to absorb immediate and delayed edema fluid accumulation at the laser-treated site; the omentum having an enormous capacity to absorb edema fluid.[8,19] Another reason for wrapping the omentum around the cord transection site was to increase vascularization in this area. The final steps in this experimental surgical procedure was to immobilize the vertebral column by fixing two long stainless steel plates on both sides of the dorsal spinal processes, which extended above and below the operation site.

The results of the above experiment were successful in that 7 of 15 cats with complete spinal cord reconstruction and OT to the area had return of somatosensory evoked potentials (SEPs) at the end of 2 months after surgery, but none of the control cats (without OT) had return of SEPs. The cats with the postoperative return of SEPs demonstrated the presence of axons that crossed the transection site in a longitudinal fashion. This finding was not observed in control cats. Unfortunately, the cats with positive SEPs and evidence of axonal growth at the transection site has no return of motor function. However, the experiment did show that the transected spinal cord had the capacity to heal, but the procedure was abandoned since it had no therapeutic clinical significance.

By the early 1990s, a new and much simpler experimental operation had been developed to promote axonal regeneration in the spinal cord that hopefully would lead to the return of motor function distal to a spinal cord transection site. The new procedure in cats involved filling the gap (3-6 mm) resulting from complete spinal cord transection with collagen (Zyderm, Collagen Corp., Palo Alto, Calif) which acted as a bridge between the divided proximal and distal spinal cord stumps.[2,3]

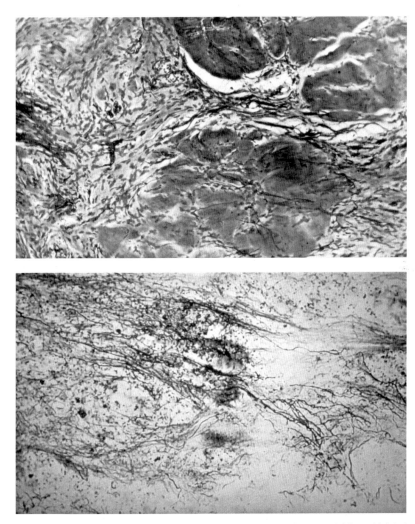

Figures 6.1A Axons in center of collagen bridge. **B:** Axons exiting distal end of collagen bridge, which is in the process of breaking up. Axons connect to distal neurons.[3-5]

In order to vascularize and introduce neurotransmitters and nerve growth factors into the collagen bridge, which we believed might prove critical for creating a favorable environment for axonal regeneration, a pedicled omental graft was placed on the bridge, which also covered the adjacent proximal and distal spinal cord stumps. It was subsequently shown that vascular perfusion, which originated from the omentum into the collagen bridge, resulted in a 58% increase in spinal cord blood flow[3] compared to control animals, with a 3 to 1 increase in blood vessel density counts into the bridge as compared to controls.[2] Of interest was the finding of immunoreactive catacholaminergic axons that crossed through the collagen bridge and continued well down into its distal cord stump at a growth rate of 1 mm day^{-1}, a phenomenon not seen on control animals. Of particular importance was the ability of some cats with OT to have coordinated hind-forelimb walking when hind-limb support was provided. This ability was well documented on film.

At the end of the experiments, the animals were sacrificed and their spinal cords were grossly and histologically examined. The observation was made that the longitudinal extent of the collagen bridge was now shorter than the length of the collagen bridge that was originally created between the stumps of the divided cord. Additionally, on histologic examination, it could be seen that the collagen material itself was breaking up and being absorbed at both ends of the collagen bridge (*Figures 6.1A and 6.1B*). This observation suggested that the spinal cord was reconstructing itself in a longitudinal manner.

CASE REPORT

The patient is a 24-year-old woman who was involved in a high-speed skiing accident on January 3, 1993, at which time she struck a stone wall, which resulted in a dislocation fracture at T6-T7, with fractures of the vertebral arches at T6 on the left and T7 on the right. Magnetic resonance imaging (MRI) shortly after injury showed what was described as a complete anatomical transection of her spinal cord at the T6-T7 level (*Figure 6.2*). On January 13, 1993, the patient's vertebral column was surgically stabilized using metal plates and after 5 months of physiotherapy, she was discharged to her home. The orthopedic plates were removed from her back 1 year later.

Over the next 3 years, she continued to have complete motor loss, beginning at the T6-T7 level with an associated sensory loss at that level. However, she stated that on rare occasions she felt the sensation of light touch on isolated areas of her legs. She had no other sensory findings but had moderate spasticity of both legs. She had no bladder or urinary awareness, and controlled these functions with

intermittent bladder catheterization and a bowel regimen requiring suppositories.

At 39 months after injury, the patient underwent reconstruction of her divided spinal cord using the same surgical techniques that had been successfully used by us in the cat; namely, filling the transection gap between the divided cord stumps with a collagen matrix after which an intact omentum pedicle was placed directly on the underlying collagen bridge.[3]

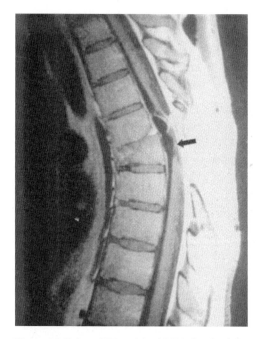

Figure 6.2 Enlarged T1 weighted MRI showing burst fracture at T6 and T7 with total disc extrusion. Arrow points to originally described complete spinal cord transection. Limited posterior spinal cord connection was not appreciated on immediate post-injury (non-enlarged) MRI.

Preoperative

The patient had complete motor loss below the T6-T7 level. Because of her claim that she had an occasional sensation of light touch in her lower legs in spite of her initial MRI, which was reported as a total anatomical transection of the spinal cord, a review of the MRI taken at the time of her injury was radiographically reinterpreted following enlargement as showing a contiguous connection of a small portion of her posterior spinal cord (*Figure 6.2*).

Operative procedure

The technical plan for the operation was to remove the scar that was expected to have developed between the divided ends of the spinal cord and replace it with an omental-collagen bridge. It was believed that the scar tissue that would be found at operation in and around the spinal cord separation would be not much larger than the transection gap seen on the patient's initial MRI. This was found not to be the case.

The rationale for using the omentum-collagen preparation to bridge the spinal cord gap was twofold. The collagen matrix would be the scaffolding structure through which axons could grow, with the omentum overlying the collagen bridge being the source of additional blood flow to the proximal and distal spinal cord stumps and to the collagen matrix.[1,11,12] In addition, neurochemials[14,15] and nerve growth substances

known to be produced by the omentum[16] would be expected to perfuse into the reconstructed area and provide additional support for axonal regeneration.

The patient was placed in a supine position and a midline abdominal incision was made and carried into the peritoneal cavity. The omentum was then removed from the transverse colon and stomach by a technique previously reported.[20,21] After the omentum had been lengthened into a long intact pedicle, the abdominal wound was closed and the patient repositioned in a prone position on the operating table. With the patient in this position, the intact pedicled omental graft was brought around the flank through a subcutaneous tunnel to the middle of the back. A laminectomy was then carried out between T6-T8, with exposure of the spinal cord at the lower portion of T5 and the upper portion of T9. Following this, the dura mater was opened and a massive block of scar tissue was seen between T6-T8 that had resulted from the fibrotic reaction that had developed between the separated stumps of the spinal cord. The extent of the scar formation found at operation was much greater than expected (*Figure 6.3*) based on the post-injury MRI.

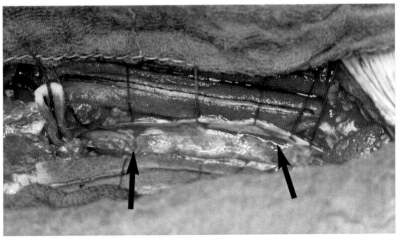

Figure 6.3 Area between arrows depicts spinal cord disruption between T6-T8. Spinal cord transection region composed almost entirely of firm scar tissue.

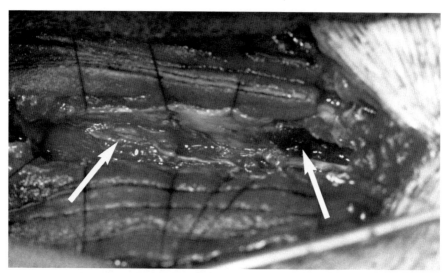

Figure 6.4 Note absence of spinal cord tissue between T6-T8 (arrows) following excision of scar tissue. Sutures hold dural edges apart.

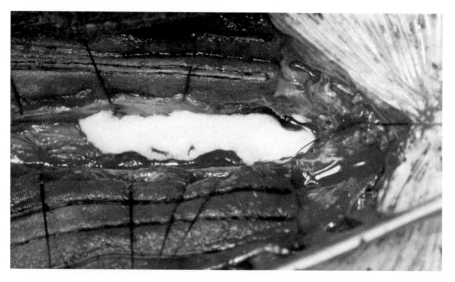

Figure 6.5 Operative photo showing collagen filling extensive spinal cord defect between T6-T8.

Using an operating microscope, the scar tissue between T6-T8 was removed, which left a very large spinal cord defect that measured approximately 1.6 inches (4 cm) in length. Deeply positioned between the upper and lower spinal cord stumps was the presence of a small ribbon of connected spinal cord tissue. It was estimated by three observers that approximately 90% to 95% of the spinal cord was absent between T6-T8 (*Figure 6.4*).

The extensive defect between the upper and lower portions of the almost totally transected spinal cord was filled with collagen (Zyderm). Approximately 4 cc of collagen was needed to fill the extensive spinal cord defect that separated the proximal and distal spinal cord segments (*Figure 6.5*). The collagen had been kept refrigerated at a temperature of 4°C but was removed from the refrigerator 1 hour before surgery in order to allow it to warm to room temperature. The collagen was delivered to the extensive spinal cord defect through a small syringe and allowed to polymerize (harden), which took approximately 30 to 40 minutes. After the hardening process had taken place, the omentum was placed directly on the collagen bridge and carefully sutured to the cut edges of the dura (*Figure 6.6*). Overlying muscle and fascial layers of the back were then carefully approximated over the omentum-collagen bridge. The skin was closed in a routine fashion without drainage.

Postoperative course

The patient underwent omental-collagen reconstruction on April 2, 1996, which was 39 months after her spinal cord injury. The operation was uneventful, as was her postoperative course. Prior to her hospital discharge, she had an MRI that showed the omental-collagen bridge to be in place with no adverse effects (*Figure 6.7*). She was discharged on her 10th postoperative day and over the next 2 months, she recuperated from her operation.

Approximately 3 months after surgery on June 26, 1996, she began a rehabilitation program that consisted of 1 hour a day of swimming and passive exercises. Prior to surgery, the patient had complete absence of abdominal, low back, hip, and leg muscle movement. She also had no sexual feelings during intercourse. By September 1996, which was now 6 months after surgery, she claimed to be aware of muscle activity in her legs when

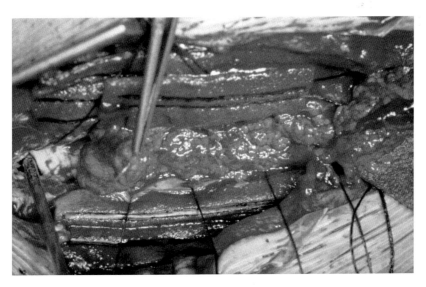

Figure 6.6 Operative photo showing pedicled omentum overlying the collagen bridge (arrows). Edges of omentum are carefully attached to the cut edges of the dura with a closely placed running suture.

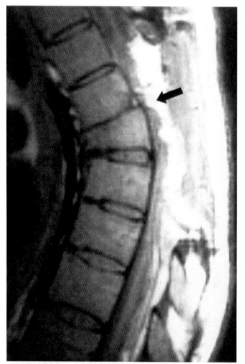

Figure 6.7 T1 weighted MRI showing collagen bridge and overlying omental flap (arrow) in place between spinal cord separation at T6-T8.

they were being passively moved. By November 1996, 8 months after surgery, she claimed that she experienced gluteal muscle activity that extended into her legs. By the following month, her physiotherapist began to feel leg muscle activity, especially around the knees, when the patient attempted to actively move her legs.

By January 1997, minimal activity of her toes was noted. On March 24, 1997, the patient was recorded as showing slight movement of her left knee, with the physiotherapist being able to feel the leg muscle contractions.

By June 1997, functional changes continued to increase. Before surgery, the patient was unable to sit without support because of complete lack of trunk and abdominal muscle strength, but she could now sit unassisted since she had regained a significant amount of abdominal muscle strength (*Figures 6.8A and 6.8B*). She could also maintain a crawl position on the floor, which was impossible before surgery since at that time she would collapse because of loss of back, trunk, and hip muscle strength (*Figure 6.9*).

She subsequently began to move her legs either alone or in combination, repetitively and on command while in a swimming pool, and on occasion can voluntarily extend her lower legs minimally (3-4 inches) from the knee to the foot while in a sitting position. She could also plantar flex her feet, especially on the right. Additionally, she could get off a chair and stand with knee support, an action that was impossible before surgery.

The patient continues to self-catheterize for bladder control. Prior to surgery, when she performed this activity, she had urine volumes of approximately 500 cc. She now claims an awareness of bladder filling when there is approximately 200 cc of urine present. She also states that she now has sexual awareness during intercourse, which she claims is intense.

An MRI taken 1 year after surgery showed a soft-tissue mass between the proximal and distal cord stumps (*Figure 6.10*). The neurologic improvements that had occurred in this patient during the first postoperative year suggested that regenerating axons had passed through this soft-tissue mass and made appropriate connections with neural tissue below the spinal cord transection site. A follow-up MRI done 24 months after surgery showed that the soft-tissue mass at the transection site had changed in configuration to a longitudinal structure, which suggests connections to the proximal and distal spinal cord stumps *(Figure 6.11).*

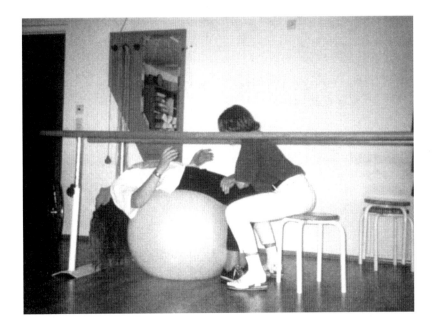

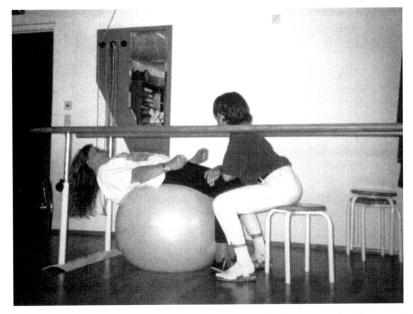

Figure 6.8A and 6.8B Marked postoperative strength of abdominal muscles that were paralyzed preoperatively.

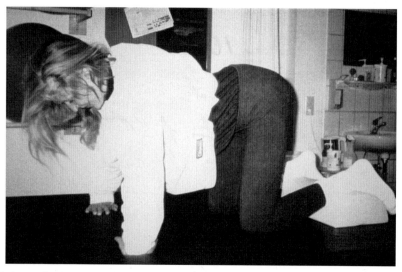

Figure 6.9 Patient on hands and knees, which could not be maintained prior to omental-collagen reconstruction of her cord because of lower abdominal muscle and hip instability.

DISCUSSION

Efforts have continued over the years to develop techniques to induce axonal regeneration following spinal cord transection that could lead to the return of motor function. A new experimental surgical procedure has been developed, which involved complete spinal cord transection with insertion of collagen into the spinal cord transection gap followed by the transposition of a pedicled omental flap that covers the collagen bridge and the proximal and distal spinal cord stumps. This surgical technique proved successful and resulted in the following findings[5] in cats, forming the basis for the operation performed on the patient reported in this chapter:

1. Increased spinal cord blood flow, which was supplied by the omentum at the spinal cord transection site.
2. Prevention of hind-limb muscle atrophy, which normally occurs with spinal cord transection in cats.

3. Outgrowth of supraspinal axons through the collagen bridge, with axonal progression into the distal spinal cord for long anatomic distances. Axonal growth occurred at the rate of 1 mm day^{-1}, a rate comparable to peripheral nerve growth.
4. Immunostaining techniques that indicated apparent synaptic contact with preganglionic sympathetic and motor neurons distal to the cord transection site.
5. Coordinated hind-forelimb locomotion following cord transection when tail support was provided.

The early results of the operation performed on the patient being reported suggest that omental-collagen reconstruction allowed her severely injured spinal cord to achieve the return of a significant degree of motor function years after injury as a result of natural healing mechanisms. It also seems reasonable to suggest, based on the patient's serial MRIs at the end of the first and second postoperative years, that an omental-collagen bridge placed in the gap at a spinal cord transection site appears to allow the spinal cord to reconstruct itself in an in-continuity longitudinal fashion.

In view of the devastating and presently incurable results following spinal cord transection, a surgical trial seems justified using an omental-collagen preparation, which could be carried out in a small number of selected paraplegic patients who have sustained a limited and relatively early anatomical transection of their spinal cord or have a marked but limited segmental cord injury or syrinx that could be excised, followed by omental-collagen reconstruction. When such a trial is attempted, it is absolutely essential that truly motivated patients be chosen because of the intensive and protracted postoperative physiotherapy that will be required following such surgery.

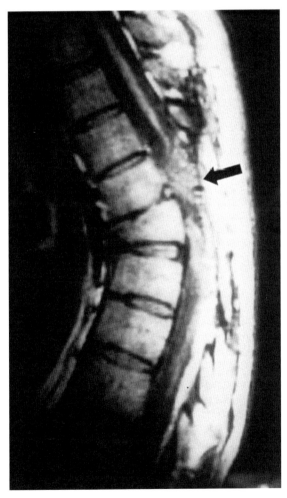

Figure 6.10 T1 weighted MRI of spinal cord 1 year after cord reconstruction. Arrow points to soft tissue mass located in spinal cord separation between T6-T8.

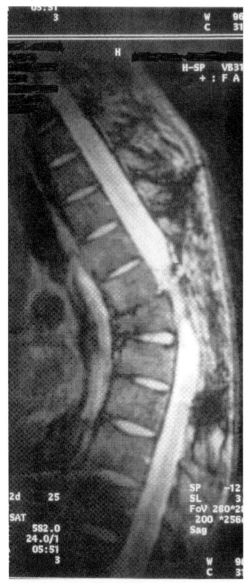

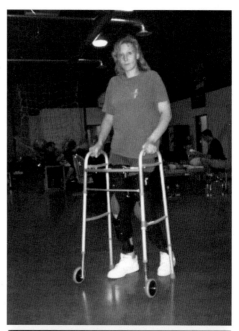

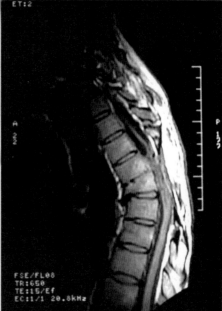

Figure 6.11 T1 weighted MRI of spinal cord 2 years after cord reconstruction. Previous soft tissue mass appears to be developing into a longitudinal structure between the proximal and distal spinal cord stumps.

Figure 6.12 A: Photo showing patient walking with a walke;r B: MRI at 6 years after surgery shows connection between proximal and distal segments of the previously divided spinal cord.

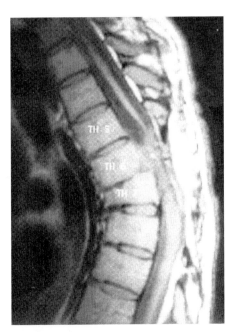

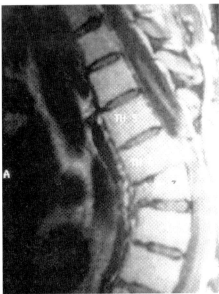

Figure 6.13 T1 weighted MRI (gadolinium enhancement on right) demonstrating a longitudinally structured connection at the site of spinal cord separation, which was reconstructed using an omental-collagen bridge.

ADDENDUM

The patient at 4 years after surgery was able to walk for extensive distances. However, she requires the use of a walker since she remains unstable and lacks balance in her walking ability *(Figure 6.12A)*. The patient's last MRI showed what appears to be a longitudinal reconstruction of her divided spinal cord *(Figure 6.12B)*.

Of neuroradiological interest is her latest MRI (taken exactly 3 years after surgery), which shows the continuing development of a longitudinal structure at the site of her spinal cord separation, which appears to be connecting the proximal and distal spinal cord segements *(Figure 6.13)*.

REFERENCES

1. de la Torre JC, Goldsmith HS. Increased blood flow enhances axon regeneration after spinal transaction. *Neurosci Lett.* 1988;94:269-273.
2. de la Torre JC, Goldsmith HS. Collagen-omental graft in experimental spinal cord transaction. *Acta Neurochir.* 1990;102:152-163.
3. Goldsmith HS, de la Torre JC. Axonal regeneration after spinal cord transaction and reconstruction. *Brain Res.* 1992;589:217-224.
4. de la Torre JC, Goldsmith HS. Supraspinal fiber outgrowth and apparent synapsis remodeling across transected-reconstructed feline spinal cord. *Acta Neurochir.* 1992;114:118-127.
5. de la Torre, JC. Goldsmith HS. Coerulospinal regeneration in transected feline spnal cord. *Brain Res Bull.* 1994;35:413-417.
6. Goldsmith HS, Duckett S, Chen WF. Spinal cord revascularization by intact omentum. *Am J Surg.* 1975;129:262-265.
7. Goldsmith HS. The omentum in spinal cord injury. In: Lee BY, Ostrander LE, eds. *Comprehensive Care of the Spinal Cord Injured Patient.* Philadelphia: W.B. Saunders; 1991:313-327.
8. Levander B, Zwetnow NN. Bulk flow of CSF through a lumbo-omental pedicle graft in the dog. *Acta Neurochir.* 1978;41:147-155.
9. Goldsmith HS, Steward E, Duckett S. Early application of pedicled omentum to the acutely traumatized spinal cord. *Paraplegia.* 1985;23:100-113.

10. Goldsmith HS, Chen WF, Duckett S. Brain vascularization by intact omentum. *Arch Surg.* 1973;106:695-698.

11. Goldsmith HS, Griffith A, Kupperman A, Catsimpoolas N. Lipid angiogenic factor from omentum. *JAMA.* 1984;252:2034-2036.

12. Goldsmith HS, Griffith A, Catsimpoolas N. Increased vascular perfusion after administration of an omental lipid factor. *Surg Gynecol Obstet.* 1986;162:579-583.

13. Zhang QX, Magovern CJ, Mack CA, et al. Vascular endothelial growth factor is the major angiogenic factor in omentum. *J Surg Res.* 1997;67:147-154.

14. Goldsmith HS, McIntosh T, Vezena RM, Colton T. Vasoactive neurochemicals identified in omentum. *Brit J Neurosurg.* 1987;1:359-364.

15. Goldsmith HS, Marquis JK, Siek GC. Choline acetyltransferase activity in omental tissue. *Brit J Neurosurg.* 1987;1:463-466.

16. Siek GC, Marquis JK, Goldsmith HS. Experimental studies of omentum-derived neurotrophic factors. In: Goldsmith HS, ed. The Omentum—Research and Clinical Applications. New York: Springer-Verlag; 1990:85-96.

17. Goldsmith HS. The First International Congress of Omentum in CNS. *Surg Neurol.* 1996;45:87-90.

18. Goldsmith HS. Acute spinal cord injuries: a search for functional improvement. *Surg Neurol.* 1999;51:231-233.

19. Goldsmith HS, de los Santos R, Beattie EJ. The relief of chronic lymphedema by omental transposition. *Ann Surg.* 1967;166:573-585.

20. Alday ES, Goldsmith HS. Surgical technique for omental lengthening based on arterial anatomy. *Surg Gyn Obstet.* 1972;135:103-107.

21. Goldsmith HS. Omental transposition to the brain and spinal cord. *Surg Rounds.* 1986;9:22-23.

CHAPTER 7

TRANSPORT OF CEREBRO SPINAL FLUID VIA OMENTUM–ALTERNATIVE TREATMENT OF HYDROCEPHALUS: EXPERIMENTAL AND CLINICAL STUDIES

BO LEVANDER

INTRODUCTION

Many techniques have been developed for the treatment of hydrocephalus since Kausch in 1908 inserted a rubber tube from the lateral ventricle of the brain into the peritoneal cavity.[1] Most of these techniques employed tubes of rubber, plastic material, or metal to drain cerebrospinal fluid (CSF) from the ventricular space into other body cavities or into a vein. Many of these shunts require mechanical valves of plastic material or metal, which are interposed along the course of the conductive tubing to promote unidirectional flow of CSF, and to prevent reflux of blood or other body fluids. A large number of complications are common with this arrangement, such as disconnection or blocking of the tubing, valve insufficiency, bacterial colonization, and outgrowing the length of the catheter.[2,3] It has also been shown that rapid decompression following ventriculoatrial or ventriculoperitoneal shunts may result in an epidural or subdural hematoma.[4] Furthermore, the rapid removal of CSF may also cause ventricular collapse with the draining cerebral shunt catheter becoming trapped between the abutting ventricular walls with high risk of occlusion of the catheter.[5] In 1963, Scarff[2] found that the incidence of severe late complications was many times greater after most operations for CSF drainage using foreign material than after techniques where foreign material was not introduced. All this indicates that the techniques in routine use at present are far from perfect and that further research for improved CSF drainage is required. The absorptive capacity within the peritoneal cavity is utilized when hydrocephalus is treated by means of a ventriculoperitoneal or lumboperitoneal shunt. The absorption by, and the transport of, fluids through the greater column has been extensively studied by Kraft et al.[6] In 1967, Goldsmith et al[7] reported that the greater omentum had been successfully transposed to an arm or a leg in order to relieve chronic lymphedema in man. This technique has been in clinical practice with good results since 1966,[8] and gave us the idea of placing a pedicle graft of the greater omentum in contact with the lumbar subarachnoid space for the absorption of CSF.

EXPERIMENTAL STUDIES

In a pilot study in rats,[9,10] a lumbo-omental shunting procedure was performed. After laparotomy, a pedicle graft of the greater omentum was mobilized and, using the operating microscope, a laminectomy was performed followed by excision of the underlying dura and arachnoid. Through a lumbar incision, the omental graft was then introduced into the spinal cord through the posterior abdominal wall and paravertebral muscles, and sutured to adjacent muscles overlying the exposed spinal cauda equine. The CSF absorption of the lumbo-omental shunt was assessed by the inulin clearance method.[10] Subsequent results showed more than a sixfold increase in inulin uptake into portal venous blood after the lumbo-omental procedure compared to control animals during a 1-hour observation period after intrathecal administration of inulin. After this preliminary study, experiments were performed using mongrel dogs and the surgical technique illustrated in *Figure 7.1.*[11]

The transport of CSF with an admixture of radionuclide through the pedicle graft was also studied. Gamma cisternography using 99Tcm-DPTA was carried out on dogs 1 to 17 months after shunt operation and on control animals. In all the dogs, the radionuclide was administered into the lumbar CSF space; at a level below the implanted omentum in the operated group. The control dogs showed a normal intrathecal cisternograph, with blood samples from their inferior vena cava showing no accumulation of radionuclide. However, the lumbo-omental shunt-operated dogs studied by the same gamma camera technique showed an accumulation within 20 minutes of radionuclide in kidneys and bladder, with no normal transport in the spinal canal moving in a cranial direction. The blood samples in the omental-shunted animals had a significantly higher level of radionuclide than in the control group.[12,13] To prove the value of an omental-lumbar shunt in the treatment of hydrocephalus, it was necessary to show its effects in hydrocephalic animals and demonstrate the existence of CSF bulk absorption from an omental graft placed in the isolated lumbar sac. For this purpose, an experimental procedure was performed on shunt-operated dogs by the infusion of mock CSF under constant pressure with continuous measurement of the inflow volume. The

pressure-flow curve showed an increased outflow of CSF in animals with lumbo-omental pedicle graft. The difference in outflow was particularly marked in perfusion of the isolated dural sac (*Figure 7.2*). Thus, while the outflow in the control animals was very low, if any, the omentum-operated animals showed CSF drainage that amounted to one third of the gross outflow from the total CSF system in the control animals. The increase in bulk flow of CSF in animals with a lumbo-omental shunt was statistically significant, and the outflow in the isolated spinal sac of control animals was virtually non-existent.[11] By microangiographic technique and by visualization through an operating microscope, an abundant network of newly formed vascular channels was observed growing from the intradural portion of the omental flap to the dura and the surrounding muscles.[13] These results are in agreement with a 1975 study by Goldsmith et al[14] on revascularization of the spinal cord in dogs. This group found that new blood vessel developed between the meninges of the spinal cord and the pedicle graft of the omentum as early as 3 days after implantation.

CLINICAL STUDIES

Early in the course of our investigation it was felt that a lumbo-omental flap could absorb lumbar CSF and thus improve a hydrocephalic condition. No untoward effects of the implantation of the greater omentum into different areas of the body had ever been reported. The greater omentum had actually been used in other studies to enhance CSF absorption, although in a different location.[14] Against this background, it was considered justified to use the lumbo-omental shunt procedure in a small series of patients with clinical hydrocephalus. The clinical part of this chapter will give a 7 to 32 year follow-up of our first four patients (in all 97 y). For surgical technique, see Levander et al[22] and *Figure 7.3.*

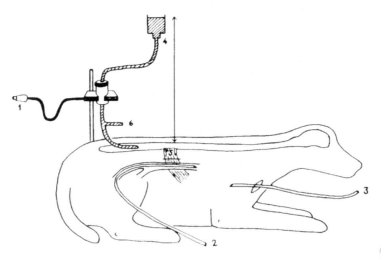

Figure 7.1 Dogs in horizontal prone position. Varying the height container with mock CSF (4) produced different levels of steady-state CSF pressure, measured through a side branch (6). An electronic drop recorder (1) measured the volume of infused fluid. Central venous pressure (3) and systemic arterial pressure (2) were recorded. The lumbo-omental flap (5) is marked with a horizontal bar at the region of clamping (see text). (From Levander and Zwetnow, *Acta Neurochirurgica*, 1978).

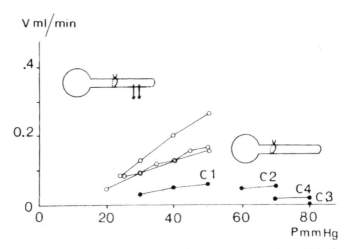

Figure 7.2 Pressure-flow curves from isolated dural sacs. Control animals C1-C4, dogs with lumbo-omental shunt open circles. No inflow of fluid occurred at 1 mm Hg and 10 mm Hg. Note the varying opening pressure and nearly horizontal slope of the curve from the control animals. No infusion occurred in animal C3, despite a cerebrospinal fluid pressure of 80 mm Hg. (From Levander and Zwetnow, *Acta Neurochirurgica*, 1978)

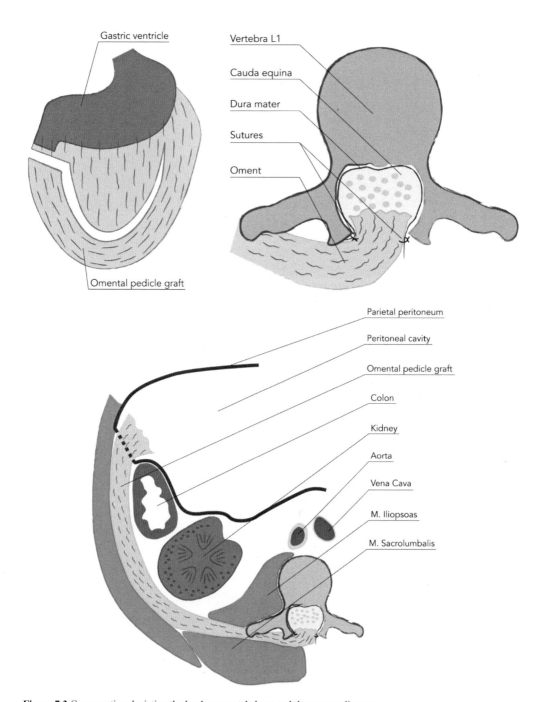

Figure 7.3 Cross-section depicting the lumbo-omental shunt and the surrounding area.

Table 7.1 Clinical history of patients

Patient	Age	Occupation	Type of brain disorder	Lumbo-omental Shunt op	Pre- or postop CT ventr. index*
RA	48	Butcher	Aneurysm-bleeding	1974	0.49-0.44
RC	27	Biological scientist	Head injury	1976	0.51-0.38
LS	35	Typesetter Photographer	Head injury	1978	0.39-0.34
KS	29	-	Congenital comm. hydrocephalus	2003	-

*The ventricular index[15] over the anterior horns calculated by computed tomography (CT).

Case reports: A total follow-up of 97 years

All of the three first patients had developed a communicating hydrocephalus (CH), two after head injury and the third after subarachnoid hemorrhage resulting from an aneurysm of the anterior communicating artery (*Table 7.1*). On admission 1 to 2 years after head injury or subarachnoid hemorrhage, which required an intracranial operation, the patients demonstrated the typical clinical picture of CH, which among other signs included unsteadiness of gait, psychomotor retardation, spatiotemporal disorientation, and deterioration of short-term memory. The diagnosis of communicating hydrocephalus was confirmed by computed tomography (CT), lumbar constant-infusion Katzman test,[16] and radionuclide cisternography. The first patient (RA) had pre- and postoperative carotid angiography combined with cerebral blood flow.

The lumbar-constant infusion test showed normal values 12 months after the shunt operation. The mental capacity of the patients was examined immediately before and 3 weeks after the operation with psychometric tests, except in Case No. 4 (KS)—Benton, Block, K.S. Memory test battery and CVB scale (the CVB scale is a Swedish modification of the Wechsler Adult Intelligence Scale).[17,18,19] The tests showed a general improvement, with a statistically significant increase of the IQ score. At testing 1 year later, this improvement was stabilized (*Table 7.2*). Case No. 2 (RC) developed bilateral subdural hematomas 7 months after the shunt operation. He was readmitted, the hematomas were evacuated, and the patient was again discharged in good condition. Eight years after the surgery, one of the patients (RA) was suffering from low back pain and sciatica, which required a lumbar CT myelogram. Two minutes after intrathecal administration of contrast media (Isopaque), the omental graft was visualized with its rapid transport of the water-soluble contrast (*Figures 7.4A and 7.4B*). His low back pain and sciatica disappeared after 2 weeks.

Table 7.2. Patient psychometric tests/IQ scores

Patient	Age	Psychometric tests/IQ score	
		Preoperative	Postoperative
RA	48	70-77	94-102
RC	27	127-133	136-142
LS	35	77-83	112-118

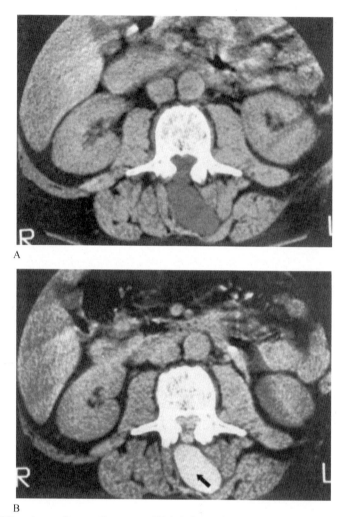

Figure 7.4 Lumbar CT myelogram 8 years after surgery. CT **A:** before and **B:** 2 min after lumbar injection of contrast media (Isopaque). Notice the rapid transport of the water-soluble contrast in the omental graft (arrow).

Case No. 4 (KS) suffered from congenital toxoplasmosis with CH. The patient was treated with a ventriculoperitonial shunt in early infancy. She then suffered repeated malfunctions, often associated with infections, and was subjected to a large number of revisions—no fewer than 82 shunt operations (*Figure 7.5*). There was a successive development of neurological deficits in the form of optic atrophy, diplopia, ataxia, and speech disturbance. At age 29, the patient was again urgently admitted with severe signs of shunt malfunction. For the first time in 3 decades, it was decided to try treatment with lumbo-omental shunting. As part of the preoperative assessment, a ventricular catheter was implanted for continuous intracranial pressure (ICP) monitoring. The original surgical technique was employed (*Figure 7.3*). The patient recovered soon after

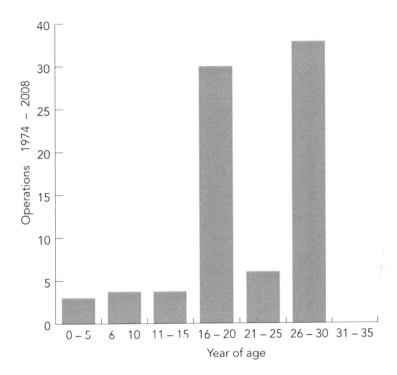

Figure 7.5 Incidence of surgical shunt interventions in 5-year periods in the 36-year-old woman with a congenital CH reported. At the age of 17, she suffered frequent skin infections and acne (*Proprionibacterium acnes* and *Staphylococus epidermis*), which caused repeted shunt malfunctions due to bacterial colonization. The lumbo-omental shunt operation was performed when she was 29 years old. Note that in the subsequent 6-year period, no further surgery was required.

surgery, and the ICP normalized. The first sign of clinical improvement was that menstruation reappeared after years of amenorrhea, presumably a secondary result of reduced stretch of the third ventricle. Subsequently, the neurological symptoms slowly subsided, headaches ceased, and she became totally independent. She even started training alpine skiing and competed in the 2008 Special Olympics World Winter Games in Boise, Idaho. She won a gold and a bronze medal.[20]

All patients tolerated well the implanted omental graft, with no infections or CSF leaks. From a preoperative condition requiring institutionalization, all patients gradually returned to independent life and to their previous or similar occupations.

DISCUSSION

Experimental and clinical studies support the assumption that a lumbo-omental shunt can be a useful method in the treatment of communicating hydrocephalus and that the rapid vascularization by the omental graft may allow the best environment for nerve root or cord regeneration (study in progress, Levander et al).[21]

These qualities of the omentum (high absorption of CSF and extracellular fluid associated with edema, and the rapid angiogenesis of central nervous system [CNS] tissue) might be of high clinical therapeutic value for syringomyelia and traumatic cord lesions in the future.[13,23]

REFERENCES

1. Kausch W. Die behandlung des hydrocephalus der kleiner kinder. *Arch Klin Chir.* 1908;87:709-796.
2. Scarff JE. Treatment of hydrocephalus: an historical and critical review of methods and results. *J Neurol Neurosurg Psychiatry.* 1963;25:1-26.
3. Rekate HL. Treatment of hydrocephalus. In: *Pediatric Neurosurgery*, 2nd ed. Philadelphia: W.B. Saunders Co; 1989: Ch 14.
4. Driesen W, Elies W. Epidural and subdural hematomas as a complication of internal drainage of cerebrospinal fluid in hydrocephalus. *Acta Neurochir.* 1974;128:847-849.
5. Naidich TP, Epstein F, Lin JP, Jircheff II, Hochwald CM. Evaluation of pediatric hydrocephalus by computed tomography. *Radiology.* 1976;119:337-345.
6. Kraft AR, Tompkins RK, Jeseph JE. Peritoneal electrolyte absorption analysis of portal, systemic venous, and lymphatic transport. *Surgery.* 1968;64:148-153.
7. Goldsmith HS, De Los Santos R, Beattie EJ Jr. Relief of chronic lympedema by omental transposition. *Ann Surg.* 1967;166:572-585.
8. Goldsmith HS, Long term evaluation of omental transposition for chronic lympedema. *Ann Surg.* 1974;128:847-849.
9. Levander B, Wennerstrand J. Omentets likvorabsorberande formaga. En ny experi-mentell shuntteknik. *Sv Lakaresallskapets riksstamma Stockholm.* 1972;269.
10. Wennerstrand J, Levander B. Lumbo-omental drainage of cerebrospinal fluid. *Acta Chir Scand.* 1974;140:9-94.
11. Levander B, Zwetnow NN. Bulk flow of cerebrospinal fluid through a lumbo-omental pedicle graft in the dog. *Acta Neurochir.* 1978;41: 147-155.
12. Levander B, Asard P. Lumo-omental shunt for drainage of cerebrospinal fluid: an experimental study in dog. I: the transport of cerebrospinal fluid from the lumbar subarachnoid space, studied by 169Yb-DTPA and a gamma camera. *Acta Neurochir.* 1978;43:1-11.
13. Levander B, Asard PE. Lumbo-omental shunt for drainage of cerebrospinal fluid: an experimental radionuclide study in dog. II: evaluation of transport routes from lumbar subarachnoid space to venous blood. *Acta Neurochir.* 1978;43:251-262.
14. Goldsmith HS, Duckett S, Chen WF. Spinal cord vascularization by intact omentum. *Am J Surg.* 1975;129:262-265.
15. Hansow J, Levander B, Liliequiest B. Size of the intracerebral ventricles as measured with computer tomography, encephalography and echoventriculography. *Acta Radiologica.* 1975; suppl 346.
16. Katzman R, Hussel R. A simple constant infusion manometric test for measurement of CSF absorption. *Neurology.* 1970;20:534-544.
17. Benton AL. The revised visual retention test. Iowa City: State University of Iowa; 1955.
18. Cronholm B, Ottosson JO. Reliability and validity of a memory test battery. *Acta Psych Scand.* 1963;39:218-234.
19. Wechsler D. *The Measurement and Appraisal of Adult Intelligence.* Baltimore:Williams and Wilkins; 1958.
20. Scandinavian Airlines System (SAS) monthly magazine, *SCANORAMA.* Nov 2008.
21. Levander B, Aldskogius H, Mellstrom A. Effect of vascularized omental tissue on peripheral nerve or cauda equine. 2010 (in manuscript).
22. Levander B, Granberg PO, Hindmarsh T. Lumboomental shunt for drainage of cerebrospinal fluid in hydrocephalus. *Acta Neurochir.* 1978;44:1-9.
23. Levander B. *Studies on the Absorption of Lumbar CSF by a Pedicle Graft of the Greater Omentum* (thesis). Stockholm; 1977: ISBN 91-7222-190-199.

ACKNOWLEDGMENT

I would like to thank Johan Werner, photographer and illustrator at the University Hospital, Jankoping, Sweden, and Professor Bjorn Meyerson, Karolinsk Institute, Stockholm, Sweden, for their assistance in creating this chapter.

CHAPTER 8

PEDICLED OMENTAL LUMBAR GRAFTS FOR LUMBOSACRAL ADHESIVE ARACHNOIDITIS

R. LAWRENCE FERGUSON, M.G. LUKEN III,
AND R. A. GETTLEMAN

INTRODUCTION

Lumbosacral adhesive arachnoiditis (LSAA) can be viewed in a variety of ways, which include:

1. A public health issue responsible for 17% of a multimillion dollar growth industry known as "the failed back syndrome."
2. An unpredictable immune response by the arachnoid to a number of offending agents such as the oil-based contrast material previously used in lumbar myelography (Pantopaque), as well as aneurysmal subarachnoid hemorrhage, trauma, meningitis, intrathecal steroids, spinal anesthesia, and the nucleus pulposus itself.[1]
3. A confusing clinical condition that is difficult for clinicians to explain,[2] for patients to understand, and for courts to resolve.
4. All of the above.

THE CLINICAL PROBLEM

The unpredictable relationship between the clinical complaints of a patient with LSAA and the patient's radiologic findings led one experienced surgeon to call this condition arachnoiditis confuscens.[2] Most patients with the condition have a clinical picture that is comparable to the discomfort they experienced before the development of arachnoiditis and, in many other cases, it was thought to be coincidental. The painful symptoms of lumbosacral arachnoiditis are in sharp contrast to the myelopathic symptoms common to arachnoiditis that occur at the cervical and thoracic regions, making the clinical differences readily apparent.[3] A study of the long-range prognosis for patients with LSAA demonstrated that life expectancy was decreased by 12 years in this group and while their symptoms were not progressive, the return to work was unlikely, and their treatment in general was disappointing. In fact, the results from surgery for patients with LSAA has been reported to be actually worse than the discomfort that occurs in the natural history of this condition.[4]

There was early enthusiasm for microsurgical decompression of lumbosacral adhesive arachnoiditis[5,6] but interest has been markedly tempered,[7,8] and it is now felt that this microsurgical procedure should not be performed to treat this condition until a method is developed to prevent the recurrence of the postoperative scar that routinely forms at the operative site.[9] The authors believe they have developed such an operation for LSAA. The surgical procedure involves the microsurgical lysis of the adhesions affecting the cauda equina and lower spinal cord, followed by the application of a pedicled omental graft. The purpose of the graft is to prevent the reformation of scar tissue and to help revascularize the cauda equina.

Prior to describing the operative technique and postoperative results of the procedure, a short review of the pathology of arachnoiditis and its pathophysiologic characteristics will be helpful in explaining the rationale for lysing adhesions and the application of a pedicle omental graft for lumbosacral adhesive arachnoiditis.

PATHOLOGY OF LUMBOSACRAL ADHESIVE ARACHNOIDITIS

The response to injury is similar in the peritoneum, the pericardium, the pleura, and the dura mater, namely, vascular damage from scar formation that prevents normal revascularization. When the cauda equina is injured, fibrous arachnoid bands in the area of injury are invaded by fibrocytes and collagen, followed by calcium depositions. This invasion of arachnoid fibrils by collagen cells causes adhesions that have a constrictive effect on the cauda equina, which results in varying degrees of ischemia. Veins in the area of injury become restricted by scar tissue, which causes a higher venous pressure that is reflected in a diminished capillary perfusion pressure in the cauda equina.[10]

PATHOPHYSIOLOGY OF LUMBOSACRAL ARACHNOIDITIS

Fibrinolytic activity was studied in 34 patients with chronic back pain. It was found that fibrinolysis was significantly impaired in patients with chronic back pain compared to matched controls and particularly in patients with proven arachnoiditis. This

study suggested that there was an underlying defect in fibrinolytic activity in some patients that leads to fibrin deposition, which can be the cause of the chronicity of many back pain syndromes.[11]

Clinical features, contrast-enhanced lumbar tomographic findings, and biochemical plasma fibrinolysis determinations were critically assessed in a study of 70 patients suffering chronic post-surgical low back and radicular pain. These patients exhibited gross functional disability and significant impairment of their plasma fibrinolytic activity compared to 84 normal control subjects. The fibrinolytic defect was attributed to a disproportionate increase in circulating plasminogen activator inhibitor-1 levels. Clinical features were also found to be slightly worse in patients who showed radiologic evidence of epidural fibrosis, with these radiologic abnormalities also showing a higher correlation in patients with decreased fibrinolytic activity. However, no significant association was noted between biochemical and radiologic abnormality in patients with low back pain, but normal biochemical values were seen in control patients as opposed to those with arachnoiditis.[12] In experimental models, ß-endorphin in the brain was severely reduced and spinal cord metencephalon significantly elevated in iocarmate-treated mice who developed arachnoiditis.[13] Additionally, brain ß-endorphins were found to be decreased in monkeys with arachnoiditis.[14] The immunogenicity of cells incorporated in the arachnoid membrane was studied utilizing a protein substance (HLA-DR). This preparation demonstrated the *in vivo* immune capability of tissue-cultured arachnoid cells, which supported the long-held view that arachnoid cells are capable of initiating and participating in an immune inflammatory reaction.[15] Additional support for an immunologic basis for arachnoiditis is found in a clinical-immunological study of rhinosinogenic arachnoiditis in patients who developed blindness associated with chronic sinus infections.[16]

RATIONALE FOR USE OF OMENTAL LUMBAR GRAFT IN ARACHNOIDITIS

After review of the pathological and pathophysiological characteristics of arachnoiditis, there are several aspects of the biology of the omentum that suggest that it may help in the control of arachnoiditis and in alleviating some of its symptoms. The omentum is derived from the spleen, and the milky spots seen in the omental apron are known to have immune functions. This would have therapeutic implications for the immune inflammatory reaction seen in arachnoiditis; however, it is the angiogenic potential of the omentum[17] and its well-documented ability to reverse ischemia in a number of conditions[18-22] that first attracted this author (R.L. Ferguson). Increased levels of nerve growth factor, noradrenalin, and endorphins are also known to be present in omental tissue.[23,24] Additionally, the omentum can absorb cerebrospinal fluid, which can explain the successful use of an omental lumbar graft to treat hydrocephalus.[25] The intense biological activity of the omentum in contrast to subcutaneous fat is also well appreciated by the authors of this publication.[26]

PREVENTION OF ARACHNOIDITIS

Prevention of arachnoiditis remains the most effective way to limit this condition. The removal of oil-based contrast agents from myelography has led to a significant decrease, but not the elimination, of LSAA as a source of failed back syndrome. Using high-resolution MRI in 129 patients symptomatic for at least 1 year after low back surgery, arachnoiditis was reported in 20% of the cases, but when patient who had oil-based myelography were excluded from this group, only 3% of the patients experienced arachnoiditis. It was concluded that arachnoiditis can occur after extradural lumbar disc surgery, which can be diffuse or confined and can be independent of the use of myelographic contrast medium.[27]

Many cases of radiologically significant arachnoiditis do not have pain. When pain is present, however, it is typically constant and burning in nature and is comparable to the pain associated with causalgia. It is poorly localized palliospinal thalamic pain that is diffuse, unlike neospinal thalamic pain, which is sharp and well localized. Because of its constancy, pain from arachnoiditis is more depressing and debilitating to patients than a more intense but short-lived pain.[1] Pain that originates from the nerve-root compression, such as caused by vertebral column stenosis or instability, should be treated before therapy is applied to arachnoiditis.

Pain in the arachnoiditis is multifactorial, with the dorsal root ganglion being the most sensitive anatomic site for the pain. Compression of the capillaries by adherent scar formation causing ischemia is the likely pathophysiologic mechanism that is instrumental in the development of pain. However, in common with other chronic pain syndromes are personality and socioeconomic factors which can obfuscate a clinical picture associated with pain phenomenon. Findings on MRI in 165 patients who had symptoms suggestive of degenerative disease were evaluated to determine if there was a relationship between abnormalities of nerve and root compression and degenerative disease of the lumbar spine in the absence of other risk factors that could cause arachnoiditis[28] included central clumping of nerve roots in 16 patients (9.7% of which was associated with spinal stenosis, $P<0.001$). While this nerve-root clumping resulted from mechanical compression, the appearance was indistinguishable from the central pattern of nerve-root adhesions that occurs in adhesive arachnoiditis. Awareness of this finding may avoid the possibility of an incorrect diagnosis of arachnoiditis in the presence of treatable vertebral canal stenosis.[28]

FAT GRAFTS IN LUMBAR SURGERY

Fat grafts have been used for many years for the desired purpose of reducing postoperative epidural and peridural defects and minimizing postoperative cerebrospinal fluid leaks.[29-31] In 1979, animal studies demonstrated that pedicle fat grafts helped to prevent scar formation.[32] Previous studies on scar prevention reported in 1955 claimed that a free autologous graft was superior to other materials for this purpose.[33] Based on such reports, a free graft composed of subcutaneous fat, which is placed on exposed dura, continues to be common practice for many contemporary spine surgeons. However, it has been shown that free fat in the subcutaneous tissue is not as biologically active as fat that is present in the omentum.[26]

It was shown conclusively for the first time in 1985 that a pedicled omental graft, when placed on an injured spinal cord in an animal, had the ability to markedly reduce the development of scar tissue at the injury site.[34] This experimental work was later confirmed.[35] Such observations regarding the omentum led, in 1986, to the first use of the pedicled omentum for the treatment of a patient with a chronically injured spinal cord.[36] Eventually, this form of surgical treatment was successfully used on a patient with post-traumatic arachnoiditis.[37]

Surgical technique

Preoperative preparation:

1. An energetic bowel prep is ordered prior to surgery. Patients with arachnoiditis develop a paralytic ileus for 3 to 4 days following surgery. We believe that this is due to the surgical manipulation on the cauda equina that occurs during the operative procedure and to the extensive prior use of codeine and other medications consumed in quantity by patients who suffer the longstanding discomfort of adhesive arachnoiditis.

2. Two broad-spectrum antibiotics are given immediately before surgery and are continued for 1 to 3 days thereafter. This is done to reduce the risk from the usual contamination that can occur in both the neurosurgical portion and the abdominal portion of the operative procedure.

Operative technique:

A laparatomy and "Goldsmith" omental dissection is performed, with the omentum being brought through a lateral incision placed in a subcutaneous tunnel that runs to the cauda equina that has been surgically exposed.[38] A careful microsurgical lysis of the cauda equina adhesions is performed in the manner described by Wilkinson,[5] after which the pedicled omental graft is placed directly on the nerve roots of the cauda equina. The dural edges are sutured to the graft in a watertight manner in order to minimize the possibility of postoperative spinal fluid leak (*Figure 8.1*). In two patients where the dura was thinned and attenuated, a 2-inch cuff was made from artificial dura. The lower edge of this cuff was stitched to the dura, with the upper edge being stitched to the edge of the pedicled omental graft.

RESULTS

To date, we have performed 25 operations involving omental grafts, of which 11 were for cerebral applications and 14 were for spinal applications. Seven of the spinal procedures were for patients with lumbosacral adhesive arachnoiditis and details are presented in *Table 8.1.*

All of the patients were female, with the youngest being 40 years old and the oldest being 70 years old. In this study, patients who had ongoing litigation were not considered

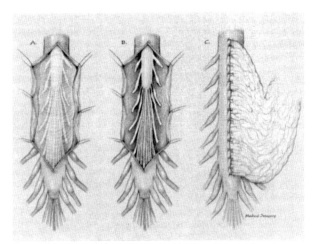

Figure 8.1 Lysis of cauda equine arachnoiditis and omental graft.

for this study because of the adverse effect litigation has shown to have on surgical results. We did the initial surgery in three patients, while four were referred by colleagues who had performed the previous lumbar surgery. Improvement in all patients was noted. Two are now working and are no longer on any pain medication. Three are functional but are still taking codeine. The remaining two patients are not working but have much reduced medication needs. It merits mention that five of these patients had private indemnity insurance, and their carriers paid for this procedure with only a simple explanation needed for the financial authorization of the operation. While patients with LSAA are rare, they are enormously costly to their insurance carriers.

Based on our understanding of the pathology of arachnoiditis, and the physiologic characteristics of the omentum, our initial good results with the use of the pedicled omental lumbar graft were not unexpected. However, because of the rarity of this condition in any single general surgical practice, it will take larger clinical trials to determine the eventual place of omental lumbar grafts in the treatment of patients with LSAA.

Table 8.1 Profile for lumbosacral arachnoiditis

Patient	Myelogram	Laminectomy	Fusions	Stimulator failure	Drug-addicted
1. BD 04/17/91	3	3	None	Yes	Yes
2. MK 04/18/91	2	2	0	Yes	Yes
3. CJ 08/17/92	2	2	Yes	Yes	Yes
4. AJ 10/21/92	4	3	0	Yes	Yes
5. SB 01/13/93	3	3	Yes	Yes	Yes
6. MJ 06/23/95	5	2	0	Yes	Yes
7. DF 11/18/96	2	3	0	Yes	Yes

REFERENCES

1. Burton CV. Adhesive arachnoiditis. In: Youmans JR, ed. *Neurological Surgery.* Philadelphia: Saunders; 1990:2856-2863.
2. Compare EL. Arachnoiditis confuscens. *Int Surg.* 1980;65:4.
3. Mooj JJA. Spinal arachnoiditis. *Acta Neurochir.* 1980;53:131-160.
4. Guyer DW. Long range prognosis of arachnoiditis. *Spine.* 1989;14:123.
5. Wilkinson HA, Schuman M. Results of surgical lysis of lumbar adhesive arachnoiditis. *Neurosurgery.* 1979;4:401-409.
6. Tomasello F, D'Avanzo R, Albanese V, Conforti R, Cioffi FA. Spinal ossifying arachnoiditis. *J Neurol Sci.* 1985;29:335-340.
7. Long DM (Chairman) Seminar (164-46AB) on the Failed Back. *AANS Ann Meet, Denver, Colorado, April 17, 1986.* (Available on audio cassette from Info-Medix, 12800 Garden Grove Blvd, Suite F, Garden Grove, CA 92643-2043, 714/530-3454).
8. Tetsworth KD, Ferguson RJL. Arachnoiditis ossificans of the cauda equina. *Spine.* 1986;11:765-766.
9. Johnson J, Matheny J. Microsurgical lysis of lumbar adhesive arachnoiditis. *Spine.* 1972;3:1.
10. Bourne IHJ. Pathology of arachnoiditis. *Roy Soc Med.* 1990.
11. Poutain GD, Keegan AL, Jayson MI. Impaired fibrinolytic activity in defined chronic back pain syndromes. *Spine.* 1987;12:83-86.
12. Cooper RG, Mitchell WS, Illingworth KJ, Forbes WS, Gillespie JE. The role of epidural fibrosis and defective fibrinolysis in the persistence of post laminectomy back pain. *Spine.* 1991;16:1044-1048.
13. Lipman BT, Haughton VM. Brain beta-endorphin and spinal cord. Enkephalin concentrations in experimental arachnoiditis. *Invest Radiol.* 1987;22:197-200.
14. Lipman BT, Haughton VM. Diminished cerebrospinal fluid beta-endorphin concentrations in monkeys with arachnoiditis. *Invest Radiol.* 1988;23:190-192.
15. Frank E, Mayfield F. Presented at: *Cong Neurol Surgeons,* Annual Meeting; 1982.
16. Mukhamedzhanov NZ, Blagoveshschenskaia NS, Simonova AV. Clinical-immunological studies in rhinosinogenic cerebral arachnoiditis. *Zhurnal Nevropatologii I Pakhitrii Imeni S-S-Korsakova.* 1990;990:98-100.
17. Williams R. Angiogenesis and the greater omentum. In: Goldsmith HS, ed. *The Omentum.* New York: Springer-Verlag; 1988:45-61.
18. Turner-Warwick R. The use of the omental pedicled graft in urinary tract reconstruction. *Trans Am Assoc Genitourinary Surgeons.* 1975;67:126-132.
19. Gue S. Omental transfer for treatment of radionecrosis of the chest wall. *Aust NZ J Surgery.* 1975;45:390-394.
20. Vineberg A. The bloodless greater omentum for myocardial revascularization. *Chest.* 1968;54:315-322.
21. Goldsmith HS, Chen WF, Duckett SW. Brain revascularization by intact omentum. *Arch Surg.* 1973;106:695-698.
22. Yazargil MG, Yonekawa Y, Denton I, Piroth D, Benes I. Experimental transplantation of autogenous omentum majus. *J Neurosurgery.* 1974;40:213-217.
23. Siek GC, Marquis JK, Goldsmith HS. Experimental studies of the omentum-derived neurotrophic factors. In: Goldsmith HS, ed. *The Omentum.* New York: Springer-Verlag; 1988:83-95.
24. Makintosh TK, Goldsmith HS. Vasoactive neurochemicals in the omentum. In: Goldsmith HS, ed. *The Omentum.* New York: Springer-Verlag; 1988:75-79.
25. Levander S, Wennerstand J. Lumbo-omental shunt for the treatment of communicating hydrocephalus. In: Goldsmith HS, ed. *The Omentum.* New York: Springer-Verlag; 1988: 207-221.
26. Bujalska IJ, Sudesh KS, Stewart PM. Does central obesity reflect 'Cushing's Disease of the Omentum.' *Lancet.* 1997;349:1210-1213.
27. Fitt GJ. Postoperative arachnoiditis diagnosed by high resolution spin echo MRI of the lumbar spine. *Neuroradiology.* 1991;37:176-180.
28. Jackson A, Isherwood T. Does degenerative disease of the lumbar spine cause arachnoiditis? *Br J Radiol.* 1994; 67: 840-847.
29. Burtgon CV. Full thickness fat grafts in the prevention of epidural fibrosis cont. *Neurosurgery.* 1984;5:1-6.
30. Lexer E. Die frien transplantation en Part 1. *Neue Deutsche Chirugie.* 1919;26:264-545.
31. Lexer E. Zwanag jahre transplantations forschung in der chirugie. *Arch Klin Chir.* 1925;38:251-302.
32. Gill GG, Sakovich I, Thompson E. Pedicled fat grafts for the prevention of scar formation after laminectomy: an experimental study in dogs. *Spine.* 1979;4:176-186.
33. Pospeeich J, Pankonk F, Stolke D. Superiority of free autologous grafts. *Eur Spine.* 1955;14:213-219.
34. Goldsmith HS, Stewart E, Duckett S. Early application of pedicled omentum to the acutely traumatized spinal cord. *Paraplegia.* 1985;23:100-112.
35. McMillan M, Staffert ES. Defective omental pedicle graft transfer on spinal microcirculation and laminectomy membrane formation in spine. *Spine.* 1991;16:176-180.
36. Goldsmith HS, Neal-Dwyer G, Arsume L. Omental transposition to the chronically injured spinal cord. *Paraplegia.* 1986;24:173-174.

37. Abrams G, Patterson A, Bothra M, Mofty AB, Taylor GM. Omental myelosin angiosis in the management of chronic traumatic paraplegia. *Paraplegia.* 1987;25:44-49.

38. Goldsmith HS. The omentum in spinal cord injury. In: Lee BV, Austrander LE, Cochran GVB, Shaw WWW, eds. *The Spinal Cord Injured Patient—Comprehensive Management.* Philadelphia: W.B. Saunders; 1991:313-329.

CHAPTER 9

APPLICATION OF OMENTAL TRANSPLANTATION TO MOYAMOYA DISEASE

JUN KARASAWA AND HAJIME TOUHO

INTRODUCTION

Moyamoya disease is an ischemic disease discovered by Japanese neurosurgeons.[1] Its onset may usually be seen by the age of 10 years. The cause still remains unknown, yet the disease begins with stenosis or occlusion at the periphery of the internal carotid artery and proximal segments of the anterior cerebral artery or the middle cerebral artery, followed by development of an abnormal vascular network that acts as a bypass in the neighborhood of the occlusion in the internal carotid artery, anterior cerebral artery, or middle cerebral artery. This vascular network looks like the rising smoke of tobacco and the condition is thus expressed as "moyamoya" (Japanese for "misty").

Moyamoya vessels, by the way of bypass, grow extremely slowly in relation to the progress of occlusion of the major vessels. Therefore, the brain may accommodate itself to the progressing ischemic condition, with some patients not exhibiting the disease even when the cerebral blood flow rate is reduced to about half. Carbon dioxide reactivity is clinically important in patients with Moyamoya disease, because conditions associated with reduction in arterial carbon dioxide partial pressure, such as crying, blowing food to cool it, rope skipping, playing the harmonica, laughing, and inflating a balloon, often provoke the symptoms. This article is concerned with 77 patients with omental transplantation performed on 79 sides out of a total of 630 patients diagnosed as having Moyamoya disease between 1973 and 1996. Ages ranged from 2 years to 56 years; there were 72 infants and 5 adults.

OMENTAL TRANSPLANTATION AND CEREBRAL BLOOD FLOW

There are two modes of surgical treatment for Moyamoya disease, direct and indirect vascular anastomosis. Indirect vascular anastomosis consists of encephalomyosynangiosis in which the temporal muscle is placed over the brain surface,[2] and encephaloduroarteriosynangiosis (EDAS) in which a non-divided superficial temporal artery flap is placed over the brain surface,[3] omental transplantation,[4] and gracillis muscle transplantation.[5] The most important factor needed for successful indirect vascular anastomosis is a lowered cerebral blood flow and an elevated oxygen extraction fraction (OEF) value, that is, the cerebral blood flow is in the state of misery perfusion. It is fortunate that Moyamoya disease has a broader region of misery perfusion than other occlusive diseases; blood circulation from the external carotid artery to the internal carotid artery may be completed when adhesion is accomplished between the superficial temporal artery flap, temporal muscle, omentum, and gracilis muscle when these structures are placed directly on the brain surface. The blood pressures of the superficial temporary artery and the occipital artery are equal to about 90% of the systemic blood pressure. On the other hand, the blood pressure on the brain surface in Moyamoya disease is about 25% to 35% of the systemic blood pressure; once vascular connections have been established with such a difference in the blood pressure, a good blood flow may be preserved as a result of the larger blood vessels becoming increasingly involved, thus inviting an increase in the cerebral blood flow rate.

Generally, the internal carotid artery is first occluded in Moyamoya disease, followed by occlusion of the posterior cerebral artery.[6]

Stenosis or occlusion of the posterior cerebral artery usually starts from the quadrigeminal segment of the posterior cerebral artery, with the Moyamoya vessels that develop at that segment contributing to the preservation of the blood flow at the periphery of the posterior cerebral artery. However, in patients who have poor development of the Moyamoya vessels or in whom the periphery of the posterior cerebral artery cannot be well visualized radiologically despite development of these blood vessels, blood flow does not run smoothly through the posterior cerebral artery and is the possible cause of symptoms such as half-blindness and unusual visual field defects. The symptom of homonymous hemianopsia can often progress to stroke instead of being confined to transient ischemic attack (TIA).[4]

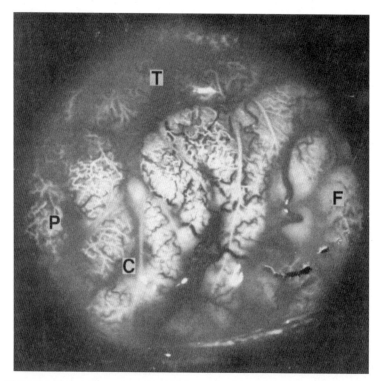

Figure 9.1 Fluorescein angiography at 13.1 sec after venous injection of the dye shows various and prolonged filling. F, frontal lobe; T, temporal lobe; C, central sulcus.

Vascular occlusion in Moyamoya disease first occurs at the distal part of the internal carotid artery and the proximal part of the anterior or middle cerebral artery, with the occlusion moving steadily toward its periphery as time passes. Small Moyamoya vessels, which are consequently created at those areas of occlusion, may help maintain the peripheral blood flow. Hence, there is a very high vascular resistance down to the cortical artery in contrast to a low perfusion blood pressure for the brain tissue.[7] This explains the absence of ischemic foci at the central region of the brain of patients with Moyamoya disease and the presence of wedge-like infarctions on their brain surface. Complexity of the blood flow on the brain surface may be illustrated by fluorescein angiography in which the arrival of the dye to the brain surface is variable at different sites (*Figure 9.1*).[8] In some patients,

therefore, the extent of ischemic progression varies at different sites of the brain; in such cases, variation in reduction of the cerebral blood-flow rate can be seen. Thus, there may be various pathological conditions of cerebral ischemia even throughout the same brain; in such cases, there may also be variation in carbon dioxide reactivity (*Figures 9.2 and 9.3*).[9] This indicates that hypercapnia may not always be ideal during anesthesia. Normocapnia is important as a factor in cerebral blood flow in Moyamoya disease.

Whether omental transplantation is indicated or not is decided on the basis of symptoms, cerebral angiography, examination of the cerebral blood flow by means of single photon emission computed tomography (SPECT), and examination of the cerebral blood-flow reserve by acetazolamide,[10] which is performed at the time of tomography.

Y.S.

7 y.o.

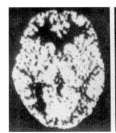 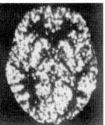

		PaCO$_2$ 42		PaCO$_2$ 32		CO$_2$ Reactivity	
		Rt.	Lt.	Rt.	Lt.	Rt.	Lt
Temporal	gray	110	106	49	36	6.1	7.0
Frontal	gray	55	61	14	13	4.1	4.8
	white	28	18	4	12	2.4	0.6
Occipital	gray	111	112	60	74	5.1	3.8
	white	39	50	19	22	2.0	2.8
Parietal	gray	97	113	48	43	4.9	7.0
	white	36	36	19	15	1.7	2.1
Thalamus		134	133	68	60	6.6	7.3
Putamen		118	115	86	52	3.2	6.3
Caudate nucleus (head)		117	110	86	63	3.1	4.7
Cerebellum hemisphere		190	212	54	58	13.6	15.4
vermis		177		44		13.3	

Figure 9.2 Xenon CT/CBF study, Normal CO$_2$ reactivity.

S.H.

13 y.o.

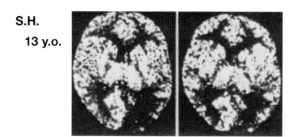

		PaCO$_2$ 44		PaCO$_2$ 36		CO$_2$ Reactivity	
		Rt.	Lt.	Rt.	Lt.	Rt.	Lt
Temporal lobe		75	65	90	65	-1.9	0
Frontal	gray	76	68	42	39	4.3	3.6
	white	22	23	13	17	1.1	0.8
Occipital	gray	78	23	79	39	-0.1	-2.0
	white	21	13	16	14	0.6	-0.1
Parietal	gray	77	100	67	105	1.3	-0.6
	white	32	32	30	27	0.3	0.6
Thalamus		119	97	115	93	0.5	0.5
Putamen		86	111	110	123	-3.0	-1.5
Caudate nucleus (head)		80	91	67	109	1.6	-2.3
Cerebellum		64		58		0.8	

Figure 9.3 Reverse CO$_2$ reactivity at some sites.

OMENTAL TRANSPLANTATION IN MOYAMOYA DISEASE

Harvesting the omentum

A median incision is made from the xiphoid process down to the umbilicus. Upon laparotomy, the greater omentum of the stomach will be seen directly under it. The gastroepiploic artery and vein may be seen running in parallel with the greater curvature of the stomach; in addition, a large number of thin blood vessels may be seen communicating between the artery and the stomach and between the stomach and the vein (*Figure 9.4*). these blood vessels are coagulated by the bipolar coagulator and divided, allowing the stomach to be separated from the gastroepiploic artery and vein. Both ends of the gastroepiploic artery are ligated with silk thread, and the artery and vein are removed in 1-cm lengths from the fat tissue.

At this point, the size of the greater omentum that is needed for the transplantation is cut by scissors while being coagulated by the bipolar coagulator. Finally, the gastroepiploic artery and vein are divided, and an elastic tube for irrigation is inserted into the artery and ligated. Heparin-added saline is injected through it to wash out blood components from the blood vessels within this piece of the greater omentum, which is then immersed and preserved in heparin-added saline.

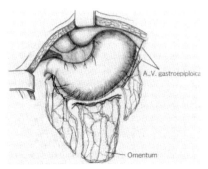

Figure 9.4 (above) An omentum fragment is isolated with the gastroepiploic artery and vein being attached.

Figure 9.5 (right) In the case of PCA ischemia, craniotomy is performed with the patient in the prone position in such a way that the occipital lobe may be exposed with the transverse sinus coming to the bottom.

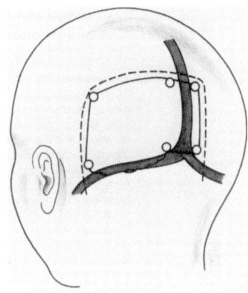

Anastomosis between the epicranial artery/vein and the gastroepiploic artery/vein

In the case of insufficiency of the anterior cerebral artery, a coronal incision is made so that the frontal branch of the superficial temporal artery may be fully exposed, and after the flap is reversed, a bone opening covering both sides of the frontal region is created, and then the superficial temporal artery and vein are separated in 1-cm lengths from the flap, and a rubber dam is laid down

In the case of insufficiency of the posterior cerebral artery, anastomosis is made in the prone position; an arched skin incision is made from the origin of the mastoid beyond the median line so that the occipital artery may be included in the flap, while the bone opening should go beyond the median line with its bottom reaching the transverse sinus (*Figure 9.5*). If there is no infarction detected in the occipital lobe by computed tomography (CT), bilateral craniotomy should be performed. The occipital artery and vein coming into the flap from the posterior side of the mastoid should be identified and removed from the flap in about 1-cm lengths, and then a rubber dam is laid down (*Figure 9.6*). It should be noted that the artery can be easily identified by its pulsations in the frontal and occipital regions, whereas the vein is often difficult to discover.

Initially, two clips are placed on the superficial temporal artery or the occipital artery under the surgical microscope, and a longitudinal incision of about 0.8 to 1.2 mm is made over the clipped interval. Following irrigation of this blood vessel with heparin-added saline, it is connected to the gastroepiploic artery by 8 to 12 stitches using 10-0 monofilament nylon, and after systemic administration of heparin, the clips are removed. The gastroepiploic artery will then pulsate strongly, changing the color of the blood vessels within the greater omentum to red and causing blood to drip from the gastroepiploic vein. The artery is clipped again, followed by placement of two clips on the superficial temporal vein or the occipital vein, with the interval between the clips being incised and connected with the stump of the gastroepiploic vein by 6 to 8 stitches (*Figure 9.7*).

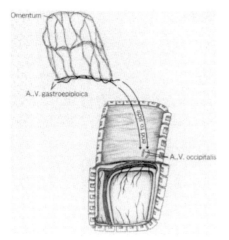

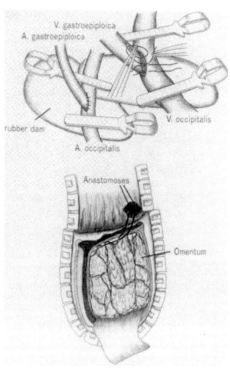

Figure 9.6 (above) The occipital artery and vein are exposed from the flap in about 1-cm lengths.

Figure 9.7 (right) Sutures are made between the occipital artery and the gastroepiploic artery and between the occipital vein and the gastroepiploic vein with 10-0 monofilament nylon using the surgical microscope.

Next, the clips on the vein are removed, and if no leakage of blood is observed, the artery is unclipped. Once the blood flow is resumed within the greater omentum, the superficial temporal vein or the occipital vein will usually bulge outward (*Figures 9.8 and 9.9*).

The dura mater is incised and opened, after which the greater omentum is spread over the brain surface (*Figure 9.7*). The dura mater is then positioned in such a way that a sizable coverage over the brain is achieved and then stitched in place. After an epidural drain is placed, the bone grafts are fixed at several spots over the bone around the craniotomy. The operation is concluded when the scalp is sutured in a double-layer fashion.

If an appropriate superficial temporal vein or the occipital vein cannot be identified, the ascending vein on the brain surface at the site of the craniotomy should be used.

Postoperative control

Because this operation is associated with incomplete closure of the dura mater, cerebrospinal fluid is liable to pool under the skin. A cerebrospinal fluid collection is likely to appear when the operation is made in the occipital region since the wound is beneath the cranial space. The cerebrospinal fluid collection lowers the pressure of the cerebrospinal fluid, occasionally inducing retching and vomiting soon after the operation. It is recommended that the epidural drain should be removed and compression bandage be applied the next day. The greater omentum has an effect of absorbing fluid. As long as the blood flow is maintained within the greater omentum, the cerebrospinal fluid can be absorbed through the liquid-absorbing effect of the greater omentum, leading to the subcutaneous resolution of cerebrospinal fluid collection in 3 to 7 days.

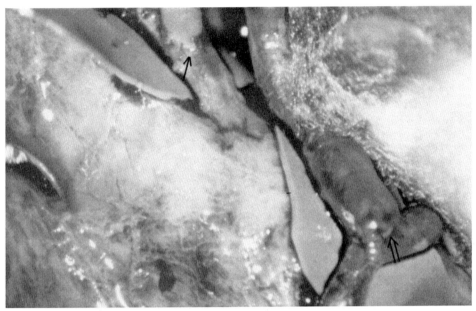

Figure 9.8 (See color section.) Occipital artery-gastroepigastric anastomosis (↑), and occipital vein-gastroepigastric vein anastomosis (↑↑).

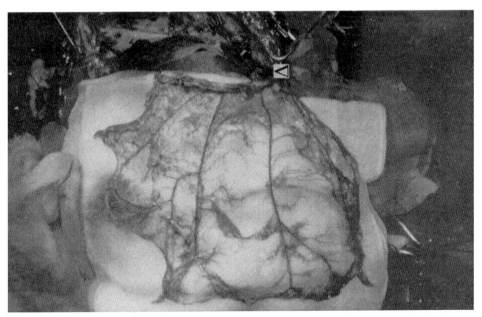

Figure 9.9 (See color section.) When clips are removed upon completion of anastomosis, the blood starts flowing again through the blood vessels within the omentum, making them red. Δ indicates the site of anastomosis.

Angiography conducted soon after the operation will visualize the superficial temporal artery and/or occipital artery, gastroepiploic artery, various blood vessels within the greater omentum, gastroepiploic vein, superficial temporal vein and/or occipital vein, and the external jugular vein. After a lapse of 1 to 3 months, angiography will visualize superficial temporal artery/occipital artery, gastroepiploic artery, anterior cerebral artery or posterior cerebral artery, superior sagittal sinus, and sigmoid sinus, which probably coincides with the arrest of progression of neurologic symptoms or their improvement.

CASE REPORT

Case 1: MK, a 9-year-old female patient

At the age of 1 year, crying was associated with palsy on the right half of the body, subsequently followed by development of TIA with palsy on the left half of the body. At age 2, these symptoms gradually became worse. With bilateral superficial temporal artery-middle cerebral artery (STA-MCA) anastomoses, TIAs ceased and her palsy symptoms improved.

At age 8, gait disturbance occurred. Angiography failed to visualize the anterior cerebral artery on either side (*Figure 9.10*). At age 9, omental transplantation to both frontal lobes was performed. This resulted in resolution of TIAs and improvement of symptoms, but a mild reduction of intelligence remained. Postoperative angiography of the external carotid artery successfully visualized the middle cerebral artery from the parietal branch of th superficial temporal artery (STA) and the anterior cerebral artery from the frontal branch (*Figures 9.11 and 9.12*).

Case 2: MI, an 8-year-old male patient

At age 5, the patient developed palsy of all limbs with increased palsy of the upper and lower limbs bilaterally whenever he cried. He was treated by bilateral EDAS at another hospital and, as a result, his TIAs were reduced. At age 8, he was admitted to our hospital because palsy of all limbs had occurred together with a speech disorder that was induced by crying. Angiography failed to visualize the left middle cerebral artery from the left STA, so we conducted a left STA-MCA anastomosis.

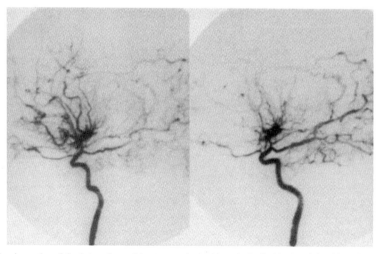

Figure 9.10 Angiography of the internal carotid artery on both sides. **A:** Left side; **B:** right side. The anterior cerebral artery on both sides is only poorly visualized.

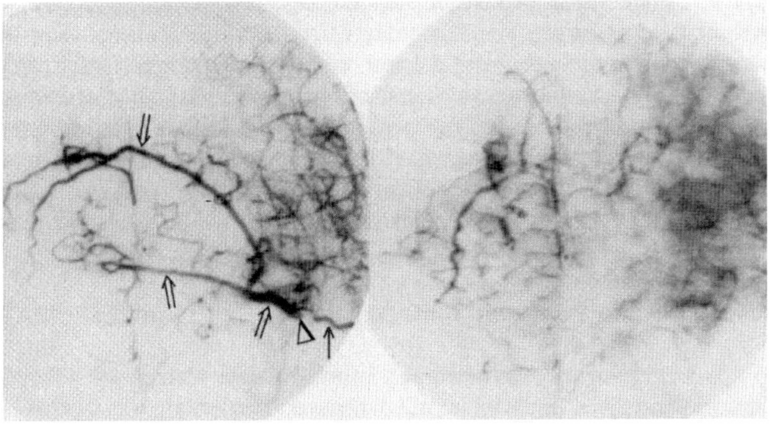

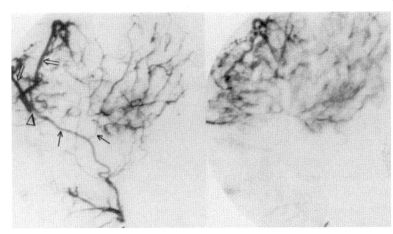

Figure 9.11 Angiography of the left external carotid artery. Anteroposterior view. **A:** Arterial phase; **B:** late arterial phase. The anterior cerebral artery on both sides is visualized from the frontal branch of the STA (↑) through the gastroepiploic artery (↑↑). Δ indicates the site of anastomosis.

Figure 9.12 Angiography of the left external carotid artery. Lateral view. **Left**, arterial phase; **Right**, late arterial phase. The anterior cerebral artery is visualized from the frontal branch of the STA (↑) through the gastroepiploic artery (↑↑) while the middle cerebral artery is visualized from the parietal branch of the STA (↑) and the meningeal artery. Δ indicates the site of anastomosis.

However, as his episodes of paraparesis did not improve, we performed omental transplantation to the left frontal lobe. After the surgery, TIAs became less frequent and completely disappeared after 1 year, making the patient self-composed with an increased ability to read and comprehend.

Preoperative angiography almost completely failed to show the anterior cerebral artery (*Figure 9.13*). However, postoperative angiography of the external carotid artery demonstrated anterior cerebral artery blood flow from the frontal branch of STA through omentum vessels and middle cerebral artery flow from the parietal branch of STA and the meningeal artery (*Figure 9.14*). An increased blood flow of the anterior lobe was seen with SPECT (*Figures 9.15 and 9.16*).

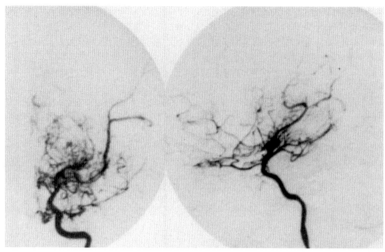

Figure 9.13 Angiography of the left internal carotid artery. The anterior cerebral artery is not visualized.

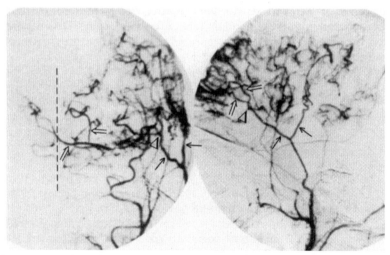

Figure 9.14 Anteroposterior view (left) and the lateral view (right) in angiography of the left external carotid artery. The anterior cerebral artery is visualized from the frontal branch of the STA (↑) through the gastroepiploic artery (↑↑) while the middle cerebral artery is visualized from the parietal branch (↑) and the meningeal artery. Δ indicates the site of anastomosis. Broken line: median line.

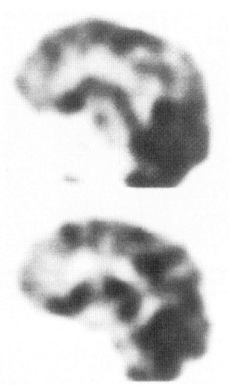

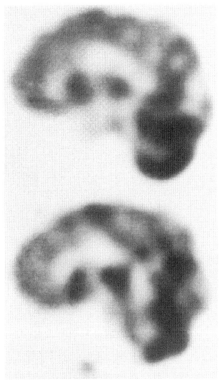

Figure 9.15 Sagittal view of the preoperative SPECT. The right cerebral hemisphere (top) and the left cerebral hemisphere (bottom) showing a decreased blood flow in the frontal lobe.

Figure 9.16 Sagittal view of the postoperative SPECT. The right cerebral hemisphere (top) and the left cerebral hemisphere (bottom) showing an increased blood flow in the frontal lobe.

Case 3: SL, a 14-year-old female patient

At the age of 11 years, she began to have TIAs, including a right hemiparesis and a speech disorder when she was scolded into crying. Similar episodes occurred from time to time thereafter. At age 13, she had additional attacks of TIAs along with neurologic left hemiparesis. Superficial temporal artery-middle cerebral artery anastomosis was performed on the right and left sides. Subsequently, her symptoms of TIA sharply decreased. Six months later, she became aware that she had an irritating focus in the left field of vision. At the age of 14, she had frequent episodes of blindness in her left field of vision lasting for several minutes on each occasion. Angiography of the vertebral artery demonstrated occlusion of the right posterior cerebral artery (*Figure 9.17*). Omental transplantation was performed on the right occipital lobe using the right occipital artery. After the operation, her TIAs, as manifested by left-sided blindness, disappeared while angiography of the right occipital artery visualized the posterior cerebral artery and part of the middle cerebral artery through the omentum (*Figures 9.18 and 9.19*).

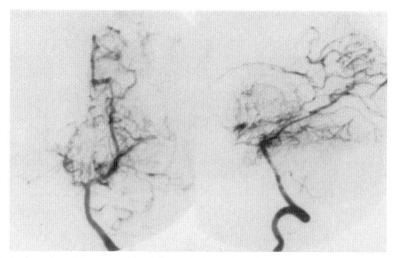

Figure 9.17 Angiography of the preoperative left vertebral artery. Anteroposterior view (left) and the lateral view (right). The periphery of the right posterior cerebral artery is not visualized.

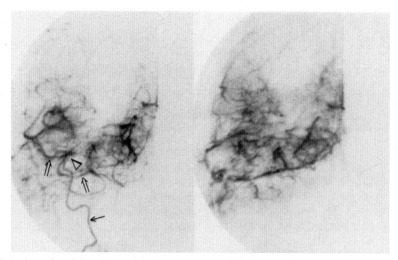

Figure 9.18 Angiography of the right occipital artery. Late arterial phase (left) and capillary phase (right) in the anteroposterior view. The posterior cerebral artery and part of the middle cerebral artery are visualized from the occipital artery (↑) through the gastroepiploic artery (↑↑). Δ indicates the site of anastomosis.

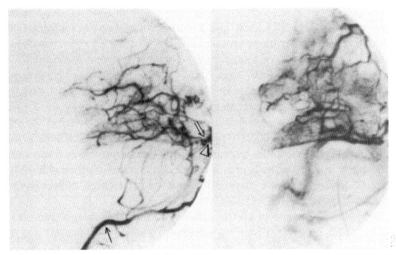

Figure 9.19 Angiography of the right occipital artery. Lateral view: arterial phase (left). Venous phase (right). The posterior cerebral artery and part of the middle cerebral artery are visualized from the occipital artery (↑) through the gastroepiploic artery (↑↑). The contrast agent is seen eliminated through the sigmoid venous sinus. Δ indicates the site of anastomosis.

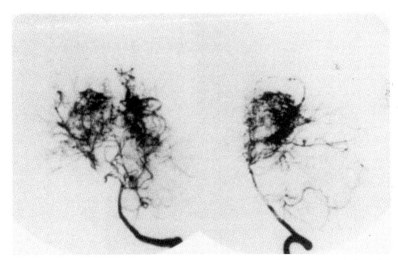

Figure 9.20 Angiography of the left vertebral artery. Anteroposterior view (left) and the lateral view (right). Stenosis at the proximal posterior cerebral artery on both sides. Occlusion at the quadrigeminal segment, where Moyamoya vessels may be seen, but the distal posterior cerebral artery is not visualized.

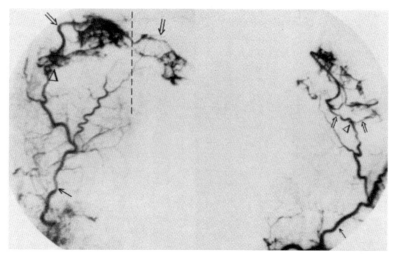

Figure 9.21 Angiography of the right occipital artery. Arterial phase in the anterior-posterior view (left). Arterial phase in the lateral view (right). The posterior cerebral artery on both sides is visualized from the occipital artery (↑) through the gastroepiploic artery (↑↑). Δ indicates the site of anastomosis. Broken line: median line.

Case 4: TA, a 6-year-old female patient

At the age of 3 years, she went blind for 30 seconds while blowing to cool hot noodles. At age 4, she developed left hemiparesis. She was treated by bilateral EDAS at another hospital. After the operation, she continued to have episodes of poor eyesight lasting for about 1 minute once every month or so. Angiography of the left vertebral artery demonstrated occlusion of the posterior cerebral artery on both sides (*Figure 9.20*). Omental transplantation was performed on the occipital lobe using the right occipital artery. After the operation, she had no further attacks of ocular symptoms.

Postoperative angiography of the occipital artery successfully visualized the posterior cerebral artery (*Figure 9.21*). Single photon emission computed tomography demonstrated an increased blood flow in the occipital lobe (*Figures 9.22 and 9.23*).

RESULTS OF OMENTAL TRANSPLANTATION

We report on 54 cases of ischemia in the frontal lobe and 25 cases in the occipital lobe. Two cases had symptoms involving both lobes. There were 28 cases who exhibited lowered intelligence.

Angiography following omental transplantation succeeded in allowing extensive radiological visualization of the frontal lobe (more than two thirds of the lobe visualized) in 18 cases, good visualization (about one half of the lobe visualized) in 26 cases, poor visualization (part of the lobe visualized) in 6 cases, no visualization in 3 cases, and no postoperative angiography in 1 case. For the occipital lobe, angiography succeeded in wide visualization in 12 cases, good visualization in 9 cases, poor visualization in 1 case, no visualization in 1 case, and no postoperative angiography in 2 cases (*Table 9.1*).

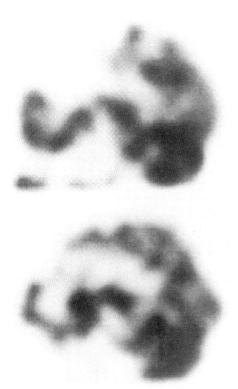 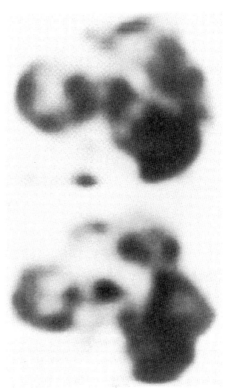

Figure 9.22 Sagittal view of the preoperative SPECT. The right cerebral hemisphere (top) and the left cerebral hemisphere (bottom). A decreased blood flow may be seen in the frontal lobe and the occipital lobe.

Figure 9.23 Sagittal view of the postoperative SPECT. The right cerebral hemisphere (top) and the left cerebral hemisphere (bottom) showing an increased blood flow in the occipital lobe on both sides.

Consequently, neurological symptoms involving the frontal lobe group were classified as markedly improved in 41 cases, improved in 6 cases, and unchanged in 6 cases, with one death. The corresponding results of the occipital lobe group were markedly improved in 16 cases, improved in 6 cases and unchanged in 3 cases (*Table 9.2*).

The clinical outcome of all the patients were further categorized into three groups: good, moderate disability, and severe disability. Of interest was the persistence of five cases of homonymous hemianopsia in the group considered "good." Except for this finding, they remained normal.

For the frontal lobe group, 33, 12, and 8 cases, respectively, were considered good, moderate, or with severe disability, with one postoperative death due to renal insufficiency. The corresponding figures for the occipital lobe group were 16, 7, and 2 cases, respectively (*Table 9.3*).

Table 9.1 Area of cerebral revascularization

	Excellent	Good	Poor	None	*
Frontal lobe	18	26	6	3	1
Occipital lobe	12	9	1	1	2

Excellent: More than 2/3 of the lobe is visualized. Good: About 1/2 of the lobe is visualized.
Poor: Part of the lobe is visualized. *Angiography was not obtained after omental transplantation.

Table 9.2 Early results: 3 months after omental transplantation

	Good	Moderate	No effect	Death
Frontal lobe	41	6	6	1
Occipital lobe	16	6	3	

Table 9.3 Clinical outcome more than 1 year after omental transplantation

	GR	MD	SD	Death
Frontal lobe	33	12	8	1
Occipital lobe	16	7	2	

GR, good recovery; MD, moderate disability; SD, severe disability.

DISCUSSION

It was Goldsmith who first used the omentum for the treatment of ischemic symptoms involving the brain and spinal cord. He placed it over the brain surface by way of an intact pedicled omental graft that was placed in a subcutaneous tunnel developed up the chest to the brain.[11,12] Subsequently, Yasargil and Yonekawa[13,14] isolated the omentum as a tissue fragment supplied by an epigastric artery and vein and placed over the brain surface, after which they were anastomosed to an artery and vein of the scalp. These experiments were performed in dogs and monkeys and subsequently the blood flow to the brain through the omentum was clearly demonstrated by post-mortem histology or by post-mortem angiography.

Ischemia of the internal carotid artery may be treated by STA-MCA anastomosis, which can improve the blood flow in the region of the middle cerebral artery but has little effect on increasing the blood flow in the region of the anterior and posterior cerebral arteries. Ischemic symptoms originating from the anterior cerebral artery begin with occlusion of the internal carotid artery. A dorsal callosal artery of the posterior cerebral artery serves as collateral circulation. If occlusion of the posterior cerebral artery begins at this time, a reduction in the blood flow of the dorsal callosal artery takes place. If the dividing ridge of the anterior cerebral artery is forced to move behind the precentral lobes because of reduced blood flow, neurologic symptoms develop.[15] These symptoms include dyskinesia of the lower limbs, sensory disturbance, urinary/fecal incontinence, lack of facial expression, reduction of intelligence, and decreased spontaneous movement. This accounts for the fact that relapses after STA-MCA anastomosis are often accompanied by paralysis of the lower limbs. Ocular symptoms associated with occlusion of the posterior cerebral artery may be improved by omental transplantation onto the occipital lobe.

There were 11 cases in which postoperative

selective angiography resulted in "poor" or "not patent" visualization (*Table 9.1*), but some of the patients were found to have spontaneous anastomoses from the meningeal artery to the middle cerebral artery, which usually developed after operation for Moyamoya disease. Early postoperative symptoms resolved in 41 cases in the frontal lobe group and in 16 cases in the occipital lobe group (*Table 9.2*). Symptoms remained unchanged in 9 cases.

With regard to the eventual clinical outcome, 33 cases of frontal lobe omental transplantation and 16 cases of occipital lobe omental transplantation were completely cured, although 5 cases of those cured patients had persistent visual disturbances, which had no negative effects on their activities. These 49 cured patients consisted, prior to surgery, of 42 cases of TIA, 2 cases of minor stroke, and 5 cases of stroke. Out of the 19 cases (12 plus 7 cases with moderate disability in Table 9.3), 17 of these patients had mental deterioration after surgery. Those patients classified as having severe disability can carry out activities with difficulty and walk with supporting devices. Of the 10 cases with severe disability (8 plus 2 cases in Table 9.3), 7 suffered from intelligence disorder resulting from a preoperative stroke.

Comparison of an intelligence disorder with CT findings showed cerebral transplantation was less effective with a large cerebral infarct, and the possibility of improvement was less when earlier cerebral ischemia eventually led to cerebral infarction.

In summary, omental transposition in our hands for Moyamoya disease proved most effective in the absence of preoperative stroke and mental deficits.

REFERENCES

1. Takeuchi K, Shimizu K. Hypoplasia of the bilateral internal carotid arteries [in Japanese]. *No to Shinkei.* 1957;9:37-43.
2. Kredel FE. Collateral cerebral circulation by muscle graft. Technique of operation with report of 3 cases. *5th Surg.* 1942;11:235-244.
3. Matsushima Y, Fukai N, Tanaka K, et al. A new surgical treatment of moyamoya disease in children: a preliminary report. *Surg Neurol.* 1981;15:313-320.
4. Karasawa J, Touho H, Ohnishi H, Miyamoto S, Kikuchi H. Cerebral revascularization using omentum transplantation for childhood moyamoya disease. *J Neurosurg.* 1993;79:192-196.
5. Touho H, Karasawa J, Ohnishi H. Cerebral revascularization using gracilis muscle transplantation for childhood moyamoya disease. *Surg Neurol.* 1995;43:191-198.
6. Karasawa J, Touho H, Kawaguchi M. Moyamoya disease: diagnosis and treatment. *Neurosurg Quart.* 1996;6:137-150.
7. Okada M, Shima T, Matsumura S, Nishida T. Pathophysiological studies in moyamoya disease by rCBF and cortical artery pressure measurements in comparison to those in ICAS or MCA occlusion [in Japanese]. *No to Shinkei.* 1988;40:899-903.
8. Takeuchi S, Ishii R, Tsuchida T, Tanaka R, Kobayashi K, Ito J. Cerebral hemodynamics in patients with moyamoya disease: a study of the epicerebral microcirculation by fluorescein angiography. *Surg Neurol.* 1984;21:333-340.
9. Kuwabara Y, Ichiya Y, Sasaki M, et al. Response to hypercapnia in moyamoya disease. Cerebral response to hypercapnia in pediatric and adult patients with moyamoya disease. *Stroke.* 1997;28:701-707.
10. Touho H, Karasawa J, Ohnishi H. Preoperative and postoperative evaluation of cerebral perfusion and vasodilatory capacity with 99mTc-HMPAO-SPECT and acetazolamide in childhood moyamoya disease. *Stroke.* 1996;27:282-289.
11. Goldsmith HS, Chen WF, Duckett SW. Brain vascularization by intact omentum. *Arch Surg.* 1973;106:695-698.
12. Goldsmith HS, Duckett S, Chen WF. Prevention of cerebral infarction in the monkey by omental transposition to the brain. *Stroke.* 1978;9:224-229.
13. Yasargil MG, Yonekawa Y, Denton I, Piroth D, Benes I. Experimental intracranial transplantation of autogenic omentum majus. *J Neurosurg.* 1974;39:213-217.
14. Yonekawa Y, Yasargil MG. Brain vascularization by transplantation omentum: a possible treatment of cerebral ischemia. *Neurosurgery.* 1977;1:256-259.
15. Touho H, Karasawa J. Ohnishi H. Hemodynamic evaluation of paraparetic transient ischemic attacks in childhood moyamoya disease. *Neurol Res.* 1995;17:162-168.

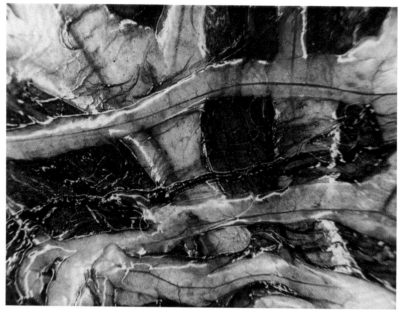

Figure 3.1 (See page 38.) Omental lymphatics absorb dye within 30 seconds after immersion in India ink solution.

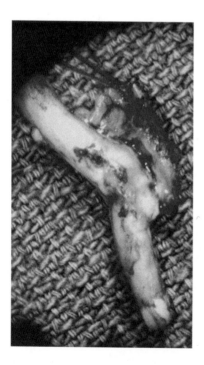

Figure 3.2 (See page 39.) Circumferential scar formation has developed several weeks following a standard 400 g cm^{-1} injury to cat spinal cord. Note dense scar at point of impact with persistent fluid accumulation in area where still-edematous spinal cord has herniated into laminectomy site

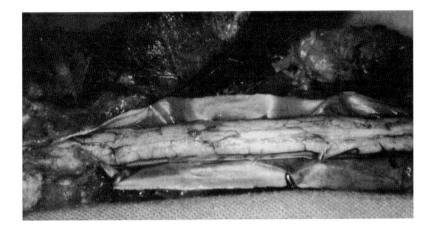

A

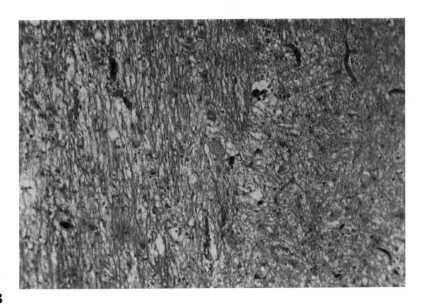

B

Figure 3.6 (See page 42.) Omental-spinal cord segment of cat removed en bloc. Dye markers injected into an omental artery are apparent **A:** on spinal cord surface and **B:** in deeply located spinal cord capillaries.

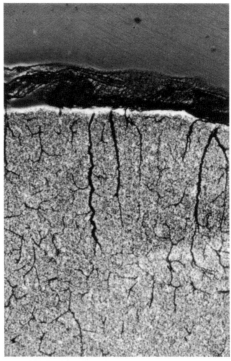

Figure 3.8 (See page 43.) Omentum placed on brain shows blood vessels filled with India ink penetrating directly into underlying brain tissue. The blood-brain barrier is broken.

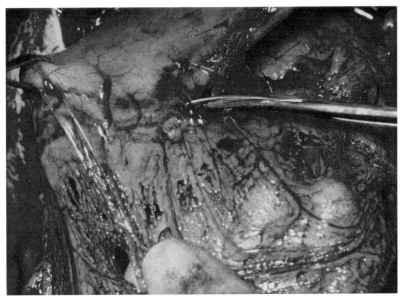

Figure 3.10 (See page 45.) Second major surgical maneuver is to remove the omentum from proximal portion of the greater curvature of the stomach. This is tedious because of the numerous small blood vessels connecting the stomach to the omental apron.

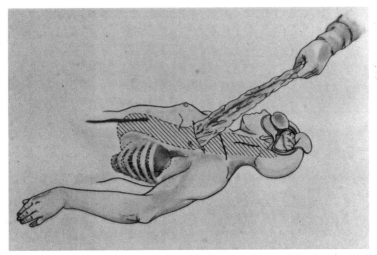

Figure 3.12 (See page 47.) Omentum is brought up through a subcutaneous tunnel to the exposed brain.

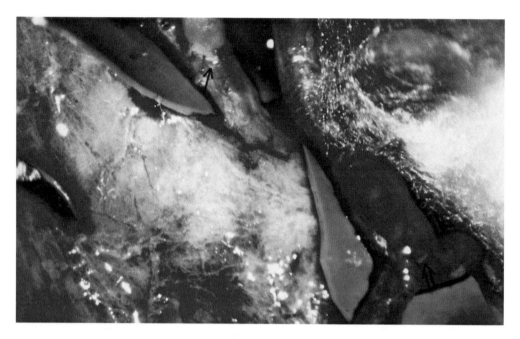

Figure 9.8 (See page 117.) Occipital artery-gastroepigastric artery anastomosis (↑), and occipital vein-gastroepigastric vein anastomosis (↑↑).

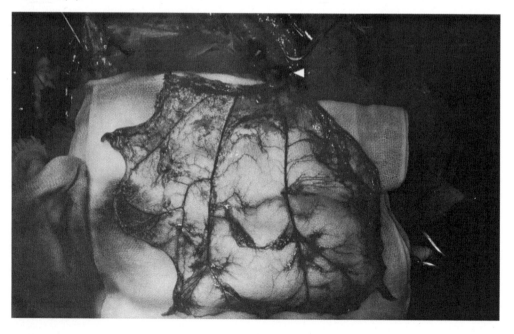

Figure 9.9 (See page 117.) When clips are removed upon completion of anastomosis, the blood starts flowing again through the blood vessels within the omentum, making them red. Δ indicates the site of anastomosis.

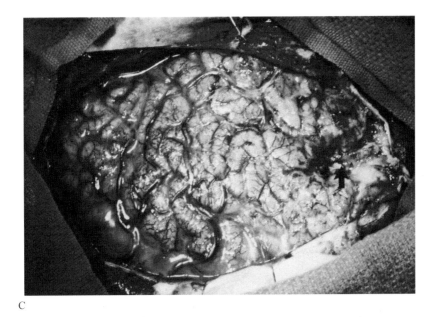

C

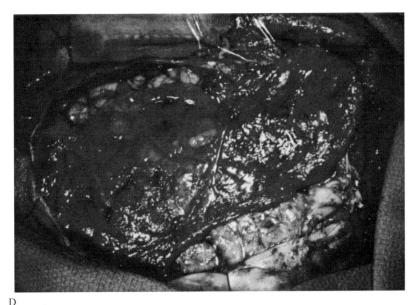

D

Figure 10.1 (See page 139.) C: Right cerebral hemisphere exposed for omental transposition. Arrow indicates small area of prior infarct. **D:** Omentum transposed to cerebral cortex after opening arachnoid.

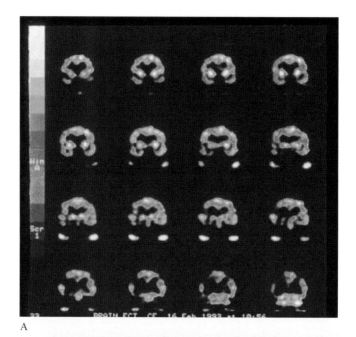

A

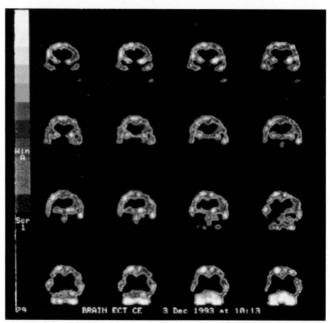

B

Figure 15.4 (See page 191.) **A:** Preoperative SPECT scan. Coronal slices with images displayed in an anterior to posterior position with color scale on right side. A major preoperative perfusion defect is seen in right parietal-occipital location. **B:** Postoperative SPECT examination 10 months after surgery. Reperfusion has occurred in right parietal-occipital area. (From Goldsmith HS. *Neurol Res.* 1996;18:103-108).

AD1 HMPAO SPECT

Post-op 4 months   Post-op 15 months

Post-op 23 months   Post-op 42 months

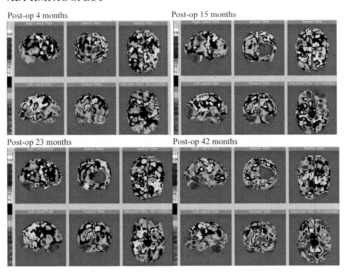

AD2 HMPAO SPECT

Post-op 4 months   Post-op 14 months

Post-op 20 months   Post-op 39 months

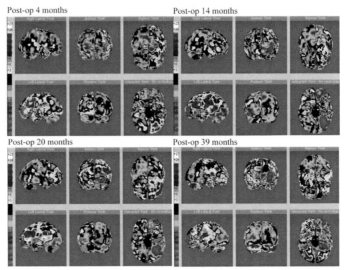

Figure 16.4: (See page 204.) Changes in cortical activities measured by SPECT. The changes in cortical activity for patients AD1 and AD2 were studied with quantitative HMPAO SPECT neuroimaging for up to 41 months. We standardized the longitudinal changes in regional brain HMPAO SPECT activity by dividing the percent change by the standard deviation of test-retest values (σ=5.25%). Patients AD1 and AD2 showed a maximal increase in cortical activity of four standard deviations (21%), plus showed increased cortical activity of one to two standard deviations above preoperative baseline for between 22 and 41 months in areas underneath, adjacent to, and directly contralateral to the omentum. Since the cortical activity of other areas decreased by 20%-27% over 41 months, we hypothesize that the omentum delivers its effect to directly underlying and trans-synaptically connected cortical areas. The changes in the CDRSS, MMSE, and NPI values are consistent with the observed increases in HMPAO SPECT cortical activity.[10]

CHAPTER 10

OMENTAL TO CEREBRAL TRANSPOSITION FOR THE TREATMENT OF CEREBRAL ISCHEMIA

JEFFREY A. LEE AND GARY K. STEINBERG

INTRODUCTION

Omental grafts have been successfully used for revascularization of ischemic organs and post-traumatic reconstruction.[1,2] Its uses include reconstruction of scalp defects and complicated wounds, salvage of ischemic limbs, and reduction of lymipedema.[3-5] However, the technique of omental grafting was not applied to revascularizing the brain until 1973.

EXPERIMENTAL RESULTS

In 1973, Goldsmith and colleagues first described pedicled omental transposition to the surface of the brain in dogs.[6] Vascular anastomoses between the brain and the omentum were demonstrated via fluorescein and India ink injections. Remarkably, staining with dye markers in deep portions of the brain, including the contralateral cerebral hemisphere, were confirmed histologically. The following year, free omental transposition was performed by Yasargil in dogs via microsurgical end-to-end and end-to-side anastomoses of the gastroepiploic artery and vein.[7] Graft patency rates approached 70%.

In 1975, Goldsmith and colleagues reported that omental transposition to the canine brain 1 to 18 months prior to complete occlusion of the middle cerebral artery (MCA) prevented cerebral infraction.[8] Extracerebral blood flow delivered to the brain via the omentum supplied sufficient blood to prevent stroke. They confirmed their results in monkeys in 1977, showing omental transposition 4 to 6 weeks before MCA occlusion prevented hemiparesis and infarct.[9] Yasargil and Yonekawa also demonstrated attenuation of infarct size in dogs using free omentum transplantation 2 to 3 months before MCA occlusion.[10] In addition, Goldsmith and colleagues showed that omentum placed directly over the spinal cord could lead to blood vessel development at the omental-spinal–cord interface.[11] Together, these results suggested omental transposition might be a useful technique for cerebral and spinal cord revascularization.

DeRiu, Viale, and colleagues measured blood flow in rabbit brain tissue using a modified inhaled hydrogen clearance technique. Pedicled omental grafts placed 3 months prior to MCA occlusion minimized stroke by maintaining collateral blood supply and limiting the decline of cerebral flow.[12] They later showed normal patterns of somatosensory evoked potentials (SEPs), with only a mild (25%) drop in regional cerebral blood flow (rCBF), thus functionally preserving cortical electrical activity.[13]

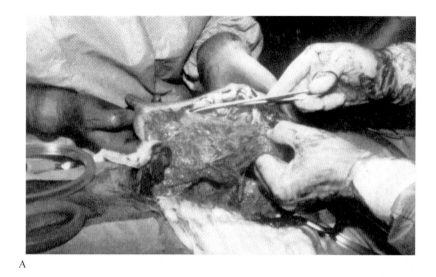

A

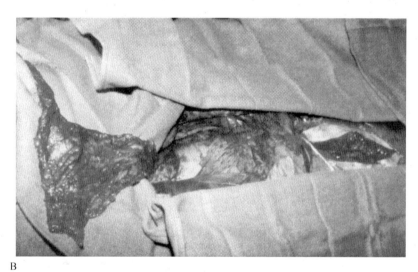

B

Figure 10.1 A: Harvesting of pedicled omentum from abdomen, maintaining its vascular supply. **B:** Omentum tunneled subcutaneously along the chest wall.

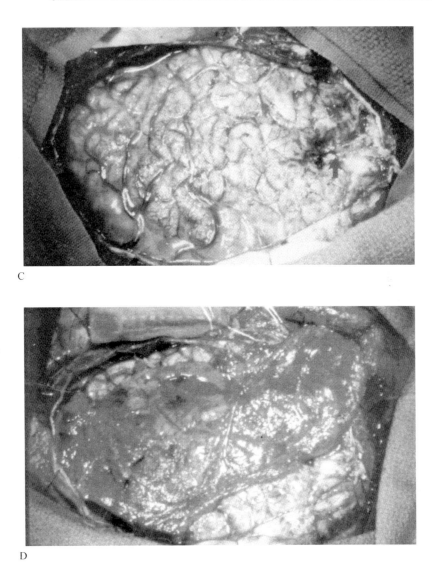

C

D

Figure 10.1 (See color section.) C: Right cerebral hemisphere exposed for omental transposition. Arrow indicates small area of prior infarct. **D:** Omentum transposed to cerebral cortex after opening arachnoid.

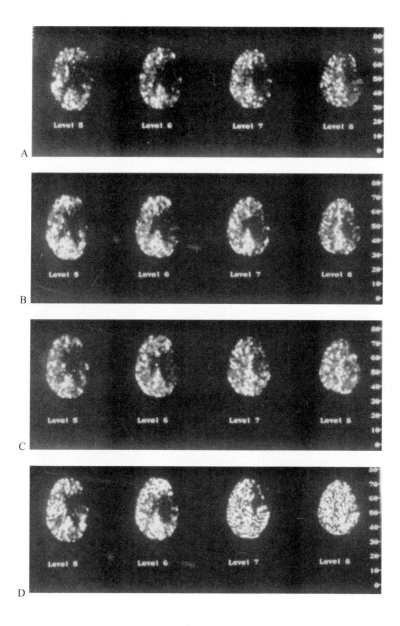

Figure 10.2. 64-year-old male with occlusive disease and prior left parietal infarct. **A:** Xenon CT without acetazolamide prior to omental transposition. **B:** Xenon CT after acetazolamide prior to omental transposition. Note impaired hemodynamic reserve in the left hemisphere. **C:** Xenon CT without acetazolamide 4 months following omental to left hemisphere pedicled graft. **D:** Xenon CT after acetazolamide 4 months following omental to left hemisphere pedicled graft. Note markedly improved hemodynamic reserve.

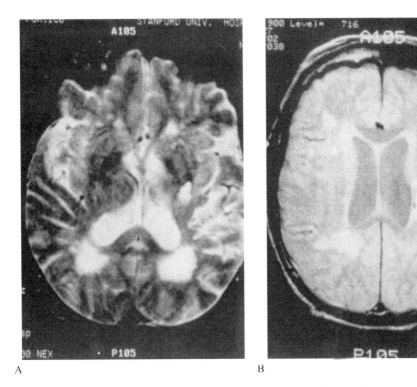

A   B

Figure 10.3 A: MRI of ischemia brain before omental-to-cerebral transposition. **B:** MRI of brain after omental-to-cerebral transposition. Arrow indicates omental graft.

MECHANISM OF CEREBRAL PROTECTION AGAINST ISCHEMIA

Goldsmith and colleagues have hypothesized that the mechanism underlying cerebral protection for omental transposition may be threefold. First, the additional source of blood brought to the brain by ingrowth of omental vessels may improve flow to the ischemic penumbra: viable but non-functional neurons at the borders of a cerebral infarct. Second, omentum may absorb vasogenic edema, resulting in decreased interstitial tissue pressure and a reciprocal rise in capillary perfusion pressure. In spinal cord injury models, omentum placed on the cord shortly after injury decreased scar formation, possibly by absorption of edema and fibrinogen.[14] Decreased conversion of fibrinogen to fibrin would be expected to result in decreased scarring. Third, various nutritive factors are produced by omentum, including angiogenic substances, neurotransmitters, nerve growth factors, and gangliosides. The angiogenic substance may act as a stimulus for developing widespread collateral circulation from the omentum to the brain.

OPERATIVE TECHNIQUE

Goldsmith has reported the surgical technique used to elongate and transpose pedicled omentum to the brain.[14] Initially, the omentum is separated from the transverse colon. Proximal and central attachments to the greater curvature of the stomach are removed. Gastroepiploic vessels are left intact within the omental apron. In order to gain increasing length of omentum, the left gastroepiploic vessels are divided, and the omentum is partially divided while preserving its arterial and venous connections along the periphery. After sufficiently lengthening, the omentum, in order to allow it to reach the brain without tension, is tunneled subcutaneously or retrosternally along the chest wall and neck, behind the ear, to beneath the base of a scalp flap. A craniotomy is performed. The dura is opened and small areas of arachnoid membrane are opened. The omentum is placed directly on the brain and secured to the surrounding dura with interrupted sutures.

For free omental transplantation, omentum is removed from the abdominal cavity. The parent gastroepiploic artery and vein are ligated and divided. A thin piece of omentum is excised, including a 4- to 5-cm length of parent artery and vein with branches to the arcade complex with its gastroepiploic vessels. The sheet of omentum is fashioned to include the arcade complex and its blood supply. A craniotomy is performed, and the superficial temporal artery and vein prepared. Using the microscope and 10-0 suture, an end-to-end or end-to-side anastomosis of the gastroepiploic vein and superficial temporal vein is performed, followed by an end-to-end or end-to-side anastomosis of the gastroepiploic artery and superficial temporal artery.[7]

CLINICAL STUDIES

In 1979, Goldsmith first reported the results of omental transposition in patients. Three aphasic patients 8, 30, and 66 months following a dominant hemispheric ischemic stroke underwent pedicled omental transposition to the brain. One patient showed only minor subjective and objective improvements in mental and physical capabilities. Two patients showed subjective improvement in speech, confirmed by language and psychometric examinations. Somatosensory evoked potentials over the dominant hemisphere were increased, and initial delays in brainstem auditory evoked responses (BAERs) improved. There were no complications.[15]

Herold and colleagues used positron emission tomography (PET) to measure regional cerebral blood flow, blood volume, and fractional oxygen consumption in four stroke patients prior to 6 months following omental transposition. There was no change in these physiological parameters postoperatively. Either blood flow through the transposed omentum was not sufficient to increase flow to the critically perfused area, a brain-to-omentum anastomosis failed to form, or the changes were beyond the resolution capability of the PET scanner.[16]

Goldsmith and colleagues reported a statistically significant increase in regional cerebral blood flow in four to six patients 5 years after omental transposition for cerebral ischemia. Postoperative blood-flow values, recorded by the Xenon-133 inhalation method, were increased over infracted areas of brain upon which omentum had been placed, as well as in areas of the ischemic hemisphere without omental placement and the contralateral hemisphere. Of the five patients who demonstrated preoperative flow values below normal for age, four showed final cerebral blood flow within normal limits for their age. Three of the patients with improved blood-flow values demonstrated some improved neurological function.[17]

Yoshioka et al have performed free omental transposition in four patients with ischemic cerebrovascular disease, in hopes of increasing the collateral blood flow to the brain and restoring cerebrovascular reserve capacity.[18] All four patients, ages 47 to 63 years, suffered from cerebral ischemia, including transient ischemic attack (TIA), reversible ischemic neurological deficit (RIND), or stroke, and demonstrated impairment of hemodynamic reserve using cerebral blood flow studies with acetazolamide challenge prior to surgery. All four patients showed clinical improvement, as well as increased perfusion reserve capacity by CBF study following omental to cerebral transposition. Patent gastroepiploic arteries were demonstrated on postoperative angiography. No patient experienced further recurrent ischemic episodes.

Karasawa and colleagues reported free omental transplantation to brain in a single patient with Moyamoya disease in 1980. The patient presented with impairment of recent memory, left hemiplegia, right hemiparesis, and blindness. Angiography revealed obstruction of the proximal posterior cerebral and terminal portions of the internal carotid arteries bilaterally. Anterior and middle cerebral arteries were only slightly visible through the basal Moyamoya vessels. Two months after free omental transplantation, temporal and occipital arteries were visualized angiographically via a right external carotid injection. Eighteen months later, central, parietal, and temporal arteries were visible through the transplanted omentum via a right external carotid angiogram.[19]

Karasawa and colleagues performed free omental transplantation in 30 of 400 children with Moyamoya disease who had previously been treated with superficial temporal artery-middle cerebral artery (STA-MCA) anastomosis, encephalomyosynangiosis (EMS), or encaphaloduroarteriosynangiosis (EDAS) for anterior circulation ischemia. Patients, ages 2 to 17 with persistent anterior and/or posterior cerebral artery ischemic symptoms, including paraparesis and visual disturbances, were further treated with omental transplantation. Seventeen patients with monoparesis, paraparesis, and/or urinary incontinence were treated with unilateral and bilateral omental transplantation to the anterior cerebral artery territory. Eleven patients with visual symptoms were treated with unilateral or bilateral omental transplantation to the posterior cerebral artery territory. Two patients had symptoms associated with both anterior and posterior cerebral artery territories and were treated with dual omental transplantations. Three months postoperatively, all patients with omental transplantation to the anterior cerebral artery territory showed neurological improvement, while 11 of 13 patients with omental transplantation to the posterior cerebral artery territory showed neurological improvement. Nausea and vomiting was the only reported complication.[20]

A single patient with Moyamoya disease has been reported[21] in whom an initial STA-MCA bypass failed to control ischemic symptoms despite a patent anastomosis. A subsequent pedicled omental transposition to the right cerebral cortex resulted in a dramatic improvement of the patient's symptoms over a 2½ year follow-up. Postoperatively, deep venous thrombosis was a complication.

The senior author has performed either pedicled or free omental to cerebral transposition in 17 patients suffering prior stroke or TIAs in addition to prior stroke (*Table 10.1*). Seven patients had Moyamoya disease and 10 had atherosclerotic or thromboembolic occlusive cerebrovascular disease. There were 6 males and 11 females; ages of patients ranged from 9 to 70 years old. The mean clinical follow-up was 3.4 years. No patients suffered a subsequent stroke or TIA ipsilateral to the omental-cerebral transposition. One child with Moyamoya disease showed almost complete resolution of his daily TIAs. Eleven patients remained neurologically stable while six patients showed modest improvement. The six who improved were younger (mean age 34 years compared with 51 years). Four of seven patients with Moyamoya disease improved clinically and functionally as compared with 2 of 10 patients with occlusive cerebrovascular disease. Minor complications included subgaleal fluid collections, subdural hygromas, temporary worsening in preoperative neurologic deficits, transient seizures, ventral hernia, and wound dehiscence. The use of a postoperative lumbar subarachnoid drain has significantly reduced the incidence of postoperative subgaleal and subdural hygromas.[22]

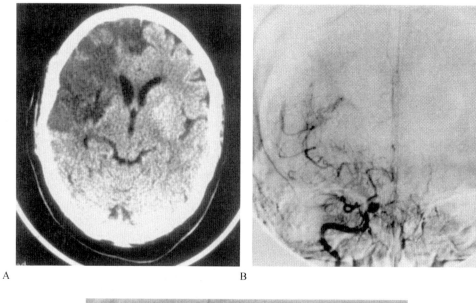

A   B

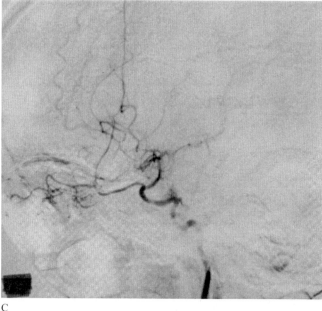

C

Figure 10.4 A: CT of brain demonstrating right frontoparietal infarct prior to omental transposition. **B:** Cerebral angiogram, right carotid injection. AP view demonstrating focal high-grade stenosis of supraclinoid internal carotid artery and resultant poor filling of the anterior and middle cerebral arteries. **C:** Cerebral angiogram, right carotid injection. Lateral view demonstrating focal high-grade stenosis of supraclinoid internal carotid artery and resultant poor filling of the anterior and middle cerebral arteries.

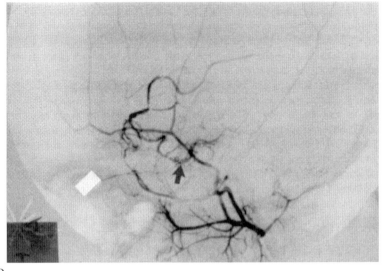

D

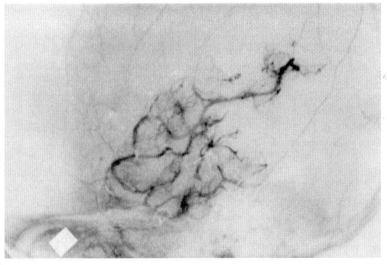

E

Figure 10.4 D: Early phase right lateral cerebral angiogram after free omental-to-cerebral transposition demonstrating omental graft filling via superficial temporal artery-gastroepiploic artery anastomosis (arrow). **E:** Later-phase right lateral cerebral angiogram after free omental-to-cerebral transposition demonstrating middle cerebral artery vessels filling.

Table 10.1 Omental-to-cerebral transposition and transplantation for cerebral ischemia. Stanford Series, 1991–1995.

Patient	Age	Sex	Diagnosis	Preoperative neurologic deficit	Prior surgery	Graft type	Complication	Clinical outcome
A.D.	36	F	Moyamoya	Aphasia Visual field deficit Short-term memory loss	Left EDAS Left STA-MCA	Free	Wound dehiscence	Improved
T.D.	33	F	Occlusive	Left hemiparesis Left homonymous hemianopsia		Free		Improved
B.R.	42	F	Moyamoya	Right hemiplegia Right homonymous hemianopsia Aphasia Seizures	Right STA-MCA	Free	Subgaleal CSF collection	Stable
T.B.	59	M	Occlusive	Right hemiplagia Right homonymous hemianopsia Aphasia Short-term memory loss		Free		Stable
H.R.	70	F	Occlusive	Left hemiparesis		Free	Subgaleal CSF collection	Stable
B.G.	42	F	Moyamoya	Left hemiparesis Seizures Short-term memory loss	AVM resection	Pedicle	Subdural CSF collection	Improved
J.D.	57	M	Occlusive	Right hemiparesis Aphasia		Pedicle		Stable

Patient	Age	Sex	Disease	Presentation	Prior surgery	Omentum	Complication	Outcome
M.B.	60	F	Occlusive	Right hemiparesis Aphasia		Free	CSF leak	Stable
B.H.	39	M	Occlusive	Left hemiparesis Seizures		Pedicle		Improved
H.Z.	64	M	Occlusive	Right hemiparesis Aphasia		Pedicle		Stable
J.W.	62	F	Occlusive	Right hemiparesis Aphasia		Pedicle	Wound dehiscence	Stable
E.S.	76	M	Occlusive	Right hemiparesis Aphasia		Pedicle	Ventral hernia	Stable
C.S.	41	F	Moyamoya	Left hemiparesis	Left STA-MCA	Free	Subdural CSF collection	Stable
J.L.	47	F	Moyamoya	Right hemiparesis Aphasia	Right STA-MCA Right EDAS	Free		Improved
A.B.	24	F	Moyamoya	Left homonymous hemianopsia Seizures Memory loss	Bilateral STA-MCA	Free		Stable
L.D.	11	F	Occlusive	Left hemiparesis		Free		Stable
R.H.	9	M	Moyamoya	Right hemiparesis Aphasia TIAs	Bilateral EDAS Right STA-MCA Right EMS	Free		Improved

Moyamoya, Moyamoya disease; Occlusive, occlusive cerebrovascular disease; STA-MCA, superficial temporal artery to middle cerebral artery bypass; EDAS, Encephaloduroarteriosynangiosis; EMS, encephalomyosynangiosis.

CONCLUSIONS

Omental-cerebral transposition can be performed safely with low risks. We prefer using a free omental graft rather than a pedicled graft because of the reduced morbidity associated with the abdominal surgery and tunneling procedure. Although no prospective, randomized, controlled studies have been conducted, small retrospective patient series and anecdotal reports suggest that cerebral revascularization using omentum to cerebral transposition may be useful in preventing future stroke or TIAs in patients with Moyamoya disease or occlusive cerebrovascular disease.

Omentum to cerebral transposition may improve chronic neurologic deficits in young patients and in those with Moyamoya disease. Moyamoya patients are considered for omental-brain revascularization after they have failed prior revascularization attempts, including STA-MCA anastomosis and EDAS. Patients with symptomatic occlusive cerebrovascular disease are candidates for omental-cerebral transposition if they are young and continue to suffer ischemic episodes or stroke despite maximal medical therapy. Although somewhat controversial, in our experience, elderly patients do not show clinical improvement after omentum to cerebral transposition.

ACKNOWLEDGMENTS

This work was supported in part by funding from Bernard and Ronni Lacroute (G.K. Steinberg) and the William Randolph Hearst Foundation (G.K. Steinberg).

REFERENCES

1. Browing FS, Eastwood DS, Price DJ, Kester RC. Scalp and cranial substitution with autotransplanted greater omentum, using microvascular anastomosis. *Br J Surg*. 1979;66:152-154.
2. Hoshino S, Hamada O, Iwaya F, Takahira H, Honda K. Omental transplantation for chronic occlusive arterial diseases. *Int Surg*. 1979;64:21-29.
3. Furnas H, Lineweaver WC, Alpert BS, Buncke HJ. Scalp reconstruction by microvascular free tissue transfer. *Ann Plast Surg*. 1990;24:431-444.
4. Panje WR, Pitcock JK, Vargish T. Free omental flap reconstruction of complicated head and neck wounds. *Otolaryngol Head Neck Surg*. 1989;100:588-593.
5. Goldsmith HS, de los Santos R, Beattie EJ Jr. Relief of chronic lymphedema by omental transposition. *Ann Surg*. 1967;166:573.
6. Goldsmith HS, ChenWF, Duckett SW. Brain vascularization by intact omentum. *Arch Surg*. 1973;106:695-698.
7. Yasargil MG, Yonekawa, Y. Experimental intracranial transplantation of autogenic omentum majus. *J Neurosurg*. 1974;39:213-217.
8. Goldsmith HS, Duckett SW, Chen WF. Prevention of cerebral infarction in the dog by intact omentum. *Am J Surg*. 1975;130:317-320.
9. Goldsmith HS, Duckett SW, Chen WF. Prevention of cerebral infarction in the monkey by omental transposition to the brain. *Stroke*. 1977;9:224-229.
10. Yonekawa Y, Yasargil MG. Brain vascularization by transplanted omentum: a possible treatment of cerebral ischemia. *Neurosurgery*. 1977;1:256-259.
11. Goldsmith HS. Brain and spinal cord revascularization by omental transposition. *Neurol Res*. 1994;16:159-162.
12. De Riu PL, Falzoi A, Papavero L, Rocca A, Viale GL. Local cerebral blood flow after middle cerebral artery occlusion in rabbits following transposition of omentum to the brain. *J Microsurg*. 1980;1:321-324.
13. DeRiu PL, Rocca A, Falzoi A, Carai M, Papavero L. Physiological function after middle cerebral artery occlusion in rabbits with neovascularization of the brain by transposed omentum. *Neurosurgery*. 1980;7:57-60.
14. Goldsmith HS. Brain and spinal cord revascularization by omental transposition. *Neurol Res*. 1994;16:159-162.
15. Goldsmith HS, Saunders RL, Reeves AG, Allen CP, Milne J. Omental transposition to brain and stroke patients. *Stroke*. 1979;10:471-472
16. Herold S. Frackowiak RSJ, Neil-Dwyer G. Studies on cerebral blood flow and oxygen metabolism in patients with established cerebral infarcts undergoing omental transposition. *Stroke*. 1987; 18: 46-51.

17. Goldsmith HS, Cosso M, Pau A, et al. Regional cerebral blood flow after omental transposition to the ischemic brain in man. A five year follow-up study. *Acta Neurochir.* 1990;106:145-152.

18. Yoshioka N, Tominaga S, Suzuki Y, et al. Vascularized omental graft to brain surface in ischemic cerebrosvascular disease. *Microsurgery.* 1995;16:455-462.

19. Karasawa J, Kikuchi H, Kawamaura J, et al. Intracranial transplantation of the omentum for cerebrovascular Moyamoya disease: a two-year follow-up study. *Surg Neurol.* 1980;14:444-449.

20. Karasawa J, Touho H, Ohnishi H, Miyamoto S, Kikuchi H. Cerebral revascularization using omental transplantation for childhood Moyamoya disease. *J Neurosurg.* 1993;79:192-196.

21. Havlik RJ, Fried I, Chyatte D, Modlin IM. Encephalo-omental synangiosis in the management of Moyamoya disease. *Surgery.* 1992;111:156-162.

22. Lee JA, Steinberg GK. Benefits and limitations of omental-to-cerebral transposition for patients with cerebrovascular disease. *Annual Meet AANS.* 1997;65: 12.

CHAPTER 11

OMENTAL TRANSPOSITION TO THE ISCHEMIC BRAIN: A CRITICAL REVIEW OF 60 PATIENTS

R. MRÓWKA, S. HENDRYK, AND D. LATKA

INTRODUCTION

Various surgical treatments for ischemic cerebral disease have been performed in the past, with transposition of the omentum to the surface of an ischemic brain being a relatively new operative procedure for this condition.[1] This surgical operation is intended to protect the ischemic brain by developing a collateral circulation from an extracranial source— namely, the omentum. Earlier attempts at providing additional cerebral blood flow (CBF) to an ischemic brain consisted of laying a pedicled fragment of the temporal muscle on the surface of the brain, a procedure called encephalomyosynangiosis (EMS).[2] There have been modifications of this surgical technique developed by Japanese surgeons, which include encephaloduroarteriosynangiosis (EDAS)[3] and encephaloduroarteriomyosynangiosis (EDAMS).[4] The main goal of these procedures was to improve blood flow to the brain through the growth of blood vessels originating from the temporal muscle in EMS and in the other surgical procedures from additional blood flow from the superficial temporal artery, which most likely passes through small galeal branches that supply ischemic brain tissue. The effectiveness of these various operations have been confirmed clinically and angiographically and by measurement of regional CBF, mainly in patients with Moyamoya disease.[4] However, the length of time it takes for a significant number of blood vessels to grow into the brain can make these operations beneficial for some patients with limited cerebral ischemic, as in transient ischemic attacks, but not for patients who have already sustained a completed stroke.

Yasargil and Donaghy proposed a new microsurgical approach in 1968 to revascularize the brain by using a superficial temporal artery (STA) anastomosis to the middle cerebral artery (MCA), or an STA-MCA in the attempt to prevent, and as a possible treatment for, a stroke.[5] In spite of initial enthusiasm for the procedure, the operation fell into disrepute when it was shown to be ineffective by controlled clinical trials.[6]

The transposition of the omentum to an ischemic brain was first reported by Goldsmith, in animals in 1973[1,7,8] and in man in 1979.[9] Since that time, thousands of such operations have been performed over a 20-year period but relatively few surgeons have had clinical experience with this surgical procedure, which is finding increased acceptance.[10]

MATERIALS AND METHODS

During the period from 1989 to 1993, members of our Department of Neurosurgery have transposed the pedicle omentum to the brain of 60 post-stroke patients[11,12] (*Figures 11.1 to 11.3*).

Almost all the patients who underwent omental transposition following their stroke were deeply hemiparetic or hemiplegic. Patients were selected for surgery on the basis of their clinical examination, angiography, and CT scan. Omental transposition was performed after a period of medical treatment in which there was no apparent neurological improvement. Following their cerebral infarction, 46 patients were operated 2 weeks to 3 months after their stroke; 5 patients at 3 to 6 months and 9 patients, 6 months to 4 years later (*Tables 11.1 and 11.2*).

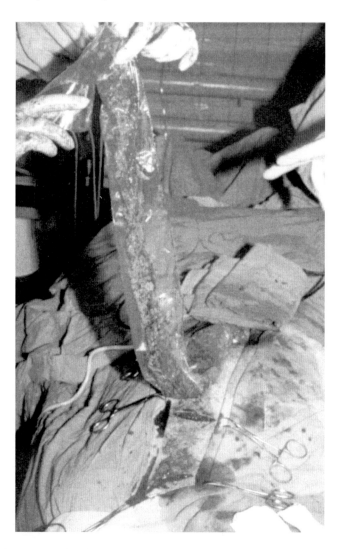

Figure 11.1 Transposing the omental pedicle up through the subcutaneous tunnel to the brain. The pedicle is covered with plastic sleeve irrigated with saline to ease its passage through the tunnel.

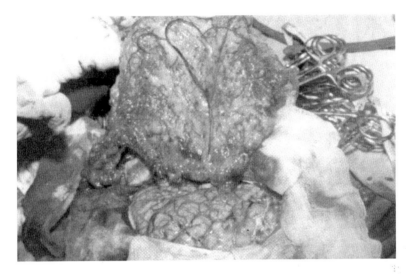

Figure 11.2 Cranial portion of operation. Omentum about to be placed directly on brain surface.

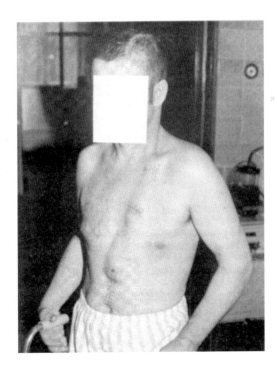

Figure 11.3 Early postoperative photograph showing omentum in subcutaneous tunnel with placement on brain.

Table 11.1 Omental transposition to the brain in 60 patients. Clinical characteristics, diagnostic criteria, and clinical results.

Sex: Male, n=55; Female, n=5	Clinical characteristics
Age: 23-66 years	PRIND (n=5); CS: (n=55)
CT results	Angiographic results
Low-density area in basal ganglia, capsula interna, and MCA territory (n=48)	Occlusive form (n=53)
	Other form (n=6)
Low density area in cortical and subcortical regions (n=6)	No angiography (n=1)
Low density area in capsula interna (n=6)	
Clinical results	
Very good (n=14); Good (n=19);	
Fair (n=13); Lack of improvement (n=9);	
Death (n=5)	

PRIND, prolonged reversible ischemic neurological deficit; CS, completed stroke.

Table 11.2 Time interval between stroke and surgery

Time of surgery	Number of patients
From 2 weeks to 1 month	18
Between 1 month to 2 months	21
Between 2 months to 3 months	7
Between 3 months to 6 months	5
From 6 months to 4 years	9

Neurologic assessment (**A**) and disturbances of speech (**B**) were carefully assessed.

A: Grade of neurological improvement (very good, good, and fair). Very good: full or almost full range of movement in lower limb enables the use of the limb alone or in auxiliary form in everyday life activity. Good: considerable range of movement in lower limb enables walking with assistance, and considerable limitation of movement in upper limb; limb had been totally useless before surgery. Fair: appearance of slight movements, mainly in large joints, in one or both limbs with no possibility of movement either with or without assistance.

B: Improvement of speech (very good, good, and fair). Very good: slight disturbances of speech causing no essential difficulty in understanding. Good: moderate disturbances making it somewhat difficult to converse; good understanding and full gesture contact preserved. Fair: considerable disturbances making it somewhat difficult to converse; good understanding and full gesture contact preserved.

Neurologic deviations from normal were graded on a scale of 0 to 5. All patients underwent long-term follow-up, which included the performance of a CT 1 month to 4 years after surgery. Statistical analysis of differences between pre- and postoperative results were performed using a Student unpaired t test. Differences were considered statistically significant when $P<0.05$.

Table 11.3 Relationship between improvement of speech and hemiparesis in the group of 12 patients observed up to 4 years after surgery

Results	Number of patients
Greater improvement of speech	3
Greater improvement of hemiparesis	1
Speech and hemiparesis equally improved	8

Table 11.4 Comparison of speech disturbances and grade of improvement in 12 patients observed up to 4 years after surgery

Number of patients	Before operation	After operation	Time interval between stroke and surgery
1	Good	Very good	2-5 months
2	Fair (mixed aphasia)	Very good	1-5 months
3	Completely asphasic	Good	11 months
4	Good	Very good	6 months
5	Fair	Very good (after operation, worsening of speech within 10 days, then speech improved)	3 months
6	Good	Very good (after operation, worsening of speech within 10 days, then speech improved)	3-5 months
7	Completely asphasic	Very good	5 months
8	Fair	Very good	1-5 months
9	Fair	Very good (after operation, worsening of speech within 3 days, then speech improved)	2 years
10	Completely aphasic	Very good	1 year
11	Completely aphasic	Good	3 weeks
12	Good	Very good	24 days

RESULTS OF TREATMENT

Of the patients who were available for long-term study, differing grades of neurological changes were observed following their stroke. Nine patients demonstrated no improvement following surgery in part due to complications that occurred during operation and in the postoperative period. Five patients died following the procedure. Of the remaining patients in the long-term follow-up of omental transposition to the post-infarcted brain, both motor and speech improvement was seen in 12 patients, especially in their speech recovery, which was quite apparent (*Tables 11.3 and 11.4*).

If clinical improvement occurred after operation, it first began to appear 7 to 30 days after surgery. Improvement of hemiparetic and hemiplegic symptoms began in the proximal joints and moved to distal joints over a period of time. The functional improvement in proximal and distal joints occurred in the shoulder or hips at 15±5 days, in the elbows and knees at 14±7 days, and in the palm and foot (if there was any improvement) at 22±7 days.

Beneficial neurological changes occurred more often in patients who were operated upon within 2 months of suffering a stroke (*Table 11.5*). Of 33 patients who were operated upon within this period, 22 showed satisfactory results (66%), with the remaining 11 patients (33%) exhibiting no neurological improvement following surgery. Twenty-two other patients were operated more than 2 months after their stroke, with neurological benefit occurring in half the cases (50%), while the remaining 11 patients exhibited no improvement (50%). The differences in neurological improvement were found to be statistically significant if omental transposition to the brain was carried out within 2 months of stroke ($P<0.05$), with clinical improvement being observed to be greater in proximal joints and less so in the hand and foot, findings that were statistically significant ($P<0.01$). Twenty-three patients were followed for up to 4 years after surgery with their neurological state remaining stable during this

time. Four patients died during this period as a result of systemic arteriosclerosis (*Table 11.6*).

Surgical results were very impressive in some patients during our experience, especially when we took into consideration the age of the patient and the length of time from their stroke to the time of surgery. Age was an extremely important criteria for neurological improvement since of 27 patients who were age 50 or less at the time of their operation, 20 showed good to very good results (74.1%). Of the remaining 7 patients who were 50 years of age or younger, fair results, lack of improvement, or death occurred in 25% (*Table 11.7*).

Table 11.5 Results of treatment

Time of surgery	Satisfactory results	Unsatisfactory results (the cases of death have been excluded)
Surgery <2 months after stroke Number of patients=33	n=22 (66.7%)	n=11 (33.3.%)
Surgery >2months after stroke Number of patients=22	n=11 (50.0%)	n=11 (50.0%)

Table 11.6 Early results after surgery and follow-up investigations up to 4 years in 23 patients

Early results (up to 30 days after surgery)	Results of follow-up investigations
Satisfactory results n=16 (69.6%)	Satisfactory results n=15 (93.8%): died n=1 (6.2%)
Unsatisfactory results (fair and lack of improvement) n=7 (30.4%)	Satisfactory results n=3 (42.9%): unsatisfactory result (lack of improvement) n=1 (14.2%): died n=3 (42.9%)

Table 11.7 Results of treatments depending upon the age of patients

Age of patients at surgery	Satisfactory results	Unsatisfactory results
Patients below 50 n=27	n=20 (74.1%)	n=7 (25%)
Patients above 50 n=33	n=13 (39.4%)	n=20 (60.6%)

Patients over the age of 50 exhibited less neurological improvement following omental transposition to the brain. Of the 33 patients in this age group, the neurological results of 13 (39.4%) were satisfactory (very good and good), but in 20 (60.6%) were unsatisfactory (*Table 11.7*). When neurological results proved beneficial after surgery, regardless of the age of the patient, the improvement continued indefinitely. However, if the neurological states did not improve early after surgery, only half of this group showed any improvement during their extended postoperative follow-up period (*Table 11.7*).

DISCUSSION

The negative neurological results reported in 1986 in the article "International Randomized Trial for EC-IC Bypass Surgery" markedly curtailed the indications for this surgical procedure.[6] In our experience over a 12-year period between 1979 and 1990, our Department of Neurosurgery performed more than 300 extracranial to intracranial (EC-IC) bypass procedures. We believe the main reason the operation failed in patients with a completed stroke was due to occlusive processes in major cerebral arteries in addition to arteriosclerotic accumulations occurring in small cortical arteries, which were often visible at the time of operation. Extracranial to intracranial operations were performed to increase blood flow through large unobstructed vessels, but since blood tends to flow to areas of least resistance and not to areas of the brain where vascular obstruction is present and where the additional blood is needed, the blood flow from an EC-IC bypass was insufficient in effectively perfusing areas of cerebral ischemia.

Another reason, in our opinion, as to why EC-IC bypass operations failed to reach expectation was that a bypass anastomosis itself may eventually become involved in an arteriosclerotic process. In a long-term study we

conducted in 81 patients with a completed stroke who had undergone an EC-IC bypass, 32 anastomoses eventually became occluded.[13] These findings were in patients with a completed stroke (CS) in comparison to 44 patients who received an EC-IC operation for prolonged reversible ischemic neurological deficit (PRIND). In this later group of patients who were followed for a long period after their EC-IC bypass procedure, only 5 of the 44 PRIND patients went on to develop obstruction at their EC-IC anastomosis. This result was of statistical significance ($P<0.01$) and of clinical interest since all the EC-IC procedures were performed at our institution by the same neurological team under similar conditions in relatively comparable patients.

The authors believe that the principle cause for the majority of strokes is the involvement of small blood vessels within the cerebral cortex and/or subcortex, which are supplied by major cerebral arteries. The advantage of using the omentum in strokes and transient ischemic attacks (TIAs) is that the omentum resides as a blanket on the brain from which grow a host of new blood vessels that penetrate vertically and deeply into the underlying brain tissue.[14] The development of new blood vessels is much less likely to occur following an EC-IC bypass in ischemic cerebral areas that are distal to the EC-IC anastomosis. In this situation, the increased blood flow to the brain following the EC-IC procedure will have the tendency to flow to unobstructed blood vessels that are in areas of the brain where there is decreased need for blood and minimal or absent neurological symptoms of cerebral ischemia.

Another reason for the benefit of omental transposition to the brain of a stroke patient may be that penumbral neurons located around the cerebral infarction may be stimulated to make new axonal connections because of the stimulus of increased blood flow[15] and the presence of biologically active substances that are known to be present in omental tissue[16-19] and are apparently protective of an ischemic brain.[20,21]

These beneficial factors following omental placement on the brain cannot be met with an STA-MCA bypass, which has been shown experimentally to deliver less blood to the brain than omental transposition.[20] Additionally, the increased CBF originating from the omentum may remain indefinitely, which we found did not occur following an EC-IC bypass.

CONCLUSIONS

Omental transposition was more effective in the post-stroke state when the patient was 50 years of age or less ($P<0.01$).

Our optimal results following omental transposition were obtained when a stroke patient was less than 50 years of age and the operation was performed within 2 months following cerebral infarction.

REFERENCES

1. Goldsmith HS, Chen WF, Duckett SW. Brain vascularization by intact omentum. *Arch Surg.* 1973;106:695-698.
2. Henschen C. Operative revascularization des zurkulatorisch geschdigten gehirn durch auflage gestilter muskellappen (Encephalo-myo-synangiosis). *Langen Beck Arch Klin Chir.* 1950;264:392.
3. Matsushima Y, Fukai N, Tanaka K, et al. A new surgical treatment of Moyamoya disease in children. *Surg Neurol.* 1981;15:313-320.
4. Kinugasa K, Mandai S, Kamata I, et al. Surgical treatment of Moyamoya disease: operative technique for encephalo-duro-arterio-myo-synangiosis, its follow-up, clinical results and angiograms. *Neurosurgery.* 1993;32:527-531.
5. Yasargil MG. Anastomosis between superficial temporal artery and middle cerebral artery. In: Donaghy MP, Yasargil MG, eds. *Microvascular Surgery.* Stuttgart: Thieme; 1967:11-127.
6. EC-IC bypass study group. Failure of extracranial-intracranial bypass to reduce the risk of ischemic stroke: Results of an international randomized trial. *N Eng J Med.* 1985;313:1191-1200.
7. Goldsmith HS, Duckett S, Chen WF. Prevention of cerebral infarction in the dog by intact omentum. *Am J Surg.* 1975;130:317-326.
8. Goldsmith HS, Duckett S, Chen WF. Prevention of cerebral infarction in the monkey by omental transposition to the brain. *Stroke.* 1978;9:224-229.
9. Goldsmith HS, Saunders RL, Reeves AG, Allen CD, Milne J. Omental transposition to the brain of stroke patients. *Stroke.* 1979;10:471-472.
10. Goldsmith HS. First International Congress on Omentum to the CNS. *Surg Neurol.* 1996;45:87-90.
11. Mrowka R, Pieniazek J, Dobkiewicz A. Surgical treatment of patients with completed stroke by transposition of omentum on ischemic brain. *Jahrestagung der Deutschen Gesellschaft fur Neurochirurgie Frankfurt A/Main.* May 10-13;43:1992.
12. Mrowka R, Pieniazek J, Dobkiewicz A. Reason and prospects of surgery by transposition of omentum on the brain in patients after ischemic stroke on the basis of authors' experience. *XI Int Symp Microvascular Surgery for Cerebral Ischemia*; November 22-27 1992; Hospital Ramon y Cajal, Madrid, Spain.
13. Hendryk S, Mrowka R. Follow-up study in patients with ischemic brain syndrome treated by extra-intracranial arterial anastomosis. The relation between angiographic bypass visualization and clinical course of the disease. *Ann Acad Med Sci.* 1995;29:235-247.
14. Goldsmith HS. Brain and spinal cord revascularization by omental transposition. *Neurol Res.* 1994;16:159-162.
15. Goldsmith HS, Bacciu P, Cossu MA, et al. Regional cerebral blood flow after omental transposition to the ischemic brain in man: a five year follow-up study. *Acta Neurochir (Wien).* 1990;106:145-152.
16. Goldsmith HS, Griffith AL, Kupferman A, Catsimpoolas N. Lipid angiogenic factor from omentum. *JAMA.* 1984; 252:2034-2036.
17. Goldsmith HS, Marquis JK, Siek G. Choline acetyl transferase activity in omental tissue. *Br J Neurosurg.* 1987;1:463-466.
18. Goldsmith HS, McIntosh T, Vezina RM, Colton T. Vasoactive neurochemicals identified in omentum. *Br J Neurosurg.* 1987;1:359-364.
19. Siek G, Marquis JK, Goldsmith HS. Experimental studies of omentum-derived neurotrophic factors. In: Goldsmith HS, ed. *The Omentum—Research and Clinical Applications.* New York: Springer-Verlag; 1990:83-95.
20. Azzena GB, Campus G, Mameli O, et al. Omental transposition on transplantation to the brain and superficial temporal artery-middle cerebral artery anastomosis in preventing experimental cerebral ischemia. *Acta Neurochir (Wien).* 1983;68:63-83.
21. Pau A, Sehrbundt-Viale E, Turtas S. Effect of omental transposition to the brain on the cortical content of norepinephrine, dopamine, 2-hydroxytryptamine and 5-hydroxyindol-acetic acid in experimental cerebral ischemia. *Acta Neurochir (Wien).* 1982;66:159-164.

CHAPTER 12

OMENTAL TRANSPOSITION FOR TREATING THE SEQUELAE OF VIRAL ENCEPHALITIS: A LONG-TERM FOLLOW-UP OF 54 CASES

WEI-LIE WU, SHUNG-QING XU, MING LIU, XU-MING HUA, AND J. ZHONG

INTRODUCTION

Epidemic encephalitis B (EEB), commonly called Japanese B encephalitis, is an acute inflammatory disease of the brain caused either by direct viral invasion or from hypersensitivity of the brain initiated by the virus. The virus can attack the spinal cord as well as the brain.

The sequelae of EEB usually involves disorders of motion, speech, and mental processes. Until 1980, there was no known treatment for this neurologic disorder. Since that time, our group began to transpose the intact pedicled omentum to the brain of patients with EEB, and we report here the clinical results that have occurred following this surgical procedure and discuss the indications for the operation.

MATERIAL AND METHODS

Fifty-four patients were studied: 26 males and 28 females ranging in age from 14 to 42 years (median 23.4 years). The length of time that transpired from a patient's EEB infection to the time of omental transposition to the brain ranged from 2 to 28 years (median 14.2 years). The length of time that patients were followed after surgery ranged from 5 to 13.2 years

(median 6.8). Documentation of the patients' neurological status was recorded as follows:

A. Evaluation of muscle strength recorded in a prospective fashion when the patient was seen on admission, at 2 weeks after surgery and at long-term follow-up. Classification of motor strength was based on a grade of 0 to 5 (1, absent; 1, trace; 2, active motion; 3, active motion against gravity; 4, sufficient strength to counteract resistance; 5, normal strength).
B. Evaluation of speaking ability recorded pre- and postoperatively on tape if the patient suffered from incomplete motor aphasia.
C. Skin temperature of all limbs taken pre- and postoperatively.
D. Careful follow-up evaluation of patient's ability to work and/or manage his own care.

CLINICAL FEATURES

Motor function

Each patient had previously been diagnosed and treated during the acute stage of the disease and discharged from the hospital with a definite diagnosis of EEB. The most marked symptom of these post-encephalitis patients was motor impairment.

Of the 54 patients in this study, all but one had spastic paralysis, with muscle tension being invariably increased. Thirty three of these cases had incomplete unilateral paralysis while 20 other patients had bilateral involvement with increased severity on one side. Except for an additional patient, all had hyperactive reflexes, with 44 exhibiting pathologic reflexes. Abnormal limb positioning was present in the form of adduction, hyperextension, and rotation of the upper limbs with equinovarus positioning of the lower limbs being frequently observed.

Various degrees of motor activity and emotional stress had a deleterious effect on some patients in terms of their muscle coordination and/or disturbances in their speech. Both of these features were markedly lessened when the patient was tranquil. When the patient was asleep, these symptoms disappeared. Of the 54 patients in this study, muscle-strength examination was normal in 1 patient, grade 2-3 in 39, and grade 3-4 in the remaining 14 cases.

Speaking ability

Motor aphasia was present in 19 cases, of which 6 were complete. There were 13 other patients whose motor aphasia was incomplete. Their speaking disabilities were characterized by phonation, which was not clear enough to be understood, or by their inability to pronounce anything other than single words.

Intellectual competency

All patients in this study had some degree of intellectual deficiency. Seven of these patients were demented with complete inability to care for themselves. Sixteen other patients had what

was classified as an intermediate defect in their intellectual capacity since they had the ability to do simple calculations and answer simple questions. In addition, their intellectual status was much lower than expected for their age. The remaining 31 cases had what was considered to be only slight intellectual disability since they had the ability to write, distinguish objects, express their opinions, and partially manage their daily activities.

Sensory disorders

Sensory disorders were considered of limited importance to the patients as compared to their motor, speech, and intellectual status. Therefore, sensory recordings were not performed in a routine and standard fashion.

Operative technique

Under adequate general anesthesia, an upper midline incision is made.[1,2] The peritoneal cavity is entered and the first step in the operation is to remove the omentum from its attachments to the transverse colon. Following this, the omentum is removed from the greater curvature of the stomach, leaving the gastroepiploic vessels within the omental apron. The omentum is then markedly elongated by a surgical technique following which the lengthened and still-intact omental pedicle is placed within a subcutaneous tunnel that is made up the chest and neck, up to the cranium.[3]

A craniotomy is performed at which time a 9x7 cm bone flap is made in the temperoparietal-frontal area. The dura is opened using a horseshoe incision, which allows the dura to be reflected from the frontal area. The omentum, which exits from the subcutaneous tunnel behind the ear, is placed below the bone flap required for the craniotomy and laid directly on the arachnoid membrane. Thickened arachnoid tissue is removed when possible, with every effort made to prevent bleeding. The cerebral cortex is covered by the omentum, which is then anchored with several interrupted sutures to the edge of the incised dura. To prevent the omentum from being compressed by the overlying bone as the omentum goes down onto the brain surface, a piece of the replaced bone is clipped off with a rongeur, to prevent compression on the underlying omental pedicle. All incisions are then closed in a routine fashion.

In preparing the brain to receive the omental placement, consideration is given to the area of the brain to be exposed, which is chosen in relation to the patient's neurological dysfunction. For example, a patient with hemiplegia and motor aphasia should have the omentum cover the motor area, the speech center, and as much of the frontal areas as possible. If the arachnoid is thickened in these areas, every effort is to be made to remove as much of this fibrotic membrane as possible from the underlying brain prior to the omental placement. Removing the thickened arachnoid helps allow for vascular proliferation at the omental-cerebral interface.

RESULTS

Motor function

Muscle tension associated with spasm was noted to decrease rapidly after surgery. This finding usually began on the first or second postoperative day and became quite obvious after 4 to 5 days. This muscle relaxation resulted in improved function of the affected limbs. Generally, it was noted that muscle tension increased slightly between postoperative days 7 and 10, but this tension decreased by the end of the second postoperative week, leading to a further gradual decrease in muscle tension with increased muscle strength. Optimal muscle strength was

noted between 1 and 3 months postoperatively.

Thirty-four cases (62.6%) attained what was considered good postoperative results as measured by decreased muscle tension and increased muscle force of over one grade (*Figure 12.1*). Patients with equinovarus deformity improved considerably with their subsequent ability to touch their heel to the ground while walking. Patients in this group were able to manage their activities, with 14 of the patients being able to return to work. Several patients attained remarkable strength by 6 months following surgery.

Fourteen cases (25.8%) attained what was considered only minimal improvement as evidenced by a slight (less than one grade) change in muscle force associated with persistent high muscle tension.

Six cases (11.1%) had no improvement following surgery.

Speech

Of the six patients who had complete aphasia prior to surgery, three showed a progressive improvement by the end of the first postoperative week. These improvements were manifested by pronouncing words that were unclear but understood in the utterances of single words and broken sentences. One patient developed the ability to say a few basic words. Two patients showed no speech improvement from their surgery.

Thirteen patients had partial aphasia before surgery. Of this number, eight developed remarkable improvement as manifested by increased clarity in speaking. Five other patients showed little improvement.

Intellectual capacity

Of the 54 cases in this study, 32 showed postoperative improvement in intellectual capacity. Five of these patients improved to the point that they were able to resume their education 1 to 2 years following surgery. Nine cases had noticeable improvements in writing and expression (*Figure 12.2*). One patient began to learn English at home; another began to paint. However, intellectual improvement was slow and at times did not become obvious until 1 to 2 years after surgery.

Miscellaneous changes

Epilepsy: There were 12 patients who had epileptic seizures prior to surgery as a result of their post-encephalitic condition. No postoperative changes occurred in 8 of these 12 cases. Of the four remaining cases, three had fewer seizures and one patient stopped his medication and had no further seizures over a 10-year follow-up period.

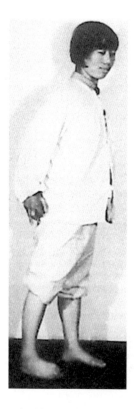 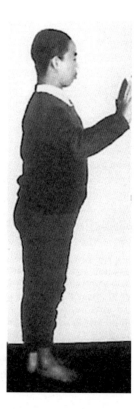

Figure 12.1 Left: Preoperative photograph of a 25-year-old housewife 14 years following an attack of EEB. Severe gait abnormality due to equinovarus deformity of right leg and foot. Note functionless right hand, which was firmly spastic in a claw-like position. **Right**: patient 3 weeks after omental transposition to left cerebral hemisphere. Loss of spasticity on right side of body has eliminated equinovarus deformity of leg leading to normal gait. Arm and hand movement have markedly improved.

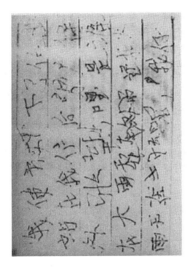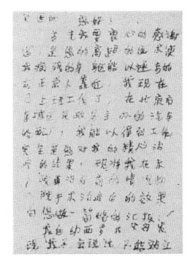

Figure 12.2 Left: Preoperative handwriting of a 23-year-old man 5 years after an attack of EEB. **Right:** Postoperative handwriting of patient 6 months after omental transposition to left cerebral hemisphere. Marked improvement is evident.

Anatomic nervous system: Twenty two of the 54 patients in this study had detailed skin temperatures taken of all limbs pre- and postoperatively. The neurologically affected limbs, resulting from their encephalitic condition, showed preoperative skin temperatures to be 0.4°C to 1.6°C lower compared to the normal limbs. After surgery, limb temperatures, which were taken biweekly until hospital discharge, showed a rise in temperature of 0.2°C to 1.7°C in the affected limbs compared to the normal limbs. The color of their nail beds was noted to have reddened, with 12 patients claiming subjective awareness of increasing warmth in their neurologically affected limbs. Fifteen patients noted that their heat-regulating mechanisms had improved during the winter months.

DISCUSSION

It is now known from both animal and clinical studies that omental transposition to the heart,[4] spinal cord,[5] and brain[6-8] results in the establishment of an extensive collateral vascular circulation. This study demonstrated that omental transposition to the brain is also effective in varying degrees for patients suffering the sequelae of viral encephalitis.

At operation, it was observed that 45 of the 54 patients comprising this study showed gross brain alteration with some degree of arachnoid membrane thickening and brain degeneration. Twelve cases underwent intraoperative brain biopsies. Histopathological examination of the tissue showed changes that were observed to be non-specific. Most specimens showed some degree of gliosis with varying degrees of simple neuronal degeneration. The cytoplasm in two cases was basophilic, with intravascular eosinophilic inclusions being observed. It is known that a number of chronic viral disorders are associated with degeneration of neurons. Such degeneration is characterized by contraction of the cell body, with the cytoplasm becoming more basophilic than eosinophilic. As long as the nucleus remained intact, however, these neuronal changes were reversible.[9]

It has been found that the degree of improvement that can follow omental transposition to the brain of a patient with chronic encephalitis appears to be in direct relationship to the degree of cerebral damage observed at surgery; the damage being due to the previous viral infection (EEB). Of the 54 patients being reported, 34 (62.9%) demonstrated objective evidence of good clinical improvement after surgery. It was felt that in the patients with speech problems who improved after omental transposition, their speech improvement depended to a degree on their age at the time of the encephalitic attack.

Seven of 19 patients with preoperative speaking dysfunction showed no postoperative speech improvement; three of these cases having had encephalitis during infancy before they had learned to speak. All patients who were severely demented before surgery failed to show any improvement after surgery.

Results of the patients being presented have allowed us to establish tentative guidelines for patients who would most likely benefit from omental transposition to their encephalitis-injured brain. Optimal candidates appear to be individuals with mild unilateral spastic paralysis (preferably right-sided) associated with a speaking dysfunction and only a mild intellectual deficit. Patients with bilateral spastic paralysis and severe intellectual damage showed only minor postoperative improvement. Because of these findings, we feel that omental transposition is not indicated in these latter types of patients.

The authors have seen definite improvement in a large number of patients with chronic encephalitis following omental transposition to their brain. Of major interest is that many of the clinical improvements occurred within several days following surgery even though the patient's encephalitis attack occurred many years earlier. We do not believe that these changes resulted solely from the known angiogenic activity of the omentum, which leads to increased cerebral blood flow. It is likely that the improvement seen soon after omental transposition results from biochemical changes originating at the omental-cerebral interface.

Perhaps it is a combination of angiogenic factors[10] and neurotransmitters,[11,12] known to be present in omental tissue, that might explain some of the clinical changes that have been observed in post-encephalitis patients following omental transposition to the brain.

Efforts continue to develop an effective vaccine against EEB.[13] However, for a patient who contracts this viral disease and suffers its neurological consequences, omental transposition to the brain may be of benefit.

REFERENCES

1. Alday ES, Goldsmith HS. Surgical technique for omental lengthening based on arterial anatomy. *Surg Gynecol Obstet.* 1972;135:103-107.
2. Wu WL, Meng GC, Xu SQ. Surgical technique of omental lengthening on anatomical basis. *Chinese Surg J.* 1984;2:94-96.
3. Goldsmith HS, Saunders RL, Reeves AG, et al. Omental transposition to brain of stroke patients. *Stroke.* 1979;10:471-472.
4. Vineberg AM, Shanks J, Pifarre R, et al. Myocardial revascularization by omental graft without pedicle: experimental background and report on 25 cases followed 6 to 16 months. *J Thorac Cardiovasc Surg.* 1965;59:103-129.
5. Goldsmith HS, Duckett S, Chen WF. Spinal cord vascularization by intact omentum. *Am J Surg.* 1975;129:262-265.
6. Goldsmith HS, Chen WF, Duckett S. Brain vascularization by intact omentum. *Arch Surg.* 1973;106:695-698.
7. Goldsmith HS, Duckett S, Chen WF. Prevention of cerebral infarction in the monkey by omental transposition to the brain. *Stroke.* 1978;9:224-229.
8. Goldsmith HS. Brain and spinal cord revascularization by omental transposition. *Neurol Res.* 1994;16:159-162.
9. Robbins SL, Angell M, Kumar V. *Basic Pathology.* 3rd ed. Philadelphia: WB Saunders; 1981:640.

10. Goldsmith HS, Griffith A, Kupferman A, Catsimpoolas N. Lipid angiogenic factor from omentum. *JAMA*. 1984;252:2034-2036.

11. Goldsmith HS, McIntosh T, Vezina RM, Colton T. Vasoactive neurochemicals identified in omentum. *Br J Neurosurg*. 1987;1:359-364.

12. Goldsmith HS, Marquis JK, Siek G. Choline acetyltransferase activity in omental tissue. *Br J Neurosurg*. 1987;1:463-466.

13. Wang J. The surveillance on the present situation of immune levels of 1044 children vaccinated with seven kinds of vaccines in Dali Prefecture (Chinese). *Chinese J Epidemiol*. 1994;15:150-153.

CHAPTER 13

OMENTAL TRANSPOSITION FOLLOWING ARACHNOID EXCISION TO TREAT POST-CEREBRAL ANOXIA (CEREBRAL PALSY)

WEI-LIE WU, SHUNG-QING XU, MING LIU, XU-MING HUA,
AND FENG JIANG

INTRODUCTION

There are many causes for cerebral anoxia in the young but the most common is oxygen deprivation resulting from fetal distress associated with a difficult birth delivery. Cerebral anoxia manifests itself clinically by decreased mental activity, decreased speech ability, and varying motor dysfunction throughout the body. The authors are presently unaware of any treatment for this severe neurological disorder.

From January 1991 to December 1995, we treated 125 patients with this neurological condition using an omental pedicle flap that is placed on the brain following the partial detachment of the thickened arachnoid membrane, which we have found to be present to varying degrees in all patients with the clinical manifestations of cerebral anoxia. All patients were followed postoperatively for a minimum of 2 years.

CLINICAL MATERIAL

There were 84 males and 41 females in the study who ranged in age from 11 to 35 years (average 17.2 years). Almost all patients suffered from cerebral anoxia caused at birth by prolonged labor, inspired amniotic fluid, or umbilical cord compression of the infant's neck at the time of delivery. These events lead to postpartum cerebral anoxia and cyanosis. Seventy-eight cases required postnatal resuscitative measures, with 32 cases in this series having subsequent high temperatures and convulsive seizures.

CLINICAL MANIFESTATION

Mental capacity

A major defect found in these patients was the loss of varying degrees of mental function. Also noted to a significant but lesser degree was a diminution in the ability to speak, to perform calculations, and to maintain daily life activities. These deficiencies showed a direct relationship to the degree of cerebral anoxia that occurred at the time of the infant's birth.

Motor function

There were varying degrees of motor problems in many of the patients. Forty one (32%) had marked to severe impairment of motor function, with 13 of these cases having incomplete unilateral paralysis of an upper extremity and the remaining 28 patients having incomplete hemiparesis.

Speech

Twenty-four patients demonstrated incomplete motor aphasia, which was characterized by the inability of their speech to be either partially or completely understood. Another 18 patients had impairment of their speech, which was less difficult to understand but their speech difficulty was clearly evident.

OPERATIVE PROCEDURE

The operation was performed by two separate teams since the procedure required a craniotomy and a laparotomy. The neurosurgical team made a coronal incision slightly above the frontal hairline followed by a bilateral craniotomy (*Figure 13.1*). The dura mater was then opened and the underlying arachnoid membrane inspected. Of significant importance was the observation in most cases of definite pathological changes involving the arachnoid membrane. It appeared that the more serious the anoxia, even at birth, the thicker, whiter, and greater the opacity of the arachnoid (*Figure 13.2*). Conversely, the less intense the anoxic insult at birth, the lighter in color was the arachnoid, with the membrane being quite thin (*Figure 13.3*). Many of the cases also demonstrated varying degrees of cerebral degeneration as evidenced by deepened groves between the gyri, with adhesions being present between the arachnoid and dura.

Using an operating microscope, pieces of the arachnoid membrane were carefully removed from the underlying brain by partial multiple resections of this membrane, with concentrated effort made to avoid injury to cortical blood vessels.

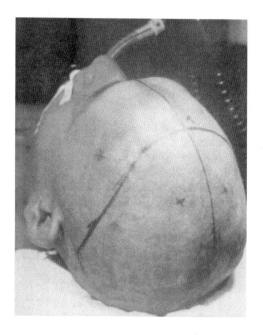

Figure 13.1 Location of craniotomy incision above the hairline.

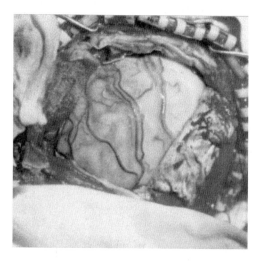

Figure 13.2 Note white, thickened, dense arachnoid membrane on right. The adjacent area of cerebral hemisphere on left had had earlier removal of thickened arachnoid membrane.

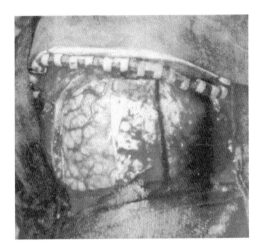

Figure 13.3 Note minimal arachnoid membrane thickening adjacent to cut dural flap. The thickness of membrane appeared to be in direct relationship to initial cerebral anoxia.

While the neurosurgical portion of the operation was being performed, abdominal surgery was being carried out at which time the omentum was surgically lengthened with its arterial and venous blood supply being maintained by way of the right gastroepiploic blood vessels, which remained intact within the omental pedicle. The technique of lengthening the omentum has been well established[1,2] and the omental pedicle was elongated to the level of the brain for either unilateral or bilateral hemispheric placement (depending on the length of the omentum). In roughly half the cases, it was possible to place the omentum on both cerebral hemispheres (*Figure 13.4*). It was felt to be very important that the motor and speech centers and as much of the frontal lobe as possible be covered with omentum.

POSTOPERATIVE FOLLOW-UP

The patients were followed after surgery for 2 to 4.2 years (median 2.7 years). The changes that were monitored were intellectual capacity,

speech improvement, mathematical problem solving, and the patients' ability to manage their daily living functions. Also studied were changes in muscle strength and tension, and pre- and postoperative computed tomography (CT) changes. Twelve of the patients in this study had cerebrovascular perfusion studies, which were measured by single photon emission computed tomography (SPECT) scans.

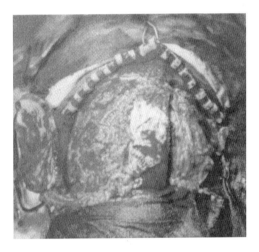

Figure 13.4 Omentum shown covering both cerebral hemispheres. Omental pedicle is entering on lower left side.

RESULTS

Motor function

Muscle tension was, surprisingly, decreased in most patients by the first and second postoperative day. This improvement continued over time. Of the 41 cases in this study who had motor function impairment, 28 (68%) recorded marked improvement with lowered muscle tension and/or the increase of muscle power of greater than one degree. Two of the patients in this group revealed no postoperative improvement in muscle strength or decrease in muscle tension.

Mental capacity

All patients had some degree of preoperative mental diminution as a result of their previous cerebral anoxic episode. Thirty-six cases (28.8%) had marked postoperative clinical improvement, which was shown by the patients' ability to return to school or become gainfully employed. Eight-two other patients (65.6%) had a moderate degree of improvement as measured by their increased ability to do mathematical problems. Seven of the patients in the study (5.6%) showed no improvement in any category.

Speech

The speech of the patients who had a preoperative speaking deficiency was evaluated postoperatively by tape recordings. Improvement was measured by increased speed of speaking and by improved clarity of phonation. Comparing pre- and postoperative tape recordings demonstrated that of the 42 patients who had preoperative speech abnormalities, 32 (76%) showed postoperative improvement.

CEREBRAL PERFUSION

Vascular perfusion before and after omental transplantation was evaluated by SPECT studies using 99mTc-ECD. This study was done on 12 omental transposition patients with 10 healthy volunteers being used as controls (Table 13.1). In the patients who had omental placement on their brain, there was preoperative evidence of scattered decreased vascular perfusion of cortical tissue in both cerebral hemispheres. The regions of decreased perfusion were seen in the parietal lobe in 11 of 12 patients, in the frontal lobe in 10 of 12 patients, in the temporal lobe in 10 of 12 patients, in the occipital lobe in 8 of 12 patients, and in the basal ganglia 1 in 12 patients. No decrease in cerebral perfusion was noted in the cerebellum of any of the patients.

Of the 12 omental transposition patients, 5 had their omentum laid on both cerebral hemispheres with 7 having unilateral hemisphere placement. The increased cerebral perfusion that was seen postoperatively was not localized to any specific areas (Figures 13.5A and 13.5B). The greatest vascular perfusion increase was noted to have developed directly under the omentum in those patients with unilateral cerebral hemisphere placement. One patient in the operative group showed no increase in cerebrovascular perfusion. The greatest postoperative increase in cerebral perfusion was noted in the parietal lobes.

Table 13.1 Comparison of semi-quantitative analysis between control group and patient group (pre- and postoperation) among patients with cerebral anoxia sequelae

| Group | Case | Left brain | | | | |
		Frontal	Temporal	Parietal	Occipital	Basal Ganglion
Control	10	0.95±0.03	0.90±0.02	0.97±0.02	0.92±0.04	0.90±0.01
Preoperation	12	0.60±0.13	0.54±0.17	0.49±0.15	0.70±0.14	0.87±0.03
Postoperation	12	0.76±0.09	0.72±0.10	0.82±0.11	0.74±0.13	0.87±0.04

| Group | Case | Right brain | | | | |
		Frontal	Temporal	Parietal	Occipital	Basal Ganglion
Control	10	0.96±0.02	0.91±0.02	0.96±0.04	0.94±0.02	0.90±0.01
Preoperation	12	0.63±0.14	0.61±0.15	0.57±0.15	0.73±0.16	0.89±0.03
Postoperation	12	0.80±0.11	0.74±0.11	0.71±0.13	0.78±0.13	0.89±0.03

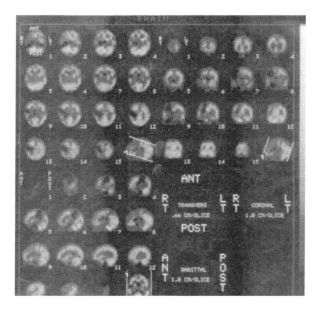

A

Figure 13.5A Preoperative SPECT scan of patient with long-term cerebral anoxia.

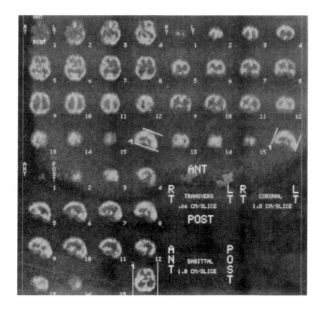

B

Figure 13.5B Postoperative SPECT scan of patient 1 year after omental transposition, showing widespread increases in cerebral perfusion.

DISCUSSION

This study, performed in patients with previous cerebral anoxia, indicated that the neurological sequelae that follow an anoxic insult can be modified many years after the incident. This strongly suggests that in addition to non-viable brain neurons that resulted from the cerebral anoxia, there remain neurons that are viable, but with decreased neuronal activity, that can later be stimulated; the so called "idling neurons."

It is known that omental tissue is replete with biological substances that are important in the function and repair of the central nervous system (CNS). These agents include angiogenic factors,[3,4] neurotransmitters,[5,6] nerve growth substances,[7] and a host of other biological agents. It seems reasonable to suspect that adding these omental agents to idling neurons that are not functioning at optimal levels would result in increased neuronal activity. This study, along with others involving long-term injury to the brain and spinal cord,[8] shows the enormous plasticity of the CNS, regardless of the number of years from the time of CNS insult or the reason for neuronal deprivation of oxygen.

One might speculate in these operated cases suffering from cerebral anoxia that the clinical improvement seen stems mainly from increased cerebral blood flow to involved neurons. The fact that neurologic improvement occurred in many cases within a few days of omental transposition would suggest that the thickened arachnoid over the brain has a constricting effect on the underlying cortical capillaries and that removing this thickened membrane would most likely increase blood flow to the cortical vessels on the underlying brain surface. This could explain the very early neurological improvement seen shortly after omental transposition. The permanent placement of the omentum on the brain would further increase cerebral blood flow in a progressive and sustaining manner. Neurobiological substances in the omental tissue might also play an important role in the clinical results we have observed following omental transposition in patients who have sustained previous cerebral anoxia.

REFERENCES

1. Alday ES, Goldsmith HS. Surgical technique for omental lengthening based on arterial anatomy. *Surg Gyn Obstet*. 1992;135:103-107.
2. Goldsmith HS. Omental transposition to the brain and spinal cord. *Surgical Rounds*. June 1986:22-23.
3. Goldsmith HS, Griffith AL, Kupperman A, Catsimpoolas N. Lipid angiogenic factor from omentum. *JAMA*. 1984;252:2034-2036.
4. Zhang QX, McGovern CJ, Mack CA, et al. Vascular endothelial growth factor is the major angiogenic factor in omentum: mechanism of the omentum-mediated angiogenesis. *Surg Res*. 1997;67:147-154.
5. Goldsmith HS, McIntosh T, Vezina RM, Colton T. Vasoactive neurochemicals identified in omentum. *Br J Neurosurg*. 1987;1:359-364 .
6. Goldsmith HS, Marquis JK, Siek G. Choline acetyltransferase activity in omental tissue. *Br J Neurosurg*. 1987;1:463-466.
7. Siek GC, Marquis JK, Goldsmith HS. Experimental studies of omentum derived neurotrophic factors. In: Goldsmith HS, ed. *The Omentum—Research and Clinical Applications*. New York: Springer-Verlag; 1990:83-95.
8. Goldsmith HS. Brain and spinal cord revascularization by omental transposition. *Neurol Res*. 1994;16:159-162.

CHAPTER 14

OMENTAL TRANSPOSITION TO BYPASS THE BLOOD-BRAIN BARRIER FOR DELIVERY OF CHEMOTHERAPEUTIC AGENTS TO MALIGNANT BRAIN TUMORS: PRECLINICAL INVESTIGATION

M.S. BERGER, P.R. WEINSTEIN, H.S. GOLDSMITH, R. HATTNER, E.Z. LONGA, AND B. PERIRA

INTRODUCTION

Primary neoplasms of the central nervous system (CNS) occur with an approximate incidence of 4.5 cases per 100,000 population annually and approximately 25% to 35% of these tumors are malignant.[1,2] Despite aggressive new approaches in treating these lesions, the mortality rate has not changed dramatically over the past 20 years. This is extremely disappointing when one considers that patients succumb to this disease due primarily to the effects of local recurrence and subsequent mass effect.[1] Malignant gliomas rarely metastasize outside the CNS[3] and, indeed, infrequently result in death due to cerebrospinal fluid dissemination and/or multicentricity. Hochberg et al[4] demonstrated that 90% to 95% of recurrences of malignant gliomas occur within 2 centimeters of the contrast-enhancing margin as depicted by computed tomography (CT) scans.

Surgery for malignant gliomas has become more aggressive in recent years because of the known focality of this disease and cytoreductive potentiation for radiation and chemotherapy.[5] However, local invasion of tumor may be subtle or involve eloquent brain regions such as language and motor cortex. Although methods have been recently developed to maximize resection and minimize

morbidity using intraoperative brain mapping,[6] malignant gliomas remain nearly impossible to cure with surgical excision alone.

The most effective therapeutic modality for malignant brain tumors is radiotherapy administered focally. There is a clear dose-response curve for patient survival.[7] However, radiotherapy by itself is not curative in the majority of malignant CNS neoplasms. As the total dose is increased, the toxic consequences of radiotherapy may develop. Radiation-induced necrosis and other adverse effects have been well described[8] and emphasize the critical relationship between total dose and fraction size in determining a good *versus* hazardous outcome. Location is also important in influencing the outcome of radiotherapy, as endocrine dysfunction and visual deterioration have been documented with radiation of the hypothalamic-pituitary axis and optic-nerve–chiasmic apparatus.[9,10] Attempts to overcome the adverse effects of radiation or to potentiate external beam therapy largely involved interstitial brachytherapy using CT-guided stereotaxic placement of high-activity radioisotopes. This technique has been quite beneficial for treating tumor recurrences and boosting external beam therapy following the initial operation, but is not often curative.[11,12]

Chemotherapy has been used in an adjuvant fashion following surgery and/or radiation and has demonstrated modest success in prolonging the mean time to tumor progression and survival. Several studies have reported a statistically significant difference in survival at 12 and 24 months when nitrosourea-based chemotherapy is added to radiation for the treatment of malignant gliomas.[13,14] However, the failure of chemotherapy to obtain or sustain a response is due to a number of factors, including inherent or acquired drug resistance and suboptimal drug delivery. Unfortunately, several drugs that are efficacious for other systemic malignancies are not used for brain tumors because of their pharmacological properties, i.e., being water soluble and non-lipophilic. This pilot study was therefore undertaken to determine if the omentum, when transposed to the brain, could increase the local concentration of the desired chemotherapeutic agents by potentiating overall delivery of nonstandard (hydrophilic) drugs, thus bypassing the intact blood-brain barrier (BBB).

MATERIALS AND METHODS

Adult New Zealand white rabbits (average weight 3.5 kg) were used in this study. The animals were pre-medicated for the procedure using ketamine (35 mg kg^{-1}) and 5 mg kg^{-1}), and subsequently intubated and anesthetized with a nitrous-oxide (60%/40%) mixture. One percent halothane was added during the initial phase of the operation for abdominal relaxation and was discontinued following lengthening of the omental pedicle.

The animals were positioned supine with their extremities stretched outward and the head turned toward the left. The head, neck, chest, and abdomen were shaved and scrubbed with Betadine solution. The omentum was isolated and lengthened according to the techniques described by Goldsmith et al[15] Briefly, a midline abdominal incision was made and the omentum was mobilized and lengthened by removing its connections with

the spleen and middle and proximal portions of the greater curvature of the stomach. The major vascular pedicle for the omentum was usually the gastroduodenal artery.

A curvilinear incision over the right side of the scalp was made and followed by a fronto-parietal craniectomy. The dura was opened and coagulated, and the arachnoid was dissected away from the pial surface. Transverse skin incisions were made in the neck and chest, and a subcutaneous tunnel fashioned. The omental pedicle was passed through the tunnel and placed directly upon the cortex. The perimeter of the pedicle was sutured to the dural margins with interrupted, absorbable sutures. All wounds were closed in a routine fashion. No neurological deficits were noted following omental transposition and the animals were fed a normal diet and observed from 4 to 16 weeks. The rabbits were then randomly assigned to experimental groups of five animals each.

CHARACTERIZATION OF VASCULAR CONNECTIONS BETWEEN THE OMENTUM AND THE BRAIN

The animal was anesthetized in the above fashion, the abdomen and chest were opened, and the superior vena cava divided. The aorta was clamped just proximal and distal to the gastroduodenal artery, and a 16-gauge angiocatheter was inserted into the isolated aorta attached to the omental pedicle. Heparinized saline was infused until the perfusate draining from the severed vena cava became clear. Following this, the neck of the rabbit was completely severed from the body, except where the omental pedicle was located as it traversed the neck.

The 30% solution of micropaque (finely dispersed barium sulphate) was injected through the angiocatheter into the omental pedicle until a total volume of 100 to 150 mL had been delivered. Therefore, the vascular contrast material was certain to perfuse the

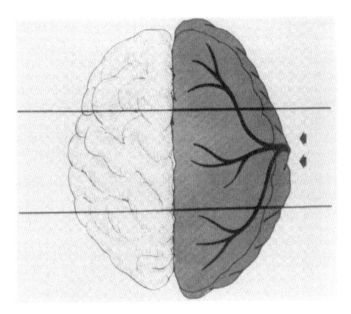

Figure 14.1 Right cerebral hemisphere is covered with omentum (arrows). The brain is then divided into three sets of mirror-image slices.

brain only via the omental vessels. Both cerebral hemispheres were immediately removed and placed in formalin prior to final sectioning.

Group I

Five rabbits that had previously undergone omental transposition were subsequently anesthetized with ketamine (35 mg kg^{-1}) and given an intravenous injection of 2 mCi technetium-99m (99Tcm) diethylenetriamine pentaacetic acid (DTPA) 1 hour prior to being sacrificed. This radiopharmaceutical agent rapidly equilibrates with the extracellular space of the brain only in regions where the BBB is disrupted.[16] It is uniquely extracted from the body via glomerular filtration and thus serves as an ideal marker for the interstitial brain space adjacent to an incompetent vasculature.

The animals were sacrificed using an intravenous injection of T-61 (1 mL), which induced immediate cardiac arrest. Prior to this, the chest was opened, the aorta clamped, and the

jugular veins divided to allow as much of the circulating blood volume to escape prior to harvesting the brain. A saline flush was also administered to potentiate depletion of the intravascular DTPA. The brain, with its attached omentum, was rapidly removed from the skull, washed with saline, and placed in liquid nitrogen to facilitate sectioning.

Both hemispheres were cut in tandem to yield three sets of mirror-image (left/right) sections *(Figure 14.1)*. The omental remnant was left attached to the cortex, the six pieces were weighed, and the radioactivity determined using the gamma scintillation counter. One animal did not receive an omental transposition, yet, following intravenous injection with DTPA, was sacrificed and processed in the same manner, thus serving as the control for the experimental groups. The right hemisphere sections were compared with the opposite hemisphere counterparts (without omentum) and a right-to-left (counts per gram tissue) ratio was expressed.

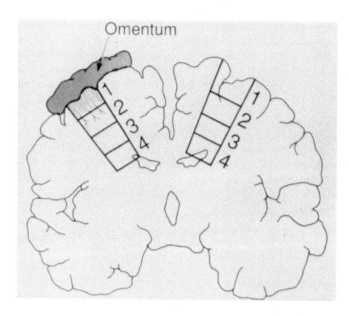

Figure 14.2 Schematic diagram of 4-mm slices (1-4) taken from the omentum-cortex interface toward the deep white matter.

Group II

The rabbits in this experimental group were prepared utilizing the same format as in Group I. After harvesting the brain and freezing it in liquid nitrogen, sequential 4-mm slices were taken from the omentum-cortex interface to deeper regions (*Figure 14.2*). Thus, 4-mm–thick brain sections directly under the omental pedicle were prepared for scintillation counting to determine the distribution of interstitial DTPA deep to the omentum. In two animals, the contralateral cortex (without omentum) was used as a control and submitted for scintillation counting. All radioactive counts were standardized to the activity detected only in the omentum and expressed as the mean percent of maximum (omentum) counts.

RESULTS

After micropaque was injected into the omental pedicle, two types of vascular connections were identified between the omentum and underlying brain. First, omental vessels were seen to communicate directly with subarachnoid surface arterial trunks (*Figures 14.3 and 14.4*). This resulted in perfusion of both cerebral hemispheres, cerebellum, and brainstem via retrograde communication with the Circle of Willis (*Figure 14.5*). Secondly, tortuous vascular channels or loops were identified to directly penetrate the brain parenchyma for a variable distance from the cortical surface (*Figures 14.6 and 14.7*). These vessels maintain the microstructure of the omental vasculature and, thus, do not have a BBB with tight endothelial junctions. A cross section of the omentum-cortex junction (*Figure 14.8*) demonstrates the micropaque-filled direct omental-penetrating channels deep to the cortical surface. The majority of these penetrating vessels are found within 4 mm of the cortex, yet, may be located as deep as 8 mm from the cortical surface.

Group I

In the control (no omentum) animal, no difference in radioactive counts could be detected when comparing the left and right hemispheres. The counts were also quite similar to the non-omentum left hemispheres in the experimental animals (*Table 14.1*). Both control hemispheres and the left side of the experimental brain showed approximately 15% of the activity found in the omentum hemispheres (right side, experimental animals). This is probably due to residual intravascular 99Tcm DTPA, despite heparinized saline perfusion and washing of the brain prior to freezing and sectioning. The experimental hemispheres (with or without omentum) were compared, and the mean right-to-left ratio was determined to be 6.11 as expressed in counts per gram tissue x10^3. The Student's paired *t* test for right (omentum) versus left (non-omentum) hemispheres was significant (*P*=0.002).

Group II

The omentum overlying the cortex was resected and counted separately. All subsequent brain sections (*Figure 14.2*) were compared to radiolabeled omentum and adjusted to yield a mean percentage of the maximum number of counts in the omental pedicle (*Table 14.2*). The number of radioactive counts was greatest in the first 4-mm section underneath the omentum. The DTPA activity was reduced by 78% in the next 4-mm segment. In the deepest segments sampled (8-16 mm), the activity was between 7% to 10% of the omentum, yet remained higher than the mean activity measured in the contralateral cortex (*Figure 14.9*). These data are consistent with the greater concentration of penetrating vascular channels in the first 4 mm of brain under the omental pedicle. As the number of direct vascular connections decreases with increasing depth from the cortical surface, less extravasated DTPA is found. This indicates that, although there may be some interstitial diffusion of the radiopharmaceutical agent away from these new omental-derived vessels, egress of DTPA, as detected in the first 4-mm brain section, is largely dependent upon leakage of DTPA into the adjacent extravascular space.

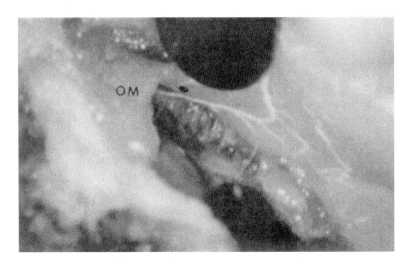

Figure 14.3 Direct omental (OM) connection to a cortical surface vessel (arrow) filled with micropaque.

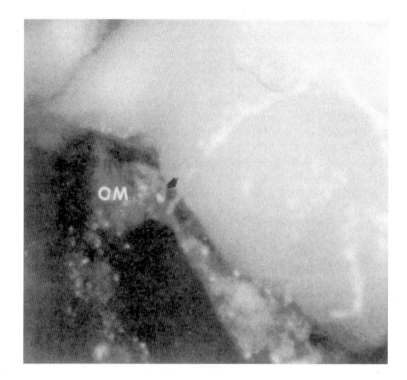

Figure 14.4 Omental (OM) to surface (arrow) anastomoses in closer detail.

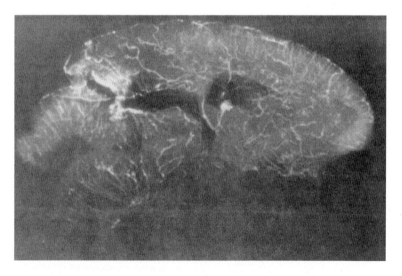

Figure 14.5 Dramatic filling of hemisphere vessels contralateral to omentum via retrograde flow through the Circle of Willis. X-ray is performed with micropaque injection into the isolated omental pedicle.

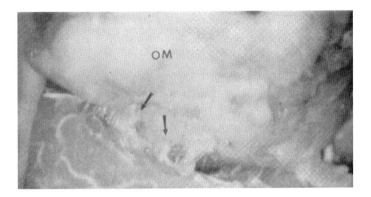

Figure 14.6 Penetrating tortuous vascular channels are seen between omentum (OM) and cortex (arrows).

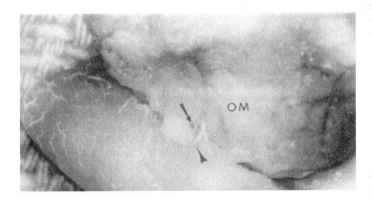

Figure 14.7 Note the S-shaped (tortuous) vessel coming from the omentum (arrow) and the direct penetration of the omental vasculature through the pial surface (arrowhead).

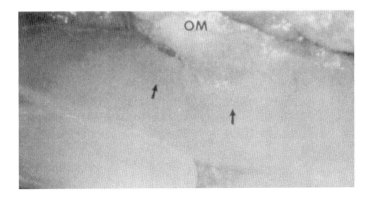

Figure 14.8 Cross-section of the omentum-cortex interface showing numerous penetrating vessels filled with micropaque (arrows) following isolated pedicle perfusion.

Table 14.1 Group I counts/gram x10^3

Hemispheres	Control	Rabbit 2	Rabbit 3	Rabbit 4	Rabbit 5
Left (L)	15.82	18.34	14.45	15.81	37.03
Right (R)	15.40	105.92	51.37	86.15	232.30
	Mean (L)	15.48			
			R/L=6.11		
	Mean (R)	118.93			

Paired *t* test, R *versus* L, *P*=0.002.
The right cerebral hemisphere, except for the control rabbit, has the omentum attached. The counts (per gram tissue x10^3) are significantly higher in the hemisphere with the omental transposition.

Table 14.2 Group II diffusion gradient

	Mean % of maximum counts	Standard error of the mean (SEM)
Omentum	100	13.2
4 mm (1)	64	9.4
8 mm (2)	14.5	4.7
12 mm (3)	7.2	4.5
16 mm (4)	10.5	
Contralateral cortex	2.6	–

Distribution of interstitial DTPA activity in sequential 4-mm sections of brain underlying the omentum. Values are expressed as the mean percent of the maximum activity of the omentum alone.

DISCUSSION

There are several factors responsible for adequate delivery of chemotherapeutic agents to malignant brain tumors, and these have been thoroughly summarized in the excellent review article by Greig.[17] After a drug is administered, it achieves a peak plasma concentration for a limited period of time, and depending upon this time versus concentration profile, the tumor is either adequately or inadequately exposed to the given agent.[18] Although local blood flow to the region of interest is a factor in drug delivery to the CNS, the critical problem that exists is the fundamental nature of the BBB in, or adjacent to, the tumor.

Although some investigators have questioned the role of the BBB and its artificial disruption for administering chemotherapy,[19,20] others have claimed a beneficial effect on bypassing the BBB to increase the blood-to-tumor drug transport kinetics. The ultrastructural anatomy of tumor blood vessels is characteristically different from the intact BBB. Tight junctions between endothelial cells are absent and the endothelial cells themselves are hyperplastic, irregular, and vesiculated.[21] There is also absence of the typical glial footplate against a disordered basement membrane.[22] However, at the tumor margin and in the brain adjacent to the tumor, this disordered vasculature is not present and drug delivery using non-lipophilic agents

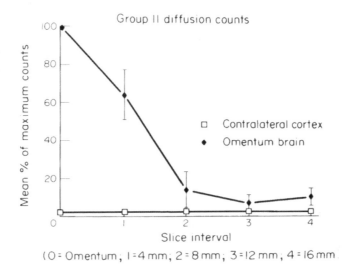

Figure 14.9 Graphic representation of data in Table 14.2.

becomes much more difficult. While it is generally accepted that the BBB is variably intact within the tumor, as evidenced by regions that enhance with contrast administration on CT scans, the brain adjacent to the tumor (BAT) represents a functionally intact barrier to overcome. As Levin et al[23] suggest, the lack of alteration in capillary permeability in the BAT is not important for lipophilic agents, but is a considerable problem when administering water-soluble drugs to treat this region of the brain when it contains infiltrating tumor cells.

Neuwelt and colleagues have refined and popularized the technique of hyperosmotic-induced BBB disruption to enhance delivery of water-soluble agents to malignant brain tumors.[24] In animal studies, Neuwelt demonstrated that methotrexate levels were significantly elevated in the hemisphere with a disrupted BBB when compared to the opposite control hemisphere.[25,26] A phase 2, multiagent trial using BBB disruption was carried out in human patients with glioblastoma multiforme. Although the control patients for this study were

taken from a historical population, the data derived indicated that the patients receiving chemotherapy following BBB disruption had a slightly longer life expectancy than the control patients who received conventionally delivered chemotherapy.[27] However, this technique is not without its problems. Seizures, transient worsening of neurological deficits due to increased intracranial pressure, ocular toxicity, and mild leukoencephalopathy have been reported with this technique.[27-29] Most importantly, several water-soluble agents are highly neurotoxic when given following BBB disruption, thus outweighing the possible benefit derived from attaining high drug concentrations using this method.[30]

Alternative approaches will thus be necessary to facilitate delivery of potentially useful water-soluble drugs to the BAT with a nearly intact or normal BBB. One technique involves the use of autogenous muscle grafts. When placed inside the brain parenchyma, the grafts become vascularized and allow passage of hydrophilic compounds into the adjacent brain via intact, permeable, muscle capillaries.[17]

The omentum has been recognized as a useful source for revascularizing ischemic regions and promoting drainage of excess fluids. Vascularized omental pedicles have been used to reperfuse ischemic extremities[31,32] and myocardium[33] with satisfying experimental and clinical results. Free omental grafts without a vascular pedicle have also been used to revascularize ischemic myocardium. In doing this, Vineberg and colleagues demonstrated diffuse capillary anatomoses between omentum and adjacent tissues with or without internal mammary artery implantation.[34] A dramatic improvement postoperatively in patients with angina was noted, yet experimental evidence from others favored the intact pedicle graft in terms of reducing mortality from acute myocardial infarction.[35]

Pedicled omentum may also serve as a rich nutritive lining for defects created following extensive carcinoma resections to promote wound healing and skin grafitng.[36] This approach is especially beneficial following radiotherapy to facilitate closure of fistulous tracts. In addition, to its revascularization capabilities, the omentum has an excellent capacity to absorb lymphedema fluid and has been used successfully in treating chronic extremity swelling following radical tissue resection including the lymphatic drainage system.

The work of Goldsmith et al[37] involving the use of omentum for absorption of chronic lymphedema resulted in the novel use of an omental pedicle by Levander and colleagues for diverting cerebrospinal fluid (CSF) away from the lumbar cistern in patients with communicating hydrocephalus. Levander demonstrated, in his experimental models, that CSF labeled with a radiopharmaceutical agent moved through the omental pedicle and into the venous system.[38] This technique was subsequently used with favorable long-term clinical results in communicating hydro-

cephalous patients, thus bypassing the need for a ventricular or lumboperitoneal shunt and avoiding all of the problems associated with these devices[39] (Levander personal communication). Other applications for the use of omentum in the CNS include cerebral revascularization, following the occurrence of completed ischemic strokes,[40,41] and improving neurological outcome in patients with spinal cord injury.[42-44] Preliminary data indicated that, for stroke patients, improvement in motor and cognitive function may occur secondary to omental revascularization of ischemic brain but not permanently damaged neurons,[45] i.e., the omentum supplies blood to the ischemic penumbra around the infarct. Omental transposition may also be effective in preventing progressive cerebral infarction in children and young adults with Moyamoya disease.[46,47] Perhaps its most effective role in treating cerebral ischemic disease will be in prevention of strokes in patients with transient ischemic attacks. Animal studies have demonstrated that when the omentum is transplanted to the brain prior to arterial occlusion, the devastating effects of cerebral infarction are prevented or lessened in a significant manner.[48,49]

The ultrastructural anatomy of the vascular networks of the omentum is different from intracranial vessels in several ways. While the endothelium in both locations is highly permeable to lipophilic molecules, the intact BBB (endothelial tight junctions) prevents passage of water-soluble, non-lipophilic compounds.[50] Mesenteric capillaries are composed of a continuous endothelial layer with distinctive gaps between the cells,[51] which are most prominent at the venous (post-capillary) end of the vessel.[52] In addition to these gap junctions, plasmalemmal vesicles have also been identified that may scrve as channels or pores that connect the inside of the vessel (luminal) with the adjacent interstitial space.[53] Whether one or both structure features exist in the mensenteric vasculature, the omentum is readily permeable to proteins and water-soluble substances including chemotherapeutic agents.[53,54] Most investigators have shown that the intercellular junctions act as the essential structural component that contributes to omental capillary permeability, thus distinguishing this vascular system from the non-fenestrated, water-impermeable endothelium of the normal cerebral vasculature.[55]

Due to its unique ability to act as a permeable membrane for fluid absorption and egress of small-to medium-size water-soluble compounds, the omentum may serve as an ideal means of bypassing the BBB in and adjacent to the primary tumor location. An added feature of omental tissue is that certain inherent lipid substances act as a strong source of angiogenesis as demonstrated in the rabbit corneal model.[56] This finding would account for the development of multiple vascular connections between the transposed omentum and the underlying brain. Together with naturally occurring tumor angiogenesis factors, the omentum could be expected to remain attached to the brain interface and provide numerous vascular channels to the tumor and adjacent infiltrated regions that would otherwise have an intact BBB. As opposed to intermittent BBB disruption with hyperosmotic agents, omental transposition to the cavity of a tumor following resection would act as a permanent source to enhance delivery of potentially beneficial chemotherapeutic agents that otherwise might not be delivered to the region of the tumor. Contrarily, the deleterious aspect of this method might be to promote extra CNS spread of primary malignant gliomas, which is usually quite rare. Thus, extensive animal research will be necessary to further define the benefits and limitations of this procedure prior to using this unique approach in patients with malignant brain tumors.

REFERENCES

1. Kun LE. Patterns of failure in tumors of the central nervous system. *Cancer Treat Symp.* 1983;2:285-294.
2. Lange OF, Oaase KD, Scheef W. Simultaneous radio and chemotherapy of inoperable brain tumors. *Radiother Oncol.* 1987;8:309-314.
3. Bloom HJG. Intracranial tumors: response and resistance to therapeutic endeavors 1970-1980. *Int J Radiation Oncol Biol Phys.* 1982;8:1083-1113.
4. Hochberg FH, Pruitt A. Assumptions in the radiotherapy of glioblastoma. *Neurology.* 1980;30:907-911.
5. Gutin PH, Levin VA. Surgery, radiation, chemotherapy in the treatment of malignant brain tumors. In: Thompson RA, Greed JR, eds. *Controversies in Neurology.* New York: Raven Press; 1983:67-86.
6. Berger MS, Ojeman GA, Lettich E. Neurophysiological monitoring to facilitate resection during astrocytoma surgery. Neurosurgical Clinics of North America. *The Role of Surgery in Brain Tumor Management.* Philadelphia: WB Saunders; 1990:65-80.
7. Walker MD, Strike TA, Sheline GE. An analysis of dose-effect relationship in the radiotherapy of malignant gliomas. *Int J Radiat Oncol Biol Phys.* 1974;5:1733-1740.
8. Sheline GE, Wara WM, Smith V. Therapeutic irradiation and brain injury. *Int J Radiat Oncol Biol Phys.* 1980;6:1215-1228.
9. Kramer S, Lee KF. Complications of radiation therapy: the central nervous system. *Seminars Roentgenol.* 1974;9:75-83.
10. Wigg DR, Murray RML, Koschel K. Tolerance of the central nervous system in photon irradiation. *Acta Radiologica Oncol.* 1982;21:49-60.
11. Bernstein M, Gutin PH. Interstitial irradiation of brain tumors: A review. *Neurosurgery.* 1981;9:341-350.
12. Gutin PH, Philips TL, Wara WM, et al. Brachytherapy of recurrent malignant brain tumors with removable high activity iodine-125 sources. *J Neurosurgery.* 1984;60:61-88.
13. Chang CH, Horton J, Schoenfeld D, et al. Comparison of postoperative radiotherapy and combined postoperative radiotherapy and chemotherapy in the multidisciplinary management of malignant gliomas. A joint RTOG and ECOG Study. *Cancer.* 1983;51:997-1107.
14. EORTC Brain Tumor Group. Evaluatoin of CCNU, W-26 plus CCNU, and procarbazine in supratentorial brain gliomas. Final evaluation of randomized study. *J Neurosurg.* 1981;55:27-31.
15. Goldsmith HS, Chen WF, Duckett SW. Brain vascularization by intact omentum. *Arch Surg.* 1973;106:645-698.

16. Hauser W, Nelson K. Technetium 99 m DTPA. A new radiopharmaceutical for brain and kidney scanning. *Radiology.* 1970;84:629-684.

17. Greig NH. Optimizing drug delivery to brain tumors. Cancer Treat Rev. 1987;14:1-28.

18. Ali-Osman F, Dougherty D, Giblin J, et al. Application of in vivo and in vitro pharmacokinetics for physiologically relevant drug exposure in a human clongenic stem cell assay. *Cancer Res.* 1988;48:715-724.

19. Heisiger EM, Voorhies RM, Basler GA, et al. Opening the blood-brain and blood-tumor barriers in experimental rat brain tumors: the effect of intracarotid hyperosmolar mannitol on capillary permeability and blood flow. *Ann Neurol.* 1986;19:50-59.

20. Warnke PC, Blasberg RG, Groothius DS. The effect of hyperosmotic blood-brain barrier disruption on blood to tissue transport in ENU-induced gliomas. *Ann Neurol.* 1987;22:300-305.

21. Long DM. Capillary ultrastructure and the blood-brain barrier in human malignant brain tumors. *J Neurosurg.* 1970;32:127-144.

22. Nystrom S. Pathological changes in blood vessels of human gliablastoma multiform. *Acta Pathol Microbiol Scand.* 1960;49:1-185.

23. Levin VA, Freeman-Dove M, Landahl HO. Permeability characteristics of brain adjacent to tumors in rats. *Arch Neurol.* 1975;32:785-791.

24. Rapaport SI. Effect of concentrated solutions on blood-brain barrier. *Am J Physiol.* 1970;219:270-274.

25. Neuwelt EA, Frenkel E, D'Agoshno AN, et al. Growth of human lung tumor in the brain of the nude rat as a new model to evaluate antitumor agent delivery across the blood-brain barrier. *Cancer Res.* 1985;45:2827-2833.

26. Neuwelt EA, Frenkel E, Rappoport S, et al. Effect of osmotic blood-brain barrier disruption on methotrexate pharmacokinetics in the dog. *Neurosurgery.* 1980;7:36-43.

27. Neuwelt EA, Howieson J, Frenkel DP, et al. A phase II trial of combination chemotherapy given in association with blood-brain barrier modification in glioblastoma patients. *Proc Am Soc Clin Oncol.* 1985;4:136.

28. Laties AM, Rappoport S. The blood ocular barriers under osmotic stress: Studies in the freeze dried eye. *Arch Ophthalmol.* 1976;94:1086-1091.

29. Neuwelt EA, Specht HR, Howieson J, et al. Osmotic blood-brain barrier modification: clinical documentation by enhanced CT scanning and/or radionuclide brain scanning. *Am J Neuroradiol.* 1983;4:907-913.

30. Neuwelt EA, Pagel M, Barnett P, et al. Pharmacology and toxicity of intracarotoid adriamycin administration following osmotic blood-brain barrier modification. *Cancer Res.* 1981;41:4466-4470.

31. Casten DF, Alday ES. Omental transfer for revascularization of the extremities. *Surg Gynecol Obstet.* 1971;134:301-304.

32. Goldsmith HS. Salvage of end stage ischemic extremities by intact omentum. *Surgery.* 1980;88:632-736.

33. Goldsmith HS. Pedicled omentum versus free omental graft for myocardial revascular-ization. *Dis Chest.* 1968;54:523-526.

34. Vineberg AM, Shanks J, Pffarre R, et al. Myocardial revascularization by omental graft without pedicle: Experiemtnal background and report on 25 cases followed six to 16 months. *J Thorac Cardiovasc Surg.* 1965;44:103-129.

35. Pffarre R, Hufnagel CA. Epicardectomy and omental graft in acute myocardial infarction. *Am J Surg.* 1968;115:589-593.

36. Abbes M. The greater omentum in repair of complications following surgery and radiotherapy for certain cancers. *Int Surg.* 1974;59:81-86.

37. Goldsmith HS, DeLos Santos R, Beattie EJ. Relief of chronic lymphedema by omental transposition. *Ann Surg.* 1967;166:573-589.

38. Levander B. Asard PK. Lumbo-omental shunt for drainage of cerebrospinal fluid: an experimental study in dogs. *Acta Neurochir.* 1978;43:251-262.

39. Levander B, Granberg PO, Hindmarsh T. Lumbo-omental shunt for drainage of cerebrospinal fluid in hydrocephalus. *Acta Neurochir.* 1978;44:1-9.

40. Yoshioka N, Tominaga S. Cerebral revascularization by omental free flap using contralateral superficial temporal vessels as recipient vessels: case report. *Surg Neurol.* 1997;45:460-465.

41. Yohioka N, Tominaga S, Suzuki Y, et al. Vascularized omental graft to brain surface in ischemic cerebral vascular disease. *Microsurgery.* 1995;16:455-462.

42. Goldsmith HS, Steward E, Duckett S. Early application of pedicled omentum to the acutely traumatized spinal cord. *Paraplegia.* 1985;23:100-112.

43. de la Torre JC, Goldsmith HS. Supraspinal fiber outgrowth and apparent synaptic remodeling across transected-reconstructed feline spinal cord. *Acta Neurochir (Wien).* 1992;114:118-127.

44. Goldsmith HS. Brain and spinal cord revascularization by omental transposition. *Neurol Res.* 1994;16:159-162.

45. Goldsmith HS, Saunders RC, Reeves AG, et al. Omental transposition to brain of stroke patients. *Stroke.* 1979;10:471-472.

46. Yonekawa Y. Experimental intracranial transplantation of omentum major in dogs: a tentative new treatment for hydrocephalus and cerebral ischemia. *Arch Jap Chir.* 1978;47:3-17.

47. Touho H, Karasawa J, Tenjin H, Ueda S. Omental transplantation using a superficial temporal artery previously used for encephalo-duroarterio-synangiosis. *Surg Neurol.* 1996;45:550-558.

48. Goldsmith HS, Duckett S, Chen WF. Prevention of cerebral infarction in the monkey by omental transposition to the brain. *Stroke.* 1978;166:224-229.

49. Goldsmith HS, Duckett S, Chen WF. Prevention of cerebral infarction in the dog by intact omentum. *Am J Surg.* 1975;130:317-320.

50. Karnovsky MJ. The ultrastructural basis of capillary permeability studied with peroxidase as a tracer. *J Cell Biol.* 1967;35:213-236.

51. Simionescu M, Simionescu N, Palade GE. Segmental differentiations of cell junctions in the vascular endothelium. The microvasculature. *J Cell Biol.* 1975;67:863.

52. Intaglietta M, Zweffach BW. Geometrical model of the microvasculature of rabbit omentum from in vivo measurements. *Circulation Res.* 1971;28:593-600.

53. Palade GE, Simionescu M, Simionescu N. Structural aspects of the permeability of the microvascular endothelium. *Acta Physiol Scand.* 1979;463:11-32.

54. Renkin EM. Transport of large molecules across capillary walls. *Physiologist.* 1964;7:13.

55. Neese TS, Karnovsky MJ. Fine structural localization of a blood-brain barrier to exogenous peroxidase. *J Cell Biol.* 1967;39:207.

56. Goldsmith HS, Griffith AL, Kupferman A, et al. Lipid angiogenesis factor from omentum. *JAMA.* 1987;252:2034-2036.

CHAPTER 15

OMENTAL TRANSPOSITION TO THE BRAIN FOR ALZHEIMER'S DISEASE

HARRY S. GOLDSMITH

INTRODUCTION

Alzheimer's disease (AD) has become one of the most devastating problems confronting medicine today, with 4 million Americans suffering from the disease that is estimated will cost up to 50 to 100 billion dollars by early in the next century.[1] Alois Alzheimer in 1907 was the first to identify the disease that now bears his name, in a 55-year-old woman who suffered from progressive dementia.[2] He observed the presence of abnormal nerve cells within the cerebral cortex, which contained tangles of fibers that are classified as neurofibrillary tangles. Also identified by Alzheimer were degenerated nerve endings that he classified as senile plaques. It remained unclear over subsequent years whether these neuropathogenic structures reported by Alzheimer were responsible for the dementia that occurred in AD. However, a direct relationship was eventually established between the number of senile plaques that are present within the cerebral cortex and an individual's cognitive performance.[3]

BACKGROUND

The neurodegenerative effects of AD are well known but the devastating cognitive results of the disease have not been clarified as to their cause. Without this knowledge, it remains difficult to develop therapeutic designs to treat the disease. Recent publications, however, have suggested that placing an intact pedicled omental graft on the brain of an AD patient led to improved cognitive and neurological function,[4] as well as neuropathological findings.[5] The operation was carried out in the hope of success based on two characteristics of the omentum: its cerebrovascular and cholingeric potential, biological activities that are deficient in AD.

Cerebrovasculature

During the mid-1960s, interest was raised in my laboratory to learn if an intact omentum pedicle could be lengthened and mobilized to reach a dog's brain with a subsequent development of vascular connections at the omental-cerebral interface. It was theorized that if this could be accomplished, it might lead to a surgical procedure that would add an extracerebral source of blood to an ischemic brain. The surgical technique for omental lengthening was developed, and the vascular connections that developed between the omentum and the brain were confirmed by injecting fluorescein and India ink into an omental artery within the peritoneal cavity that supplied the omental pedicle to the brain.[6] in order to be absolutely certain that the injected dye markers reached the brain only by way of the omental pedicle, the neck of the animal was completely severed from its body except for the intact omental pedicle coming from the peritoneal cavity. The dye markers were subsequently seen on the brain surface, in major cerebral blood vessels and in deep portions of both cerebral hemispheres. These findings of widespread cerebrovascular perfusion originating from the omentum were later confirmed by radioisotopic studies.[7]

After it had been demonstrated that vascular connections developed at the interface between the omentum and the brain (*Figure 15.1*), the next step in developing the operation was to learn whether it was possible to increase cerebral perfusion from the omentum to the brain in sufficient volume to protect the brain from the severe ischemic insult. The experimental model used to show this was accomplished by creating a cerebral infarction in the dog[8] and in the monkey[9] by ligating their middle cerebral artery (MCA). Omental placement on the brain just days prior to subsequent MCA ligation confirmed in these studies that omental transposition could supply

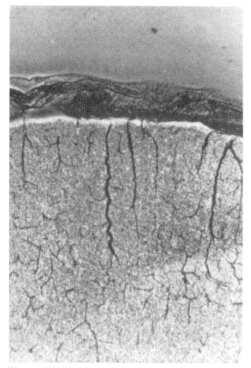

Figure 15.1 Blood vessel development at the omental-cerebral interface. Omental blood vessels filled with India ink are shown penetrating deep into underlying brain. Blood-brain barrier is broken by this development, which could allow drug therapy to the brain.

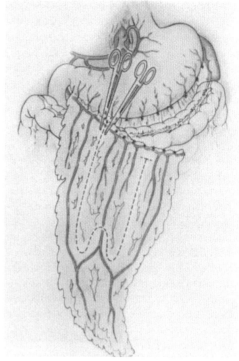

Figure 15.2 The omental apron is divided to gain increased length, with arterial supply being maintained primarily along the periphery.

sufficient extracerebral blood flow to the brain to prevent cerebral infarction. These experiments took place in the 1970s and by the 1980s, other laboratory studies from around the world also began to report favorably on the effects of transposing the omentum to the brain. These experiments confirmed that CBF was maintained by the omentum following MCA occlusion,[10] with preservation of neuronal conduction activity within the brain as measured by somatosensory evoked potentials.[11]

The original idea that the omentum might benefit patients with AD stemmed from two early experimental papers. One of these publications reported that placing the omentum on the surface of the brain prior to MCA ligation prevented the marked depression in cortical levels of biogenic amines that routinely occurs after MCA occlusion.[12] The other paper showed that protein synthesis within the brain was maintained by the omentum even in the presence of MCA occlusion.[13] These observations plus the acknowledged ability of the omentum to increase cerebral blood flow (CBF) raised the question as to whether the omentum had the biological potential to stop or at least slow down the linear destruction of neurons that is the hallmark of AD. But it was a decade before this question was addressed.

Based on favorable experiments that had accumulated from various laboratories, omental transposition was approved for human trial. It was felt that the best patients to offer the operation to were those suffering from transient ischemic attacks (TIAs). However, institutional authorities gave permission to perform the procedure only on patients who had already sustained a cerebral infarction. The operation was first carried out in 1978 on a small group of patients who had suffered a stroke years earlier.[14,15] Since that time, there have been a host of publications showing the beneficial effects of omental transposition to the brain in treating a variety of neurological conditions.[16-18]

SURGICAL PROCEDURE

A general surgeon and a neurosurgeon work as a team to transpose a pedicled omental graft to the surface of the brain. The general surgeon is responsible for performing a laparotomy, elongating the omentum into a long pedicle, and developing an extensive subcutaneous tunnel up the chest and neck to the head. The neurosurgeon is responsible for performing the craniotomy and securing the omentum on the brain.[19]

The technique for lengthening the omentum begins by separating the omentum from the transverse colon. This is followed by removing the omentum from its proximal and central attachments to the stomach, which is done directly on the greater curvature of the stomach, leaving the gastroepiploic vessels intact within the omental apron. The left gastroepiploic vessels are then divided to gain increasing omental length. In order to get sufficient length to reach the brain, the omental apron is surgically tailored, with care being taken to preserve intact at least one major artery and vein with the structure (*Figure 15.2*). At the end of the omental lengthening process, the blood vessels that maintain the vascular integrity of the omental pedicle are the right gastroepiploic artery and vein. The viability of the pedicled omental graft depends on the preservation of these vessels.

Once the omentum has been sufficiently lengthened to reach the brain without any tension, incisions are made along the chest wall, which are connected by a long subcutaneous tunnel. The omentum is brought through this tunnel, with the omentum exiting behind the ear and beneath the base of the scalp flap previously dissected in making the initial craniotomy incision on the head (*Figure 15.3*). The dura mater is opened over the cerebral hemisphere, and pieces of arachnoid membrane are carefully removed. The omentum is then laid on the brain surface and secured to the edges of the surrounding dura with absorbable

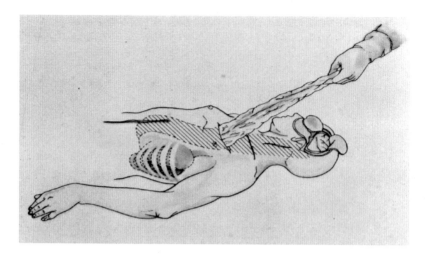

Figure 15.3 Omentum has been brought through a long subcutaneous tunnel developed between incisions along chest and anterolateral neck, where it exits behind the ear and is placed directly on the brain.

sutures. Some surgeons do not use this pedicled omentum technique but employ a free omental graft that requires microvascular anastomoses of the gastroepiploic artery and vein to the superficial temporal vessels or other vascular connections. This latter technique is more surgically demanding than the pedicled method. However, of greater significant is the tendency for a vascularized free omental graft to allow edema fluid to accumulate within the cranial vault, which I have never seen with a pedicled omental graft. I believe the reason for fluid accumulation to occur with a free vascularized omental graft is that creating a free graft markedly diminishes a major characteristic of the omentum, namely, its enormous edema-absorptive capacity. The loss of this absorption capability is a reflection of a non-functioning or poorly functioning omental graft, probably because all lymphatic vessels are divided when one takes an isolated piece of omentum and develops it into a free graft.

During the early 1980s, omentum transposition was performed with increasing frequency on the human brain, with the most common indication for the operation being to treat the neurological sequelae of patients who had sustained a previous cerebral infarction. It was never expected that omental transposition would have an effect on infarcted brain tissue but what was theorized was that increased CBF originating from the omentum might stimulate the viable but ischemic depressed neurons located in the zone surrounding the infarct (penumbra). Favorable clinical results have been subsequently published following the performance of omental transposition for post-stroke and TIA patients.[20-22]

Omentum: Alzheimer's theory

Based on favorable published experimental data and encouraging clinical results following omental placement onto a previously infarcted brain, it was theorized that the omentum might have the potential to maintain the viability of neurons still functioning in an AD patient. This seemed even more likely if the omentum could be placed on the brain early in the disease process. The main reason for believing the omentum might be helpful in this situation was

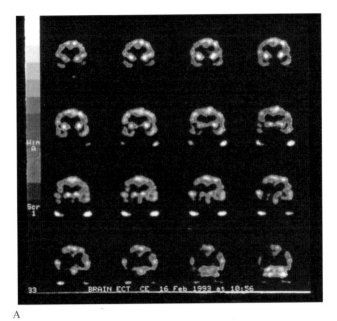

A

B

Figure 15.4 (See color section) A: Preoperative SPECT scan. Coronal slices with images displayed in an anterior to posterior position with color scale on right side. A major preoperative perfusion defect is seen in right parietal-occipital location. **B:** Postoperative SPECT examination 10 months after surgery. Reperfusion has occured in right parietal-occipital area. (From Goldsmith HS. *Neurol Res.* 1996;18:103-108.)

based on two unfavorable characteristics in AD, a decrease in CBF and depressed intracerebral cholinergic activity.

Vascular and cholinergic concepts

It has been established that there is a decrease in the CBF of AD patients but it has remained unclear as to whether diminished cerebrovascular perfusion occurs as a result of neuronal damage, which lowers the neuron's metabolic requirements, or whether the lowered CBF results in decreased neuronal activity. Recent ultrastructural studies of the AD brain have suggested the latter possibility as being the more likely because extensive architectural distortion of capillaries in the brain have been identified that may limit vital nutrient delivery to ischemic sensitive neurons over an extended period.[23] It was felt that omental transposition to an AD brain could improve this vascular situation.

Another reason for believing omentum transposition to the brain might help AD patients was based on the decrease in acetylcholine (ACh) activity that occurs in AD. This cholingeric loss is reflected in the 40% to 90% decrease in brain levels of choline acetyltransferase (ChAT), which is the enzyme that catalyzes the reaction for ACh synthesis in the brain.[24,25] Based on the report of a significant decrease in ChAT activity near senile plaque formations, which have been associated with decreased intellectual performance,[3] a pedicled omental graft, with its increased vascular and cholinergic activity,[26] was placed on the brain of an AD patient who had an 8-year history of a progressive decline in neuropsychological function. The patient, with the support of his family, elected to undergo the operation in the hope that the procedure might stabilize his mental deterioration. The operation was performed in 1993.

Postoperative course

The patient showed subjective and objective improvement in his cognitive and neurological condition for 1 year following the operation.[4] The postoperative cerebral angiogenic activity originating from the omentum became clearly evident as shown by a global increase in CBF as demonstrated by comparison of pre- and postoperative single photon emission computed tomography (SPECT) examinations (*Figures 15.4A and 15.5B*).

After the first postoperative year, the patient began to show a neurological deficit in association with deterioration in neuropsychological testing. The cognitive loss continued with a marked decline in his physical condition resulting from chronic cardiopulmonary problems. The patient died 31 months after surgery, from unrelated chronic medical problems.

Autopsy findings

An authorized autopsy confirmed the diagnosis of AD as demonstrated by the presence of neocortical senile plaques, neurofibrillary tangles, and amyloid deposition.

At the time of surgery, the omentum had been placed on the patient's right cerebral hemisphere since his cerebral perfusion deficit was most prominent on the right side of the brain and his neurological findings most prominent on the left side of his body, evidence indicating the right cerebral hemisphere to be the location most affected by the AD process. Autopsy confirmed this with increased numbers of senile plaques and neurofibrillary tangles being present in the right cerebral hemisphere as compared to the left hemisphere. This right-left brain asymmetry found at autopsy correlated with preoperative clinical and SPECT findings, which indicated greater dysfunction in the right cerebral hemisphere.

Two major neuropathological observations were made at autopsy that were totally

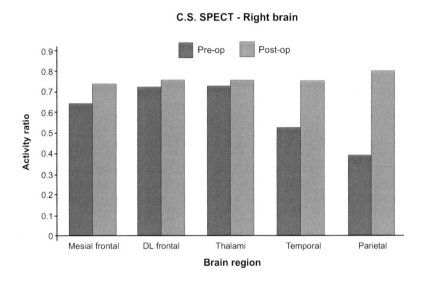

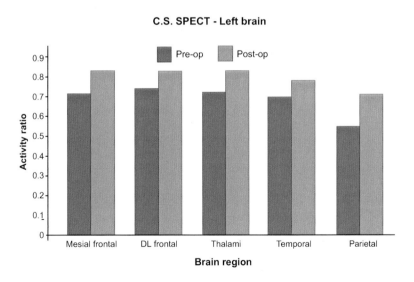

Figure 15.5 Pre- and postoperative activity ratios of cerebrovascular perfusion derived from SPECT scans (*Figures 15.4A and 15.4B*). Activity ratios compiled from measured perfusion in cerebral regions of interest compared to ipsilateral cerebellar perfusion used as a standard. Omentum placement of right cerebral hemisphere. DL frontal, deep left frontal.

unexpected.[5] One was a significant decrease in the number of senile plaques found in the cerebral cortex at the crest of the gyri subjacent to the omentum compared to an increased number of senile plaques located in the contiguous depths of the sulci (*Figures 15.6A and 15.6B*). This finding strongly suggested that the omentum played a role in this phenomenon, especially since no comparable gradient of neurofibrillary tangles was observed adjacent to the omentum.

The second significant neuropathological finding made at the time of autopsy occurred directly below the omental transplant in the upper cortical lamina. Numerous hypertrophic astrocytes were observed that contained fine granules of Prussian blue-positive cytoplasmic hemosiderin. Also noted was an inverse relationship between the presence of these hemosiderin-filled astrocytes, which are not a normal finding in AD, and a significant decrease in the number of senile plaques in the area. Careful examination of multiple cortical regions of the right and left cerebral hemispheres failed to reveal either hemosiderin inclusions or decreased numbers of senile plaque except for the area where the omentum had been located.

DISCUSSION

That placing the omentum on an AD brain could be clinically beneficial was initially based on the idea that the biological activity of the omentum might interrupt or at least slow down the progressive destruction of cerebral neurons that is observed in an AD brain. Stated in another way, would increasing CBF and possibly cholinergic activity in the brain of an AD patient enhance the neuroelectrical and neurochemical activity of still-viable neurons prior to their expected destruction? This question came into sharper focus when it was suggested that the etiology of AD was secondary to decreased blood flow to ischemic-sensitive neurons cased by an extensive

distortion of cerebral capillaries, which create abnormal hemodynamic patterns that impair the CBF and energy supply to the brain. As these cerebral capillaries, become progressively kinked, looped, and twisted in shape, it was postulated that they decrease the glucose, oxygen, and other micronutrient delivery across the blood-brain barrier and limit the egress of catabolic products from the brain.[23] The known suboptimal utilization of oxygen[27] and glucose[28] in an AD brain would be expected to cause a continuing decline of neuronal activity since glucose is the main substrate for glycolysis and oxygen is necessary for oxidative phosphorylation and adenosine triphosphate (ATP) production. As the decreased glucose and oxygen levels in the brain persist, ischemic-sensitive neurons cannot meet necessary energy demands because of decreased CBF and the lowered energy supply. This pathophysiological situation eventually leads to a slow but continuing decline in neuronal activity, which has been postulated to lead to cognitive decline and the development of senile plaques and neurofibrillary tangles.[23] Since this process is predicated on a hemodynamic abnormality caused by cerebral microvascular distortion, it was felt that omental transposition to the brain of an AD patient would improve cerebrovascular function,[29] which might increase the energy effectiveness of ischemic-sensitive neurons.

Another major reason why it was theorized that omental transposition might benefit patients with AD was to improve defective cholinergic transmission that occurs in AD. The omentum has neurotransmitters incorporated into its tissues,[30] including ChAT, which is the enzyme responsible for the formation of ACh from choline and acetyl coenzyme A and is the marker for cholingeric activity.[26] Since the omentum has ChAT activity which is depressed in the AD brain and has been correlated with decreased density of senile plaques,[3] the   question   was   asked   whether

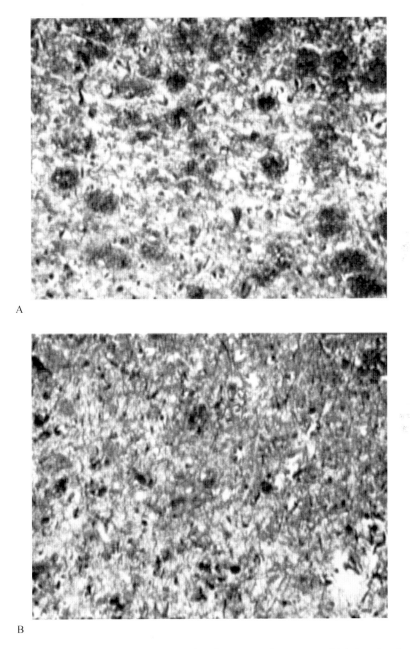

A

B

Figure 15.6 Sections of right parietal neocortex underlying the transposed omentum. (Bielschowsky silver stain, x40). **A:** Middle cortical laminae in the depth of a sulcus showing numerous senile plaques and neurofibrillary tangles. **B:** Crest of gyrus contiguous with regions shown in **A**. Conspicuously fewer senile plaques are evident. Occasional hypertrophic astrocytes containing hemosiderin are present throughout the section. (From Relkin NR, et al. *Neurol Res.* 1996;18:291-294.)

any acetylcholine in omental tissue might be transported through vascular connections at the omental-cerebral interface causing increased brain levels of acetylcholine. Even if omental ACh proved insufficient to fully supplement cerebral ACh levels, there might be partial protection since omental transposition has been shown to maintain neurotransmitter levels in the brain even in the presence of severe cerebral ischemia caused by middle cerebral artery occlusion.[31] Additionally, nerve growth substances in the omentum[32] might also benefit AD patients by increasing neurite growth into neuroactivity-deficient areas of the brain.

Other ideas were raised as to why omental transposition to the brain had the potential to help AD patients. For example, the omentum on the brain might increase cerebral ACh level simply by elevating cerebral glucose concentrations by way of the additional CBF originating from the omentum. Cerebral blood flow and glucose and oxygen metabolism are diminished in AD, with the lowest levels of glucose and oxygen, metabolism occurring in cerebral regions that have the greatest AD pathology.[27,28] Since decreased CBF is one of the earliest markers for the presence of AD,[33] even a small increase in CBF might be clinically important since hypoglycemia has been shown to dramatically decrease cerebral ACh levels.[34] Further support for this theory is suggested by the study that showed that administered glucose diminishes atropine-induced ACh depletion in the brain.[35] An increased CBF originating from the omentum might also benefit AD patients just by increasing the availability of ACh precursors (choline and acetyl coenzyme A) that are presented to the brain.

How the omentum affects the brain of AD patients awaits further elucidation. Possibilities for its actions would include facilitation of the local clearance of beta-amyloid by increasing CBF and by exerting trophic influences on local circulation, by the effect of omental macrophage activity on the microglia in the

brain, by exerting anti-inflammatory action, that the omentum is known to do, or by mechanisms that remain unknown at this time. Experience with omental transposition to the brain to treat AD has just begun.

The operation, either alone or as a delivery system for associated drug therapy, may hopefully lead to the identification of new techniques to protect Alzheimer's patients from the devastation of this neurodegenerative disease.

ADDENDUM

Three additional Alzheimer's patients have undergone omental tranposition to their brain during the past year. The last patient who underwent the operation has shown only minimal neurological improvement, but it is only 2 months since surgery and thus too soon to predict the eventual cognitive outcome.

Another Alzheimer's patient who was operated upon is a 67-year-old housewife who underwent the procedure in May 1998. During the 3 years prior to operation, a marked cognitive deterioration was noted. By the time she had surgery, she was totally unresponsive and her family categorized her as being "zombie-like."

By the second postoperative day, she became alert to her family and surroundings. By the end of the first postoperative week, she could say a few words. By the end of the first postoperative year, she has maintained a high state of alertness to people and events. She laughs at appropriate times and moves her head from side to side in order to direct her attention to people engaged in conversation. She can say words when coaxed and sing hymns along with her family. Her long-term memory has improved but her ability to speak spontaneously remains severely impaired. There is no indication, more than a year after surgery, that her cognitive improvement has lessened. This would suggest that the neurodegenerative process present in her brain

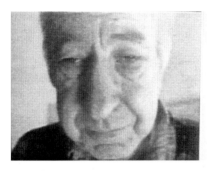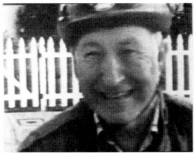

Figure 15.7 Patient (left) 1 week prior to surgery and (right) 3½ months after surgery.

has remained stable with no signs of acceleration.

The third Alzheimer's patient, who in the last year has undergone omental transposition to his brain, is a 70-year-old engineer. His cognitive condition, which began in 1993, worsened over the years and by 1995, he was involuntarily committed to a mental institution, mainly because of violent behavior associated with his condition. He underwent omental transposition in January 1999. A brain biopsy taken at the time of surgery showed pathologically, the presence of Alzheimer's disease.

Cognitive improvement in the patient was noted within the first postoperative weeks and by the third postoperative month, these changes were striking and have been carefully recorded on pre- and postoperative video tapes.

The patient now lives at home and requires no medications. His cognitive change continues to improve. However, his short-term memory remains poor. He can now read, comment on television programs, ride a bicycle, etc. I think the description of the patient by his wife at 5 months post-surgery is quite informative. "My husband has shown indefinable improvement that underlies everything else. It's just there. He's just there" (*Figure 15.7*).

REFERENCES

1. Corey-Bloom J, Thal LJ, Galasko D, et al. Diagnosis and evaluation of dementia. *Neurology.* 1995;45:211-218.
2. Alzheimer A. Uber eine eigenartige erkrangkung der himrinde. *All A Psychiatr.* 1907;64:146-148.
3. Perry EK, Perry RH, Blessed G, Bergmann K, Gibson PH. Correlation of cholinergic abnormalities with senile plaques and mental test scores in senile dementia. *Br Med J.* 1978;2:1457-1459.
4. Goldsmith HS. Omental transposition for Alzheimer's disease. *Neurol Res.* 1996;18:103-108.
5. Relkin NR, Edgar MA, Gouras GK, Gandy SE, Goldsmith HS. Decreased senile plaques density in Alzheimer neocortex adjacent to an omental transposition. *Neurol Res.* 1996;18:291-294.
6. Goldsmith HS, Chen WF, Duckett SW. Brain vascularization by intact omentum. *Arch Surg.* 1973;106:695-698.
7. Berger MS, Weinstein PR, Goldsmith HS, Hattner R, Longa EZ, Perira B. Omental transposition to bypass the blood brain for delivery of chemotherapeutic agents to malignant brain tumors. In: Goldsmith HS. *The Omentum—Research and Clinical Applications.* New York: Springer-Verlag; 1990:117-130.
8. Goldsmith HS, Duckett S, Chen WF. Prevention of cerebral infarction in the dog by intact omentum. *Am J Surg.* 1975;130:317-326.
9. Goldsmith HS, Duckett S, Chen WF. Prevention of cerebral infarction in the monkey by omental transposition to the brain. *Stroke.* 1978;9:224-229.
10. De Riu PL, Falzoi A, Papavero L, Rocca A, Viale GL. Local cerebral blood flow after middle cerebral artery occlusion in rabbits following transposition of omentum to the brain. *J Microsurg.* 1980;1:321-324.

11. De Riu PL, Rocca A, Falzoi A. Carai M, Papavero L. Physiological function after middle cerebral artery occlusion in rabbits with neurovascularization of the brain by transposed omentum. *Neurosurgery.* 1980;7:57-67.

12. Pau A, Viale ES, Turtus S. Effect of omental transposition to the brain on the cortical content of norepinephrine dopamine. 5-hydroxytryptamine and 5-hydroxyindolacetic acid in experimental cerebral ischemia. *Acta Neurochir.* 1980;51:253-257.

13. Cucca GS, Papavero L, Pau A, Viale ES, Turtus S, Viale GL. Effect of omental transposition to the brain on protein synthesis in experimental cerebral ischemia. *Acta Neurochir.* 1980;54:213-218.

14. Goldsmith HS. Omental transposition to the human brain. *Stroke.* 1978;9:276.

15. Goldsmith HS, Saunders RL, Reeves AG, Allen CD, Milne J. Omental transposition to the brain of stroke patients. *Stroke.* 1979;10:471-472.

16. Wang CC, Chao YT, Jung DA. Omentum transplantation and revascularization. In: Bignami A, Bloom FE, Bolis CG, Adeloyle A, eds. *Central Nervous System Plasticity and Repair.* New York: Raven Press; 1985:159-163.

17. Abraham J, Chandy MH, Gammon K, et al. Omental transposition to brain in patients with focal ischemia. *Ind J Surg.* 1986;48:138-142.

18. Wu WL, Meng QG, Xu SQ. Omental transposition for treating the sequelae of viral encephalitis: a surgical and follow-up study of 32 cases. In: Goldsmith HS, ed. *The Omentum—Research and Clinical Applications.* New York: Springer-Verlag; 1990:165-172.

19. Goldsmith HS. Omental transposition to the brain and spinal cord. *Surg Rounds.* 1986;9:22-23.

20. Mrowka R, Pieniazek J, Dobkiewicz A. Omental transposition to brain surface in ischemic cerebrovascular disease. *Zentralbl Neurochir.* 1990;5:166-199.

21. Luan WZ. Current status of omentum transposition to the brain in China. *Chung Hua Wai Ko Tsa Chih.* 1987;25:548-555.

22. Goldsmith HS. Brain and spinal cord revascularization by omental transposition. *Neurol Res.* 1994; 16: 159-162.

23. de La Torre J. Impaired brain microcirculation may trigger Alzheimer's disease. *Neurosci Biobehav Rev.* 1994;18:397-401.

24. Davies P, Maloney AJF. Selective loss of central cholingeric neurons in Alzheimer's disease. *Lancet.* 1976;2:1403.

25. White P, Hiley CR, Goodhardt MJ, et al. Neocortical cholingeric neurons in elderly people. *Lancet.* 1977;1:668-670.

26. Goldsmith HS, Marquis JK, Siek G. Choline acetyltransferase activity in omental tissue. *Brit J Neurosurg.* 1987;1:463-466.

27. Grubb R, Raichle M, Gado M, Eichling J, Hughes C. Cerebral blood flow, oxygen utilization and blood volume in dementia. *Neurology.* 1977;27:905-910.

28. Friedland RP, Budinger T, Koss E, Ober E. Alzheimer's disease: anterior-posterior and lateral hemispheric alterations in cortical glucose utilization. *Neurosci Lett.* 1985;53:235-240.

29. Goldsmith HS, Bacciu P, Cosso M, et al. Regional cerebral blood flow after omental transposition to the ischemic brain in man: a five-year follow-up study. *Acta Neurochir.* 1990;106:145-152.

30. Goldsmith HS, McIntosh T, Vezena RM, Colton T. Vasoactive neurochemicals identified in omentum. *Br J Neurosurgery.* 1987;1:359-364.

31. Pau A, Viale ES, Viale E, Turtus S. Effects of omental transposition to the brain on the cortical content of norepinephrine, dopamine, 2-hydroxytryptamine and 5-hydroxyindolacetic acid in experimental cerebral ischemia. *Acta Neurochir.* 1982;66:159-161.

32. Siek GC, Marquis JK, Goldsmith HS. Experimental studies of omentum-derived neurotrophic factors. In: Goldsmith HS, ed. *The Omentum—Research and Clinical Applications.* New York: Springer-Verlag; 1990;83-95.

33. Prohovnik I, Mayeux R, Sackheim HM, et al. Cerebral perfusion as a diagnostic marker of early Alzheimer's disease. *Neurology.* 1988;38:931-937.

34. Ghajar JBG, Gibson GE, Duffy TE. Regional acetylcholine metabolism in brain during acute hypoglycemia and recovery. *J Neurochem.* 1985;44:94-98.

35. Tucek S. Acetycoenzyme A and the synthesis of acetylcholine in neurons: a review of recent progress. *Gen Physiol Biophys.* 1983;2:313-324.

Chapter 16

Omentum Transposition for Treatment of Alzheimer's Disease: Clinical Outcome and Future Therapeutic Interpretation

WILLIAM R. SHANKLE AND JUNKO HARA

BACKGROUND

Surgical transposition of the greater omentum, or omentum transposition (OT), to the brain has been performed for over 30 years, with observable and measurable clinical improvement reported in case-series studies[1] for chronic or acute stroke, spinal cord injury,[2] cerebral palsy,[3] viral encephalitis,[3] Moyamoya disease, frontal temporal lobe dementia (FTLD) of the primary progressive aphasia subtype,[4] and Alzheimer's disease (AD).[5,6] While these studies were clinical case series of patients and did not meet more stringent levels of evidence criteria imposed by randomized, placebo-controlled trials case series, there have been consistent, clinically significant results in each application of OT to a disease state.

OMENTUM TRANSPOSITION FOR ALZHEIMER'S DISEASE

The first case report of OT for AD was reported by Relkin et al,[5] who demonstrated clinical improvement in behavioral and cognitive measures for up to 2 years. In AD clinical trials, the maximum duration of any placebo effect reported has been up to 6 months,[7,8] implying that treatment effects longer than 6 months are not placebo effects. Furthermore, a post-mortem autopsy of the patient showed an absence of

neuritic plaques in gyral crests, but not sulci directly underneath the omentum.

This case report was encouraging and was further evaluated by our group, which longitudinally measured behavioral, cognitive, functional, and neuroimaging outcomes in six biopsy-confirmed AD patients.[6] *Table 16.1* summarizes characteristics of these cases.

The study used a within-patient subject design to measure treatment effect, and included quarterly re-assessment of dementia severity (Clinical Dementia Rating Scale: CDRS; Dementia Severity Rating Scale: DSRS), functional capacity (activities of daily living: ADLs), behavioral problems (Neuropsychiatric Inventory: NPI), cognitive performance (Mini-Mental State Examination: MMSE), and neuroimaging (magnetic resonance imaging: MRI; HMPAO single photon emission computed tomography: HMPAO SPECT) outcomes.

Two of the six patients had postoperative complications that would have obscured the ability to measure the theraputic effect attributable to the omentum, independent of its means of delivering its effect to the brain. Patient AD3 developed acute neuroleptic malignant syndrome after being given olanzapine for post-surgical psychosis. Patient AD5 had several post-surgical complications due to a relatively thickened omentum that obstructed cerebrospinal fluid (CSF) flow (CSF hygroma, epidural hematoma).

Table 16.1: Clinical Summary of AD Cases

	Patient ID					
	AD1	AD2	AD3	AD4	AD5	AD6
Date of Surgery	8/28/2001	9/26/2001	9/28/2001	10/2/2001	10/18/2002	8/22/2003
Age at the surgery	68	69	59	76	56	69
Severity at the time of Surgery (CDRS score)	Moderate (2.0)	Moderate (2.0)	Severe (3.0)	Moderate (2.0)	Moderate (2.0)	Mild (1.0)
Side of Operation	Left	Left	Right	Right	Right	Left
Gender	F	M	F	F	M	M
Years of Education	18	18	N/A	18	18	12
Occupation	Psychologist	MFC Counselor	Exec. Secretary	School Teacher, Librarian	School Teacher	U.S. Customs Agent
Onset	1997-98	1991-94	1993	1993	1998	1998
ApoE Type	E3/E4	E3/E3	E3/E4	E2/E4	E3/E3	E3/E3
Months duration from OT to most recent visit	41	40	17	22	50	41
Date of Autopsy	n/a	5/31/2006	2/13/2003	3/9/2004	n/a	n/a

Because the focus of this chapter is on the effect of the omentum and not on potential intra- or postoperative complications, the results of the four patients whose OT surgery was not complicated by postoperative complications are presented. As discussed later, more non-invasive routes of delivery of the effect of the omentum need to be explored to make it a useful treatment that could be broadly applied. Consequently, longitudinal data will be presented for four of the six AD patients (AD1, AD2, AD4, AD6).

Figure 16.1 shows the effects of OT on dementia severity as represented by the sum of the CDRS item scores (CDRS) for patients AD1, AD2, AD4, and AD6 prior to and after OT (solid curve with data points), plus their expected post-OT scores with and without cholinesterase inhibition (solid and dashed curves, respectively). Clinical Dementia Rating Scale item scores were normalized to facilitate comparison with other measures. Five of the six patients (except AD5) showed marked improvement after OT for 22 to 41 months. At a mean of 14 ($\sigma=5$) months post-OT, normalized CDRS scores significantly improved by an average of 22% ($\sigma=10\%$), and

at 25 ($\sigma=12$) months post-OT, these scores significantly improved by an average of 39% ($\sigma=13\%$) ($P<0.0001$). Dementia Severity Rating Scale results were comparable to the *CDRS* results.

Figure 16.2 shows the effects of OT on cognition related to left hemisphere function for patients AD1, AD2, AD4, and AD6 (solid curves with square markers). The MMSE predominantly tests left hemisphere function except for the drawing task, which counts as one point only. Mini-Mental State Examination scores were normalized to facilitate comparison with other measures. Also shown are the expected normalized MMSE values for these patients if they had not received any treatment (dashed curve) and if they had received cholinesterase inhibition (solid curve). For patients whose omentum was transposed to their left hemisphere (AD1, AD2, AD6), two of them had normalized MMSE scores that were higher than that expected from cholinesterase inhibition for 30 to 42 months. For patient AD4, whose omentum was transposed to the right hemisphere, the normalized MMSE scores were worse than that expected with no treatment.

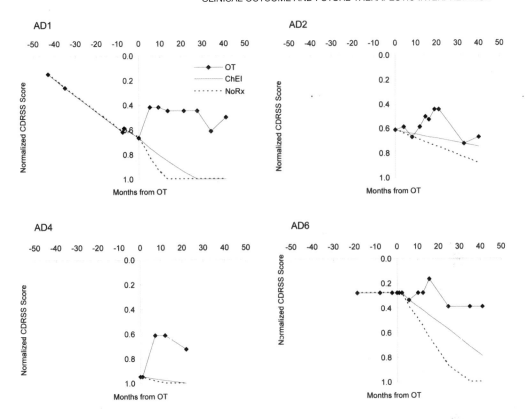

Figure 16.1 Dementia severity changes measured by CDRS. The normalized clinical dementia rating scale subscores (CDRS) for each patient (OT: solid curve with data points) were compared with their expected course attributable to ChEI (solid curve) or no ChEI therapy (no treatment: dashed curve). Larger CDRS values represent greater dementia severity. When more pre-OT CDRS data were available, they were included to more accurately estimate the expected post-OT course. No follow-up data are available for AD3.

As would be expected if OT predominantly affected the hemisphere upon which it was placed, the patients who received it on their left hemisphere did relatively better on the MMSE—a cognitive measure of left hemisphere function—than the patient who received it on the right hemisphere. The three left hemisphere OT patients had higher MMSE scores than would be obtained by cholinesterase inhibition for between 10 and 41 months.

Figure 16.3 shows the effects of OT on the NPI, a measure of behavioral problems. Neuropsychiatric Inventory scores were normalized to facilitate comparison with other measures. Two patients, AD1 and AD4, had significant behavioral problems at baseline, and their normalized NPI scores improved respectively by 16% (23 points) and 54% (78 points) for 22 and 41 months. Patients AD2 and AD6 had little change in normalized NPI scores over 40 months of follow-up.

For the above functional, cognitive, and behavioral measures, the improvements observed on all of them exceeded the maximum 6 months of improvement reported in placebo treatment arms of AD clinical trials.[7,8] Also, mild to moderately demented AD patients generally fall below their pre-

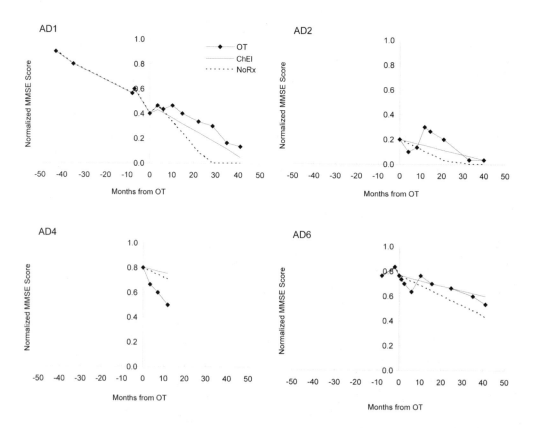

Figure 16.2 Cognitive changes measured by MMSE. The normalized Mini-Mental State Examination (MMSE) scores for each patient (OT: solid curve with data points) were compared to their expected course attributable to ChEI (solid curve) or no ChEI therapy (no treatment: dashed curve). MMSE scores were transformed to normalized values so that lower values represented greater dementia severity. When pre-OT MMSE data were available, they were included to more accurately estimate the expected post-OT course. No follow-up data are available for AD3.

treatment CDRS baseline after 6 to 9 months of cholinesterase inhibitors (ChEI).[9] In the present study, however, patients remained above their CDRS baseline for an average of 14 months.

To relate these clinical measures to changes in brain activity, we longitudinally studied patients AD1 and AD2 with quantitative HMPAO SPECT neuroimaging for up to 41 months *Figure 16.4*. We standardized the longitudinal changes in regional brain HMPAO SPECT activity by dividing the percent change by the standard deviation of test-retest values

(σ=5.25%). Patients AD1 and AD2 showed a maximal increase in cortical activity of 4 standard deviations (21%). Longitudinally, they showed increases in cortical activity of one to two standard deviations above preoperative baseline for between 22 and 41 months in areas underneath, adjacent to, and directly contralateral to the omentum. In contrast, cortical areas not in the above relations to the omentum showed decreases in tissue activity on the order of 20% to 27% over 41 months. These findings suggest that the effect of the omentum was delivered both

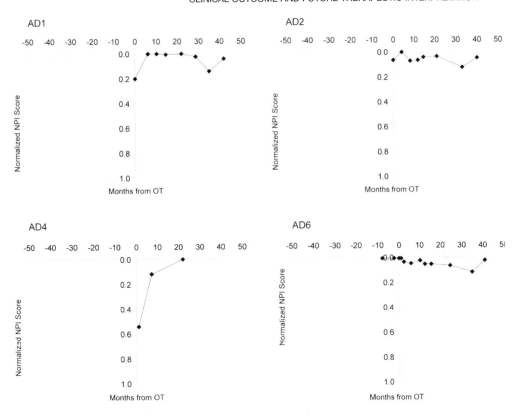

Figure 16.3 Behavioral changes measured by NPI. Normalized NPI scores were computed so that lower values represented fewer behavioral problems. There are no published data on rate of progression of NPI scores in AD. Two patients, AD1 and AD4, showed very large improvements in behavioral problems as shown by the large change in normalized NPI score toward zero. All AD patients studied showed minimal behavioral problems over the course of the postoperative follow-up as reflected by NPI scores near zero. No follow-up data are available for AD3.

locally and to tissues synaptically connected to cortical areas underneath the omentum. These findings, particularly those of MMSE performance in relation to left and right hemisphere treated patients, also agree with the observed changes in cognitive, functional, and behavioral measures.[10]

A remote effect of omentum on cortical activity relevant to AD was also observed in the HMPAO SPECT studies of AD2. At 22 months after OT, the posterior cingulate cortex showed a 20% increase in activity compared to the preoperative baseline (there is no contact between

omentum and posterior cingulate cortex). A possible mechanism for this remote effect may be synaptic connectivity between posterior cingulate and cortical areas underlying the omentum.

Of potential interest for further study is that the patterns of change in cortical activity for all patients were not linear, but, rather, appeared sinusoidal: periods of increase in cortical activity were followed by decrease and then again by increase. Such a sinusoidal pattern of change suggests local control of cortical activity by a reciprocally connected system. Such a system could be produced through

AD1 HMPAO SPECT

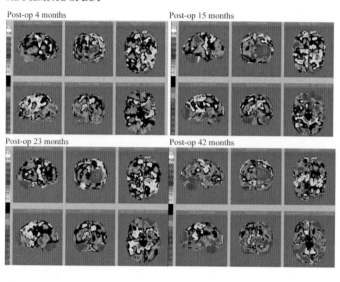

AD2 HMPAO SPECT

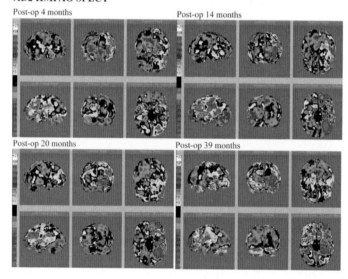

Figure 16.4 (See color section.) Changes in cortical activities measured by SPECT. The changes in cortical activity for patients AD1 and AD2 were studied with quantitative HMPAO SPECT neuroimaging for up to 41 months. We standardized the longitudinal changes in regional brain HMPAO SPECT activity by dividing the percent change by the standard deviation of test-retest values (σ=5.25%). Patients AD1 and AD2 showed a maximal increase in cortical activity of four standard deviations (21%), plus showed increased cortical activity of one to two standard deviations above preoperative baseline for between 22 and 41 months in areas underneath, adjacent to, and directly contralateral to the omentum. Since the cortical activity of other areas decreased by 20%-27% over 41 months, we hypothesize that the omentum delivers its effect to directly underlying and trans-synaptically connected cortical areas. The changes in the CDRS, MMSE, and NPI values are consistent with the observed increases in HMPAO SPECT cortical activity.[10]

locally regulated levels of neuronal fate-determining factors. The omentum has been shown to possess such factors, including brain-derived neurotrophic factor (BDNF), neurotrophin-3 (NT3) and neurotrophin-5 (NT5),[11,12] plus markers of adult stem cells and of embryonic pluripotent cells.[13] These growth factors and stem cells can stimulate synapse repair, neurogenesis, and angiogenesis.

ASSESSING THE MAGNITUDE OF OT TREATMENT EFFECT

Data from a meta-analysis of randomized clinical trials with cholinesterase inhibitors covering 7,954 AD patients provide a useful perspective regarding the degree of clinical improvement seen in the OT-treated AD patients for which adequate follow-up data were available.[14] This meta-analysis showed that only 2.4% of ChEI-treated AD patients could be expected to have the same degree of clinical improvement found in 80% of the OT-treated AD patients in the longitudinal study. Alternatively stated, OT-treated AD patients were 34 times more likely to show significant clinical improvement than ChEI-treated AD patients.

NEUROPATHOLOGIC FINDINGS

Brain autopsy findings of our three AD patients (AD2, AD3, and AD4) differ from that of Relkin,[6] who reported an AD patient who clinically improved following OT, had transposed omentum overlying the cortex at autopsy, and had marked reduction of neuritic plaques in gyral crests but not sulci only a few millimeters away and still underneath the omentum. In our patients, the omentum was severely atrophic (in contrast to Relkin's patient) and there were no differences in neuritic plaque or neurofibrillary tangle densities between sulci and crests of gyri

underneath the transposed omentum, as well as no such differences between ipsilateral and contralateral cortical areas. The most likely explanation for the neuropathologic differences between Relkin's patient and ours is attributable to three factors: 1) a shorter time to autopsy for Relkin's patient compared to patient AD2; 2) briefer viability of the transposed omentum due to infection or other postoperative complications in patient AD3; and 3) an extremely thin, fenestrated transposed omentum in patient AD4 (reduced substrate). The observed differences in neuropathologic findings between Relkin's patient and ours suggest that the transposed, vascularly intact, omentum, during its period of viability, actively influences underlying and trans-synaptically connected cortex. This hypothesis is also consistent with the observed time period when peak improvement began to decline (12-30 months post-OT) in the cognitive, functional, and behavioral measures of our AD patients.

The autopsy findings of this study and of that by Relkin do not answer whether the OT effect is mediated by reducing levels of soluble (oligomeric) and insoluble (fibrillar) beta-amyloid. While neuritic plaque load partially correlates with degree of cognitive impairment,[15] the level of soluble or oligomeric beta-amyloid appears to correlate even better.[16] Astrocytes appear to remove both soluble and insoluble beta-amyloid in AD[17] and the omentum may facilitate this process through its release of basic fibroblast growth factor (BFGF) and possibly other factors.

FUTURE THERAPEUTIC APPROACH WITH OMENTUM

As previously mentioned, the omentum—a primordial mesenchymal tissue overlying the gastrointestinal tract—contains growth factors (BDNF, NT3, NT5, bFGF, vascular endothelial growth factor [vEGF]) plus adult stem cells and embryonic pluripotent cells. In treating neurological disorders, it is beginning to be recognized that the traditional approach of neurotransmitter modulation with drug therapy has limited efficacy. Growth factors and stem cells have the capacity to stimulate general brain repair mechanisms that could ameliorate neuropathologic processes. Some early examples include nerve growth factor, which has been surgically delivered to the brains of monkeys with injury-induced cholinergic denervation and has shown therapeutic benefit,[18] and has been successfully delivered intranasally to AD animal models.[19] Insulin-like growth factor 1 has also been successfully delivered intranasally to animal models of stroke patients and shown therapeutic benefits.[20]

Like the evolution of cancer therapy, which began as monotherapy in the 1960s and 1970s, and thereafter transformed into combined therapy with greater treatment efficacy, it is increasingly being recognized that neurologic diseases trigger a variety of pathophysiologic mechanisms that can not usually be addressed by a single agent. Recent pharmacologic research on AD has shown that combination therapy with memantine and a cholinesterase inhibitor delayed AD progression over 4 years by between 33% and 60%, whereas monotherapy with a cholinesterase inhibitor (predominantly donepezil) showed a treatment effect comparable to no treatment at all.[21] This study is an early example of the potential of combination therapy for AD. The omentum is another example of a combination therapy, in which a variety of omentally derived growth factors and stem cells may provide the basis for the observed disease-modifying effect on AD progression and on clinical outcomes of other neurologic disorders. More research needs to be done to evaluate the effects of the various combinations of omentally derived factors on neurological disorders and pathophysiologic mechanisms.

REFERENCES

1. Goldsmith HS. *The Omentum: Application to Brain and Spinal Cord*. Wilton, Conn: Forefront Publishing; 2000.
2. Goldsmith HS, Fonseca A Jr, Porter J. Spinal cord separation: MRI evidence of healing after omentum-collagen reconstruction. *Neurol Res*. 2005;27(2):115-123.
3. Wu W, Xu S, Liu M, et al. Omental transposition following arachnoid excision to treat post cerebral anoxia (cerebral palsy). In Goldsmith HS. *The Omentum: Application to Brain and Spinal Cord*. Wilton, Conn: Forefront Publishing; 2000:161-168.
4. Shankle WR, Hara J, Bjornsen L, et al. Omental therapy for primary progressive aphasia with tau negative histopathology: 3 year study. *Neurol Res*. 2009;31(7):766-769.
5. Relkin NR, Edgar MA, Gouras GK, et al. Decreased senile plaque density in Alzheimer neocortex adjacent to an omental transposition. *Neurol Res*. 1996;18:291-296.
6. Shankle WR, Hara J, Bjornsen L, et al. Omentum transposition surgery for patients with Alzheimer's disease: a case series. *Neurol Res*. 2008;30(3):313-325.
7. Jann MW, Cyrus PA, Eisner LS, et al. Efficacy and safety of a loading-dose regimen versus a no-loading-dose regimen of metrifonate in the symptomatic treatment of Alzheimer's disease: a randomized, double-masked, placebo-controlled trial. Metrifonate Study Group. *Clin Ther*. 1999;21:88-102.
8. Shikiar R, Shakespeare A, Sagnier PP, et al. The impact of metrifonate therapy on caregivers of patients with Alzheimer's disease: results from the MALT clinical trial. Metrifonate in Alzheimer's Disease Trial. *J Am Geriatr Soc*. 2000;48:268-274.
9. Rogers SL, Doody RS, Pratt RD, et al. Long-term efficacy and safety of donepezil in the treatment of Alzheimer's disease: final analysis of a US multicentre open-label study. *Eur Neuropsychopharmacol*. 2000;10:195-203.
10. Shankle WR, Mena I, Hara J, et al. NeuroSPECT demonstrates increased cortical activity in Alzheimer's disease patients for at least two years after omental transposition neurosurgery. *Alasbimn*. 2006;31:AJ31-1.
11. Dujovny M, Ding YH, Ding Y, et al. Current concepts on the expression of neurotrophins in the greater omentum. *Neurol Res*. 2004:26(2):226-229.
12. García-Gómez I, Goldsmith HS, Angulo J, et al. Angiogenic capacity of human omental stem cells. *Neurol Res*. 2005;27(8):807-811.

13. Singh AK, Patel J, Litbarg NO, et al. Stromal cells cultured from omentum express pluripotent markers, produce high amounts of VEGF, and engraft to injured sites. *Cell Tissue Res.* 2008;332(1):81-88.

14. Lanctot KL, Herrmann N, Yau KK, et al. Efficacy and safety of cholinesterase inhibitors in Alzheimer's disease: a meta-analysis. *CMAJ.* 2003;169:557-564.

15. Cummings BJ, Pike CJ, Shankle R, et al. Beta-amyloid deposition and other measures of neuropathology predict cognitive status in Alzheimer's disease. *Neurobiology of Aging.* 1996;17:921-933.

16. Dodart JC, Bales KR, Gannon KS, et al. Immunization reverses memory deficits without reducing brain Abeta burden in Alzheimer's disease model. *Nat Neurosci.* 2002;5:452-457.

17. Oide T, Kinoshita T, Arima K. Regression stage senile plaques in the natural course of Alzheimer's disease. *Neuropathol Appl Neurobiol.* 2006;32:539-556.

18. Tuszynski MH, Roberts J, Senut MC, U HS, Gage FH. Gene therapy in the adult primate brain: intraparenchymal grafts of cells genetically modified to produce nerve growth factor prevent cholinergic neuronal degeneration. *Gene Ther.* 1996;3(4):305-314.

19. Covaceuszach S, Capsoni S, Ugolini G, et al. Development of a non invasive NGF-based therapy for Alzheimer's disease. *Curr Alzheimer Res.* 2009;6(2):158-170.

20. Hanson LR, Frey WH 2nd. Intranasal delivery bypasses the blood-brain barrier to target therapeutic agents to the central nervous system and treat neurodegenerative disease. *BMC Neurosci.* 2008;9(suppl 3)S5.

21. Atri A, Shaughnessy LW, Locascio JJ, et al. Long-term course and effectiveness of combination therapy in Alzheimer disease. *Alzheimer Dis Assoc Disord.* 2008;22(3):209-21.

ACKNOWLEDGMENT

This study was funded by the Omentum Research Foundation. We wish to thank Dr. Harry Goldsmith for his pioneering efforts and perseverance in demonstrating clinically beneficial effects in patients with a variety of neurological disorders.

CHAPTER 17

OMENTAL TRANSPLANTATION IN PATIENTS WITH SEVERE VISUAL DISTURBANCES DUE TO ISCHEMIA

CHRISTIANE H. MAY AND SIEGFRIED VOGEL

INTRODUCTION

The visual system is a complex structure starting with a reception of light in different wave lengths via photoreceptors in the retina, from where information is transferred over bipolar cells to the spread-out ganglion cell layer. Nerve fibers of the ganglion cells individually cross the surface of the retina and enter the optic nerve, which leads them to the optic chiasm. Here the fibers separate and represent the corresponding halves of the two retinas. Anatomically, the post-chiasmal pathway is, made up of the following parts: the optic tract, the external geniculate body, which represents a ganglion; the optic radiation; and the striate cortex, also called area V1. From there, the information goes either directly or is transduced via V2 to the specialized areas for forms (V3), for color (V4), or for movement (V5) lateral to V1.[1]

In the visual system, location-specific disturbances require location-specific treatment. For space-occupying lesions compressing the visual system, such as tumors, hygromas, hematomas, aneurysms, angiomas, granulomas, abscesses, hydrocephalus, parasitism, deformities of the cranial base, or traumatic bone dislocations, the ultimate treatment is decompression.[2,3]

More difficult is the treatment of ischemic lesion of the visual system. In fact, there is as yet no established treatment for this condition. However, there are existing methods to increase cerebral blood flow (CBF) to the brain. One of these is the superficial temporal artery to middle cerebral artery (STA-MCA) microanastomosis, first described by Donaghy and Yasargil in 1967.[4] Another is the transposition of the temporalis muscle intracranially upon the temporal cortex encephalo-myosynangiosis (EMS), first described by Henschen,[5] or the encephalo-duroarteriosynangiosis operation used by Matsushima,[6] and Kashiwagi.[7] Gracilis muscle transplantation,[8] serratus anterior muscle transplantation,[9] or the "multiple burr-hole operation"[10] are additional procedures that may lead to better CBF. Another promising operation is the transposition of the omentum onto the cerebral cortex with its vascular supply intact, first described in dogs by Goldsmith in 1973[11] and in humans in 1978.[12] The transplantation of a free omental flap to the brain surface using a microvascular technique was first described by Dong in 1982.[13]

By reviewing the literature, surgical treatment of ischemic vascular lesions of the visual system is rare and has only been described in some patients with progressive ischemia due to a chronic cerebrovascular occlusive disease; the so-called Moyamoya disease. Touho[14] had seen improvement of frequent transient visual disturbances in three patients after gracilis muscle transplantation to the territory of the posterior cerebral artery. Yoshioka[9] reported one patient with transitory episodes of homonymous hemianopia who underwent omental transposition on the left and serratus anterior muscle transplantation onto the right fronto-temporo-parietal cerebral cortex. On both sides, a good collateral circulation to the brain was shown with no further neurological events occurring. Miyamoto[15] used STA-MCA anastomosis or EMS in 38 patients who had visual field defects, decreased visual acuity, episodes of blindness, and scintillating scotoma. The procedures improved the cerebral perfusion in both the anterior and posterior cerebral circulation. However, because these two operative procedures do not lead to direct revascularization of the visual cortex, five patients with impending blindness required transplantation of the omentum to the occipital lobes in order to accomplish visual improvement.

Karasawa[16] reported that 13 patients with visual disturbances who underwent omental transplantation to an occipital lobe or lobes after bilateral STA-MCA anastomosis, EMS, or encephaloduroanteriosynangiosis had all failed to improve vision. Miyamoto[15] and Karasawa[16] stated that in all their cases after omental transplantation to the occipital region, further visual loss was stopped and functional improvement in visual field defects occurred in 15 or 18 patients with a follow-up period of 1 to 6 years.

In summary, it would seem that the best method at this time to correct blindness caused by ischemia or to prevent additional visual deficits in progressive ischemia is by omental placement on the brain. Since 1984, 32 patients in our department have undergone unilateral or bilateral omental transplantation or transpositions to the brain. Four patients had an ischemic lesion involving their visual system,

which led to visual impairment. Two of these patients had Moyamoya disease, one had bioccipital hypoxia after a pulmonary embolism, and one had optic nerve ischemia due to radiation damage.

TECHNICAL NOTES

Placing the omentum directly upon the cerebral cortex can be performed by transposition with its vascular supply intact as described by Goldsmith,[17] or as a transplantation of a free omental flap to the brain surface by a microvascular technique as described by Dong.[13] Even though either surgical technique can be done, we believe that if one is to treat the occipital cortical region, it is almost mandatory to perform a transplantation of a free omental flap because of the positioning of the patient. But to restore vision, in addition to the standard method of Goldsmith, in which the omentum is placed upon the temporoparieto-frontal cortex, the omentum may need to be wrapped around the optic nerve on both sides.

When the omentum is to be placed in the occipital area, the patient is positioned on his back and a laparotomy performed using a midline epigastric incision. A free flap of the greater omentum is removed from the greater curvature of the stomach, with preservation of the right and left gastroepiploic artery and vein. The piece of the omentum obtained should be the size of the cerebral cortex, which needs to be covered.

After closure of the abdominal wound, the patient is placed in a prone position and a broad bioccipital skin incision is made, which reaches the occipital artery and vein on both sides. A bioccipital craniotomy above the transverse sinus level is then performed and the dura opened on both sides after which the arachnoid is incised. The occipital artery and vein on one side are separated from the scalp for a distance of approximately 2 cm. After perfusing the central artery of the omentum, to confirm that the entire omental flap gets its blood supply from the artery and to wash out blood residues, an end-to-end anastomosis to the central vein in the omentum to the occipital vein is performed using four stitches of 10-0 monofilament sutures. For the omental and occipital artery, eight stitches are placed in the same end-to-end fashion. After confirmation of a good blood flow, the omentum is placed upon the bioccipital cortical surface and the interhemisphere gap after which it is fixed to the dura. The bone flap is then replaced with removal of a small piece of bone from the mediobasal side in order not to compress the anastomosed vessels connected to the omentum. During surgery, it is important to preserve the superior sagittal sinus and the bridging veins.

CASE REPORTS

Case 1 (SF)

The patient is a 22-year-old female who had pneumonia, which required a long period of immobilization at home. During this time, the patient developed a major pulmonary embolism that required cardiopulmonary resuscitation in November 1993. Because of the temporary cerebral hypoxia, the patient was comatose for 1 month and when she eventually reached consciousness, it appeared that she was blind. One month later, when she was fully awake, she was diagnosed as being cortically blind, only able to distinguish bright red and green color spots and could occasionally discriminate movements if the light was bright enough. There had been no improvement in her visual condition when she was admitted to our hospital in May 1995, 18 months after cardiopulmonary resuscitation.

Magnetic resonance imaging (MRI) demonstrated severe atrophy of the visual cortex on both sides, with the greatest involvement on

the right cerebral cortex (*Figure 17.1*). The visual evoked responses showed only minor abnormalities with a reduction in amplitude and prolonged latency.

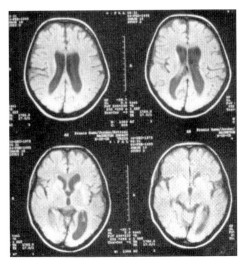

Figure 17.1 MRI images taken before omental transplantation. Severe atrophy noted in visual cortex bilaterally, greater on right side.

As the patient was cortically blind, the question arose as to whether her condition could be improved. There was no indication for an extracranial-intracranial vascular microanastomosis since she had normal perfusion of the medial and lateral branch of the posterior cerebral artery (*Figures 17.2A and B*). Since her regional CBF showed a marked reduction of cerebral perfusion in the occipital region on both sides, as shown by single photon emission computed tomography (SPECT) (*Figure 17.3*), and because encephalomyosynangiosis can only be done in the temporal region, omental transplantation was the operation performed 1½ years after her cardiopulmonary resuscitation.

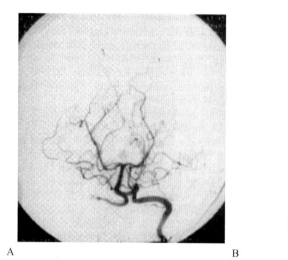
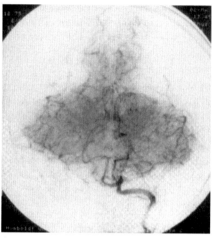

A   B

Figure 17.2 Preoperative selective left vertebral angiograms (A-P) in **A:** arterial phase and **B:** capillary phase.

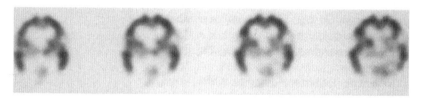

Figure 17.3 Preoperative SPECT scan demonstrating a marked reduction of perfusion bilaterally in occipital regions.

Surgery

The patient was positioned on her back, a laparotomy performed, and a free flap of the greater omentum with a central artery and vein was obtained. After closure of the wound, the patient was placed in a prone position, a biooccipital craniotomy performed, and a free flap of omentum transplanted to the occipital cortex bilaterally as previously described. The major artery and vein in the omental flap were anastomosed to the left occipital artery and vein. After confirmation of a good internal blood flow, the omentum was placed upon both biooccipital cortical surfaces and the interhemispheric gap, and fixed to the dura. The histological examination of a cortical biopsy taken at surgery revealed a marked reduction of neurons and glial proliferation, but no necrosis or porencephaly.

There were no peri- or postoperative complications.

Follow-up

In September 1995, 4 months after omental transplantation, the patient was able to detect large objects in a very small visual field when the intensity of light was strong. Seven months later (11 months after transplantation), vision could be estimated for the first time. With both eyes, she was able to recognize pictures within 1 meter. Normally these pictures can be seen at 50 meters distance.*

*All visual examinations throughout the study were performed by ophthalmologists. In Case 1, the ophthalmological examinations were carried out by Dr. Ruther, Dept. of Ophthalmology of the Charite Hospital of the Humboldt University, Berlin.

By 13 months after omental transplantation, visual fields could be estimated for the first time. She was now able to recognize moving vertical strips on a rotating cylinder. Movement as shown on drawings could be recognized. She saw moving black arrows on a piece of paper as a "pattern", but was not able to distinguish the shape of triangles, squares, and circles in black and white, but could differentiate whether they were large or small. Because her vision in a small visual field had now become permanent, the patient became well oriented to her surroundings. She could also recognize colors with different shades and could copy color patterns.

Visual examination 16 months after omental transplantation demonstrated an enlargement of the visual field (*Figures 17.4A and 17.4B*), especially involving the left eye. The patient was now able to distinguish all colors and shapes and could recognize complex structures. Visual evoked responses had also returned to normal by this time (*Figure 17.5*) and a postoperative MRI showed the correct placement of the omentum upon the bioccipital convexity of the brain over the visual cortex (*Figure 17.6*). Measurement of the regional CBF by SPECT at that time also showed an increase in perfusion in the occipital region (*Figure 17.7*).

An ophthalmological examination 18 months after omental transplantation showed further improvement of binocular vision, with the patient being able to recognize some large letters or numbers. Twenty-three months after transplantation, an 18F-fluorodeoxyglucose SPECT was performed with and without stroboscopic stimulation. There was almost no utilization of glucose in the occipital region, but there was some glucose utilization within the striate cortex, which under visual stimulation demonstrated higher glucose metabolic activity. Her vision continued to improve and on April 4, 1998, 35 months after transplantation, the visual fields of both eyes had enlarged with restoration of over 40% occurring in the left eye (*Figures 17.8A and B*). Her binocular visual acuity had also improved, but the improvement depended on the intensity of light and on the mental concentration of the patient. At present, her vision is not constantly good but she can distinguish letters and can copy pictures using the right color in the right place (*Figure 17.9*).

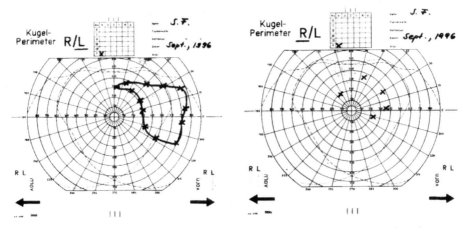

Figure 17.4 Visual field of A: left eye and B: right eye 16 months after omental transplantation.

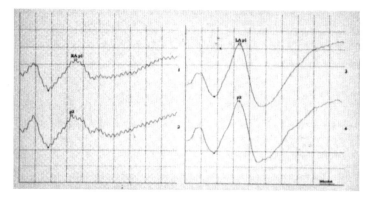

Figure 17.5 Visual evoked responses (VERs) are almost normal 13 months after omental transplantation. Photic stimuli were presented binocularly and responses obtained over the right (RA) and left (LA) occipital region. VER recorded twice on each side. Latency for p2: right hemisphere = 88 msec; left hemisphere = 84 msec. (Right occipital region #1 and #2; left occipital region #3 and #4.)

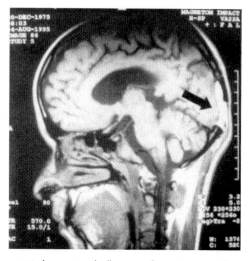

Figure 17.6 MRI demonstrating correct placement and adherence of omentum upon the occipital convexity (arrow).

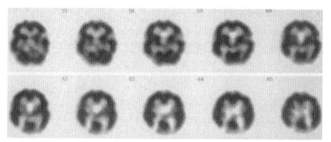

Figure 17.7 Postoperative SPECT scan 13 months after omental transplantation showing increased perfusion of both occipital lobes (see *Figure 17.3* for preoperative comparison).

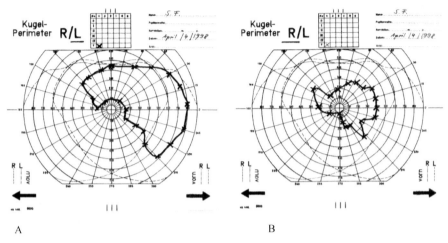

A   B

Figure 17.8 Visual field of **A:** left eye and **B:** right eye 35 months after omental transplantation.

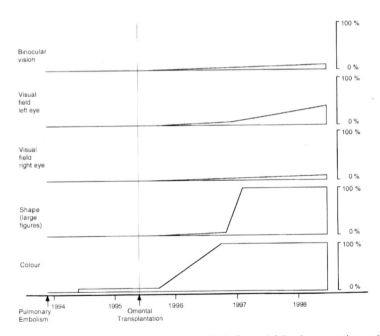

Figure 17.9 Follow-up of visual symptoms in percentage (%) before and following omental transplantation.

Case 2 (VP)

The patient is a 10-year-old girl with Moyamoya disease who had normal vision in the right eye until her third birthday (November 1990). According to her mother's information, vision in her left eye had always been relatively poor. In January 1991, the patient suddenly became blind in both eyes without any papillary reaction. Fundoscopy showed a blurred optic disk bilaterally. Papillary reaction to light returned 3 months later and she began to recognize some colors with the right eye. A month later the optic papillae were atrophic on both sides. An MRI revealed bilateral ischemic lesions in the occipital region and in the left frontal area. Cerebral perfusion showed hypoperfusion, especially in the left frontobasal region and in the parieto-occipital area bilaterally. Preoperative angiography presented a high-degree stenoses in the left internal carotid artery with an extensive collateral circulation by formation of plexiform arterioles in the basal ganglia (*Figure 17.10*). In order to obtain, hopefully, an increased blood supply to the optic chiasm and the proximal part of the optic tract, transposition of the omentum was chosen as the treatment of choice.

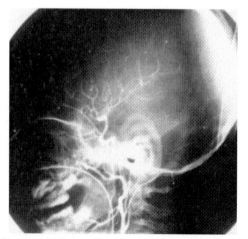

Figure 17.10 Preoperative left carotid angiogram showing a high-degree stenosis of the internal carotid artery.

Surgery

In June 1991, an intact pedicled flap of the omentum was transposed subcutaneously to the left fronto-temporo-parietal region. After a fronto-temporo-parietal craniotomy and microsurgical opening of the cisterns, the omentum was wrapped around the intracranial portion of the optic nerve on both sides, around the optic chiasm, under the frontobasal region, and directly upon the left temporo-parieto-frontal cortex. The patient tolerated the operation without any intra- or postoperative complications.

Follow-up

Cerebral perfusion increased in the left frontobasal region, as measured by SPECT (*Figures 17.11A and 17.11B*) along with angiography studies that showed an increased filling of the branches of the external carotid artery that fed the left fronto-temporo-parietal region via sprouted blood vessels (*Figure 17.12*). During the first 7 months after omentum transposition, the patient clinically improved. With her right eye, she was able to differentiate pictures with a vision of 0.02 diopter, and with the associated use of her left eye, she was able to orient herself, but the optic papillae remained atrophic in both eyes. Over the following 3 years, there was slight improvement in her vision, and by the fourth year, the vision in her left eye was now 0.02 diopter and 0.07 diopter in the right eye (*Figure 17.13*). Since that time, her vision has remained stable and there have been no further ischemic attacks.

Case 3 (HK)

The patient is a 28-year-old female suffering from Jacksonian epilepsy with focal seizures in her left arm, which began in 1990. A CAT scan demonstrated a right frontal hypodense area

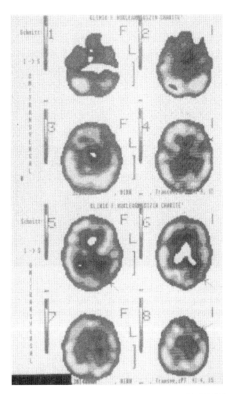

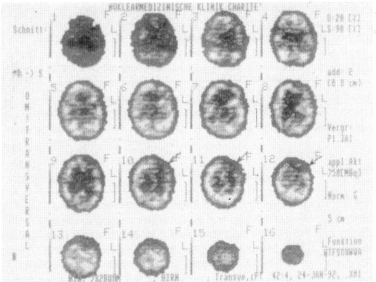

Figure 17.11 A: Preoperative SPECT scan shows hypoperfusion in left frontobasal, and to a lesser degree in parieto-occipital regions. **B:** Postoperative SPECT scan at 7 months showing increased cerebral perfusion in left frontobasal region.

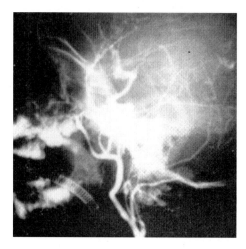

Figure 17.12 Postoperative left carotid angiogram showing an increased filling of the branches of the external carotid artery feeding the left fronto-temporo-parietal region via sprouted vessels.

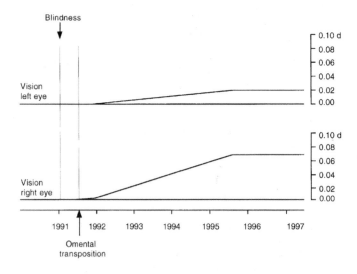

Figure 17.13 Follow-up of vision of right and left eye in d (diopter) from 1991 to 1997.

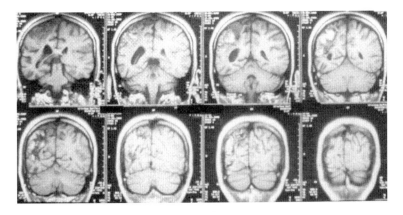

Figure 17.14 MRI demonstrating an ischemic lesion with atrophy in the right parieto-occipital area, and small lesions in the fronto-temporal regions bilaterally.

and a subsequent CAT scan in 1993 showed an additional hypodense lesion in the left parietal region. No additional clinical symptoms developed but another hypodense lesion was seen in the left frontal area on a routine MRI taken in January 1995. By October 1995, the patient developed hemiparesis and hypesthesia on her left side along with a homonymous hemianopsia to the left side. Visual evoked potentials demonstrated a prolonged latency. A subsequent MRI at that time showed ischemia and atrophy in the right parieto-occipital region in addition to the other known ischemic lesions (*Figure 17.14*). Over the following months, her hemiparesis improved, but her homonymous hemianopsia continued on the left side. Vision in the rest of the visual field remained normal. In July 1996, she had a transient ischemic attack, which caused hemiparesis on the right side.

Angiography in June 1996 revealed Moya-moya disease with occlusion of the internal carotid artery on both sides with associated collateral circulation. Measurement of the regional CBF by SPECT demonstrated small defects of perfusion in the frontoparietal regions on both sides, with a large perfusion defect in the right parieto-occipital area. These widespread areas of cerebral ischemia were the indication for omental transplantation to the brain in order to prevent further ischemic attacks and especially to prevent blindness. Surgery was carried out in August 1996, 10 months after visual symptoms had first appeared.

Surgery

The patient underwent a laparotomy followed by the harvesting of a free flap of the greater omentum with preservation of a central artery and vein, which were anastomosed to the right occipital artery and vein via microanastomosis. Following this, a large parieto-occipital craniotomy was performed on the right side, and the free flap of the omentum transplanted onto the parieto-occipital cortex and fixed to the dura. A later MRI showed the omentum had been well placed on the brain (*Figure 17.15*).

The histological examination of a cortical biopsy taken during surgery confirmed the diagnosis of Moyamoya disease with areas of astrocytic glial proliferation with underlying coagulation necrosis. There were no peri- or postoperative complications.

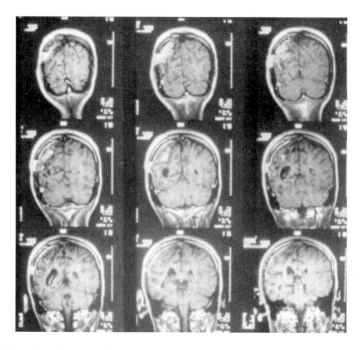

Figure 17.15 MRI 6 months after omental transplantation, showing correct placement of omentum on parietal-occipital convexity.

Follow-up

Cerebral perfusion measured by SPECT 5 months after surgery failed to show any improvement, and additional cerebral perfusion defects were not seen. Examination of visual fields 9 months after transplantation of the omentum showed improvement of the homonymous hemianopsia. The patient has continued to do well at 2 years after surgery and has had no further ischemic attacks.

Case 4 (MS)

The patient had a long history of attacks of headaches with neurohormonal disturbances and hemianopsia, which appeared in 1993. An MRI revealed a craniopharyngioma and the patient underwent local radiation using phosphorus-32 implantation seeds in August 1995. While the volume of the tumor decreased over time because of the radiation effects, the patient's vision rapidly declined, mainly on the right side. An MRI taken in May 1997 showed the almost total disappearance of tumor on the left. Her vision at that time was 0.05 diopter in a tiny area of the visual field on the right side and 0.1 diopter in the inner lower part of the visual field on the left side. Since only a small part of tumor remained, the decline of vision and the visual fields was felt to be due to ischemia resulting from radiation injury to the blood vessels supplying the optic nerve and to the optic nerve itself. Therefore, surgery for the removal of the phosphorus 32 seeds and resection of the small amount of remaining tumor in the area was carried out in addition to omental transplantation into the area.

Surgery

On June 5 1997, a pterional craniotomy on the right side was performed, and the optic chiasm exposed. The optic chiasm was surrounded by scar tissue and the optic nerves were seen to be pale and avascular. Phosphorus 32 seeds were removed and residual tumor and scar tissue excised. A free flap of omentum was transplanted and anastomosed to the right superficial temporal artery and vein via microanastomosis. After confirmation of a good blood flow within the omentum, the structure was wrapped around the optic chiasm and fixed to the dura for stabilization.

Follow-up

No complications occurred during surgery and throughout the postoperative period. Visual improvement was noted as early as the next day after surgery, which was felt to be due to better vascularization of the optic nerves because of the resection of surrounding compressive scar tissue and possibly because of vasoactive substances supplied by the omentum. There is continuing improvement in the patient's visual fields, with vision in her left eye increasing to 0.4 diopter from a pre-operative level of 0.1 diopter. Additionally, the visual field in the left eye has improved from a quarter to one half of the whole visual field. She can now distinguish all colors with the left eye. The right eye cannot recognize colors and there is no visible improvement in the visual field and vision in this eye.

CONCLUSIONS

It has been generally accepted that cortical blindness resulting from vascular occlusive disease has the potential to reverse itself to varying degrees as a result of natural healing processes.[17,18] However, the time of recovery from blindness to various levels of spontaneous recovery appears to be age-dependent, with adult recovery from blindness as a result of vascular occlusive disease occurring up to 3 months.[19-21]

The question that has remained unanswered over the years is why placement of the omentum on the ventral nervous system results in improvement in patients with neurological conditions.[22] The most reasonable explanation is that the omentum increases blood flow to any area to which it is applied.[23] As far as the ocular system itself is concerned, Goldsmith, in 1975, showed that vascular connections developed between the omentum and choroidal and retinal vessels following omental transposition to the eyeball in dogs.[24]

There are a host of neurobiological agents in the omentum that may have a direct influence, along with increased CBF arising from the omentum, on the improvement of a deteriorating visual system. These agents include neurotransmitters[25] and omental-derived nerve growth factors.[26] Of particular interest is an omental fraction of lipid origin that is highly angiogenic.[27] The presence of this angiogenic factor has been recently confirmed.[28] Also to be considered are the presence of endothelial cells in the omentum, which stimulate basic fibroblast growth factor to induce chemotactic and mitogenic activity in vascular cells that leads to angiogenesis.[29]

REFERENCES

1. Zeki SM. Das geistige abbild der welt. *Spektrum der Wissenschaft.* 1992;11:54-63.
2. Harrington DO. *The Visual Fields.* St. Louis: Mosby; 1971.
3. Huber A. Kompressions opticus neuropathie, opticustumoren. In: Huber A, Kompf D, eds. *Klinische Neuroophthalmologie.* Stuttgart: Thieme Verlag; 1998:274-283.
4. Donaghy RMP, Yasargil MG. *Microvascular Surgery.* Stuttgart: Thieme; 1967.

5. Henschen C. Operative revaskularisation des zirkulatorisch geschadigten gehirns durch auflage gestielter muskellappen (Encephalo-myo-synangiose). *Langenbecks Arch Cir.* 1950:264:392-401.

6. Matsushima Y, Fukai N, Tanaka K, et al. A new surgical treatment of Moyamoya disase in children: a preliminary report. *Surg Neurol.* 1981;15:313-320.

7. Kashiwagi S, Kato S, Yasuhara S, et al. Use of split dura for revascularization of ischemic hemispheres in Moyamoya disease. *J Neurosurg.* 1996;85:380-383.

8. Touho H, Karasawa J, Ohnishi H. Cerebral revascularization using gracilis muscle transplantation for childhood Moyamoya disease. *Surg Neurol.* 1995;43:191-198.

9. Yoshioka N, Tominaga S, Inui T. Cerebral revascularization using omentum and serratus anterior muscle flap transfer for adult Moyamoya disease: Case report. *Surg Neurol.* 1996;46:430-436.

10. Kawaguchi T, Fujita S, Hosoda K, et al. Multiple burr-hold operation for adult Moyamoya disease. *J Neurol.* 1996;84:468-476.

11. Goldsmith HS, Chen WF, Duckett SW. Brain vascularization by intact omentum. *Arch Surg.* 1973;106:695-698.

12. Goldsmith HS. Omental transposition to human brain. *Stroke.* 1978;9:272.

13. Dong YR, Lin YJ, Li YH. Transplantation of free omental flaps to the brain surface by microvascular technic for cerebral ischemic stroke. *Chung Hua Wai Ko Tsa Chih.* 1982;20:8-10.

14. Touho H, Karasawa J, Ohnishi H. Haemodynamic evaluation of paraparetic transient ischemic attacks in childhood Moyamoya disease. *Neurol Res.* 1995;17:162-168.

15. Miyamoto S, Kikuchi H, Karasawa J, et al. Study of the posterior circulation in Moyamoya disease. *J Neurosurg.* 1986;65:454-460.

16. Karasawa J, Touho H, Ohnishi H, Miamoto S, Kikuchi H. Cerebral revascularization using omental transplantation for childhood Moyamoya disease. *J Neurosurg.* 1993;79:192-196.

17. Goldsmith HS. Omental transposition to the brain and spinal cord. *Surg Rounds.* June 1986 :22-33.

18. Kupersmith MJ, Berenstein A. Neuro-ophthalmologic disorders caused by brain infarcts. In: Kupersmith MJ, Berenstein A, eds. *Neurovascular Neuroophthalmology.* Berlin: Springer-Verlag; 1993:371-386.

19. Melen O, Klein JW. Ophthalmologic manifestations of vascular diseases of the brain. In: Peyman GA, Saunders DR. Goldberg MF, eds. *Principles and Practice of Ophthalmology, Volume III.* Philadelphia: W.B. Saunders Company; 1980: pp. 2043-2087.

20. Symonds C, McKenzie, I. Bilateral loss of vision from cerebral infarction. *Brain.* 1957;80:415-455.

21. Cunningham FG, Fernandez CO, Hernandez C. Blindness associated with pre-eclampsia and eclampsia. *Am J Obstet Gynecol.* 1995;172:1291-1298.

22. Hagerty C, Licho R, Recht L. Cortical blindness after correction of symptomatic hyponatremia: dynamic cerebral dysfunction visualized using serial SPECT scanning. *J Nucl Med.* 1995;36:1272-1274.

23. Wong VC. Cortical blindness in children: a study of etiology and prognosis. *Pediatric Neurol.* 1991;7:178-185.

24. Taylor MJ, McCulloch DL. Prognostic value of VEPs in young children with acute onset of cortical blindness. *Pediatric Neurol.* 1991;7:111-115.

25. Brewster DR, Kwiatkowski D, White NJ. Neurological sequelae of cerebral malaria in children. *Lancet.* 1990;336:1039-1043.

26. Goldsmith HS. Brain and spinal cord revascularization by omental transposition. *Neurol Res.* 1994;16:159-162.

27. Goldsmith HS, Bacciu P, Cossu M, et al. Regional cerebral blood flow after omental transposition to the ischemic brain in man. A five year follow-up study. *Acta Neurochir (Wien).* 1990;106:145-152.

28. Goldsmith HS, Chen WF, Palena PV. Intact omentum for ocular vascularization. *Invest Ophthal.* 1975;14:163-165.

29. Goldsmith HS, McIntosh T, Vezina RM, Colton T. Vasoactive neurochemicals identified in omentum: A preliminary report. *Br J Neurosurg.* 1987;1:359-364.

30. Siek GC, Marquis JK, Goldsmith HS. Experimental studies of omentum-derived neurotrophic factors. In: Goldsmith HS, ed. *The Omentum—Research and Clinical Applications.* New York: Springer-Verlag; 1990:83-95.

31. Goldsmith HS, Griffith AL, Kupferman A, Catsimpoolas N. Lipid angiogenic factor from omentum. *JAMA.* 1984;252:2034-2036.

32. Levy Y, Miko I, Hauck M, et al. Effect of omental angiogenic lipid factor on revascularization of autotransplanted spleen in dogs. *Eur Surg Res.* 1998;30:138-143.

33. Bikfalvi A, Alteiro J, Inyang AL, et al. Basic fibroblast growth factor expression in human omental microvascular endothelial cells and the effect of phorbol ester. *J Cell Physiol.* 1990;144:151-158.

CHAPTER 18

PERIOPERATIVE ANESTHETIC MANAGEMENT FOR OMENTAL TRANSPOSITION TO THE CNS

THOMAS WALZ

INTRODUCTION

Omental transposition (OT) is a surgical procedure that is being performed in increasing frequency throughout the world. We have had the opportunity in our department (Anesthesiology, Critical Care, and Emergency Medicine) to treat 30 patients with OT to either their brain or spinal cord. Reported here is our personal experience in treating these patients before, during, and following their OT to the central nervous system.

PREOPERATIVE MANAGEMENT

All patients underwent a very detailed clinical history and physical examination. When indicated, special radiologic and neuroelectrical studies were performed. A preoperative conference was carried out between the anesthesia department and the surgeons involved in the case in order to coordinate the total handling of the case and to be certain that any medical or surgical problems were addressed prior to operation.

Standard laboratory tests were routinely performed. These included hemoglobin and hematocrit determination and electrolyte levels. Thrombin, prothrombin, and partial thromboplastin times were established. Four

units of blood were typed and cross-matched for the operation.

Every effort is made to decrease the use of homologous blood replacement during surgery. If patients lived close to the hospital, they were brought in over a period of several weeks to donate two to three units of blood, which were separated into fractions of red blood cells and fresh frozen plasma.

If patients came from far distances and could not donate autogenous blood, normovolemic hemodilition was carried out 30 minutes before surgery if the patient's hemoglobin level was 11 g or above. This technique was performed by taking 500 mL of blood, which was kept warm, for an early intraoperative transfusion, at a time when the coagulation factors in the blood were still highly active. This initial blood loss taken from the patient was immediately replaced with colloid fluid. It was found that the intraoperative transfusion of the patient's collected and washed red blood cells was very important in reducing the need for homologous blood replacement during the performance of OT to the central nervous system (CNS).

Preoperative electrocardiogram (ECG) tracings were carried out on all patients over 50 years of age and in younger patients if there was any indication of cardiac abnormalities. All patients operated on for spinal cord injuries, which occurred at the T10 level or higher, had spirometric testing for pulmonary function. Preoperative chest x-rays of the patients were obtained routinely in patients 60 years or older and in younger patients when a preoperative history and/or physical examination suggested that this was indicated. We have found that it is very important that the anesthesiologists and the surgeons involved with the impending surgery spend a great deal of time talking to their patients, since the surgery they are to undergo still remains controversial and so that they are made aware that there is a strong possibility (roughly 50%) that the operation they are to undergo will not result in their attaining meaningful neurological improvement. In spinal cord patients, clinical improvement is dependent on a fully committed rehabilitation program. Poor postoperative results in some patients may be a direct reflection of a lack of rehabilitation activity.

Pre-medication

All patients received sedatives the night before surgery. Our personal preference is oxazepam by mouth (10 mg). Midazolam (7.5-15 mg) was subsequently administered by mouth 40 minutes before surgery. All patients were fasted the night before surgery and any medications they were receiving prior to surgery were either continued or discontinued according to international recommendations concerning possible interaction with anesthesia agents.

INTRODUCTION OF GENERAL ANESTHESIA

Anesthesia management begins by administering fentanyl (2 µg kg^{-1} IV) followed by dihydrobenzperidol, which is used as an antiemetic agent. Anesthesia is then initiated using thiopental (4 mg kg^{-1}). Pancuronium (0.1 mg kg^{-1} IV) is also administered for its effect as a long acting nondepolarizing muscle relaxant.

Following endotracheal intubation, a nasogastic tube and a urinary catheter are inserted. In addition, an arterial catheter is placed in either the right or left radial artery in order to monitor blood pressure and to sample arterial blood gases for careful intraoperative ventilation. Two large intravenous catheters (14 gauge) are placed in peripheral veins and a central venous line is placed in either the left or right basilica vein. A rectal probe is inserted to monitor body temperature. Just prior to surgery, 2 g of Cefazolin, a basic cephalosporin, is given intravenously for antibiotic prophylaxis. Another 2 g of the antibiotic is administered 4 hours later.

INTRAOPERATIVE MANAGEMENT

General anesthesia is commenced using a balanced anesthesia technique with isoflurane and nitrous oxide in oxygen being given in a 2:1 ratio, with intermittent infusion of fentanyl (1 µg kg^{-1}) every 30 minutes. The nondepolarizing muscle relaxant pancuronium (0.02 mg kg^{-1}) is also administered every hour during the operation.

Fluid maintenance is absolutely essential during the operation as reflected by blood loss and urine production. Loss of fluid through the omentum occurs throughout the procedure and is excessive. Maintaining fluid volume is accomplished by saline infusions (5 mL kg^{-1}h^{-1}) and hydroxyethyl starch (30 mL kg^{-1}) when colloid replacement fluid is required to maintain blood pressure after major fluid loss. Potassium supplements are given during surgery if there is a need when indicated by intraoperative laboratory results.

The intraoperative use of a "cell save" lessens the need for homologous blood transfusions, but these re-transfusions of the patient's washed red blood cells contained no platelets and coagulation factors. For this reason, very early transfusions are begun of the warm blood taken from the patient immediately before surgery in order to compensate for the later loss of platelets and coagulation factors. Minimizing the subsequent need for transfused homologous blood transfusions is very important even though the risk of blood contamination is small: 1 of 4,000 transfused units for hepatitis C; 1 of 200,000 transfused units for hepatitis B; and 1 of 250,000 transfused units for HIV. Patients are very fearful of blood transfusions.

The operations are long in duration, often lasting 7 to 8 hours. Maintaining the patient's temperature at 36°C is important and can be accomplished by a special blanket that employs warm air flow and warm fluid intake, which affects heat loss.

We have treated a patient with a near-transected spinal cord with omental-collagen reconstruction of the spinal cord (see Chapter 5). In order to be assured that the patient was not allergic to the collagen, skin testing of the material was performed. Even though there was a negative skin reaction, prednisone (4 mg kg^{-1}) and H$_1$ and H$_2$ histamine receptor antagonists were given 30 minutes before implanting the collagen in order to avoid the possibility of an anaphylactic reaction caused by the collagen—a reaction that was felt to be highly unlikely.

After the surgery is completed, the patient is taken to the intensive care unit (ICU) and kept on the respirator until body temperature has returned to normal. The patient is kept in the ICU until stable, and until all laboratory results are in a normal range. The patients are sent back to the ward usually on the second and third postoperative day.

POSTOPERATIVE MANAGEMENT

All patients were placed on early postoperative respiratory exercises to avoid pulmonary problems. This is especially important in spinal cord injured patients with high cervical lesions. Early mobilization is also stressed in all patients.

The administration of heparin to prevent pulmonary emboli in postoperative neurosurgical patients remains controversial. In our patients, heparin was given only to those who were considered to be at high risk for developing pulmonary emboli or who already had a history of having previous thrombosis. Early effort was made postoperatively to prevent pulmonary emboli by encouraging passive leg exercises—dorsal and planar movement of the feet, as well as using elastic stockings.

Fortunately, there were only a few serious complications associated with omental transposition to the brain or spinal cord. Several patients who underwent spinal cord procedures complained of severe headaches for a few days following surgery, which resolved spontaneously. These headaches were felt to be due to a small CSF leak at the spinal-cord–omental interface, which quickly sealed. However, in one patient, it was necessary to control the CSF leak surgically.

One patient developed a pulmonary embolus, which resolved uneventfully under medical management. There was one death in the series in a 69-year-old post-stroke patient who developed pneumonia several days after surgery, which progressed to multi-organ failure and eventual death several weeks later.

Appendix 1

SURGICAL PERSPECTIVE

Treatment of Acute Spinal Cord Injury by Omental Transposition: A New Approach

Harry S Goldsmith, MD, FACS

Interest in the attempt to improve neurologic results after a spinal cord injury (SCI) was brought into focus by a recent article by Heimburger.[1] His article highlighted Freeman's work carried out in the 1950s, which involved successful implantation of a cut end of an intercostal nerve directly into the spinal cord of an experimental animal distal to a complete spinal cord (SC) transection.[2] The technique reportedly allowed axons to grow profusely from the end of the implanted intercostal nerve into the gray matter of the spinal cord distal to the transection site. The operation, however, is applicable only in the treatment of patients with a chronic SCI. A neurosurgical area that deserves exploration is in the evolution of new surgical approaches directed specifically toward acute spinal cord injuries because current surgical results in the treatment of an SCI have not appreciably improved over the past 50 years.

Pathophysiology of a spinal cord injury

To evaluate treatment proposals that might lead to neurologic improvement after an acute SCI, it is important to understand the pathophysiologic events that take place within a spinal cord after injury. From the moment of an SCI, there is rapid deposition of traumatic edema and blood at the injury site. This is the result of leakage of edema and blood through the porous endothelial lining of damaged capillaries located mainly in the central gray matter of the SC. The edema fluid is rich in plasma protein, which has a high osmotic pressure that attracts an increasing amount of edema fluid. As edema and blood accumulate in the injured area, they cause an extensive physical swelling of the spinal cord, which is contained within its nonyielding dura mater covering and the surrounding bony vertebral column, a condition that causes increased interstitial pressure at the site of the SCI.

As the edema expansion intensifies, the interstitial pressure within the spinal cord continues to increase, causing compression of veins in the area. This action results in an elevated venous pressure, which further

enhances the capillary extrusion of edema fluid and blood from the porous blood vessels at the injury site. Under normal conditions, extracellular edema fluid in the spinal cord drains into perivascular spaces, with eventual drainage into cerebrospinal fluid. This flow pattern is essential for edema fluid elimination because there are no lymphatics in the spinal cord. As the volume of edema accumulates after an SCI, there is eventual blockage of the central canal and subarachnoid and subdural spaces so that the normal edema drainage system within the spinal cord is compromised.

Compensatory fluid mechanics develop within the spinal cord after injury to displace edema fluid up and down the cord in an attempt to decrease expanding edema accumulation.[3] This longitudinal fluid movement, however, cannot compensate for the increasing edema volume that develops in the injury area. As the edema accumulation increases, it causes the interstitial pressure at the injury site to become excessive, resulting in capillary compression that eventually diminishes capillary perfusion to the point of total vascular occlusion. When this occurs, there can be irreversible damage to neural tissue within the SC unless circulation can be restored within 4 to 6 hours of injury.

Decompressive laminectomy and, on occasion, myelotomy, have been performed over the years in an attempt to lower the elevated SC interstitial pressure caused by an expanding edema accumulation. The uncertainty of clinical improvement that has followed these procedures, however, has failed over the years to justify their routine performance. The simple lowering of a high interstitial pressure, especially difficult with the dura mater intact, is apparently not the only factor that must be addressed in an attempt to prevent permanent SC damage. Absorption of the mixture of edema fluid and blood at the SCI site may be the critical issue if SC damage is to be minimized because it has been clearly shown in the laboratory that the presence of this material at the site of the SC-injured area leads to postinjury scar formation.[4] The presence of scar development in the spinal cord injured area has been found to be detrimental to any subsequent healing of an injured SC. This raises the question as to how these pathologic conditions might be corrected in an acutely injured SC. Omental transposition (OT) has the potential to accomplish this.

Received August 28, 2008; Revised October 21, 2008; Accepted October 23, 2008.
From the Department of Surgery, University of Nevada, Reno, NV.
Correspondence address: Harry S Goldsmith, MD, Box 493, Glenbrook, NV 89413.

ISSN 1072-7515/09/$36.00
doi:10.1016/j.jamcollsurg.2008.10.021

290   Goldsmith   Omental Transposition for Acute Spinal Cord Injury   J Am Coll Surg

---

Abbreviations and Acronyms

OT = omental transposition
SC = spinal cord
SCI = spinal cord injury

Omental transposition for spinal cord injury

It was first shown in 1973 that placing an intact omental pedicle directly on a spinal cord led to the introduction of omental blood vessels that travel through the omental-spinal cord interface and penetrate directly into the spinal cord.[5] Subsequent dye marker studies showed that these omental vessels travel down to deeply positioned capillaries in the noninjured spinal cord within 72 hours and even more rapidly when the omentum was placed on an acutely injured spinal cord.[4] It was believed that this rapid revascularization of the SC was likely from the vascular endothelial growth factor in the omentum, vascular endothelial growth factor being the most angiogenic substance in the body with its greatest concentration in omental tissue.[6] This ability to revascularize an SC shortly after injury, with continuation of this process during the healing phase of the injured SC, is an important activity of OT.

Placing the omentum on an injured spinal cord allows absorption of the mixture of edema fluid and blood within and surrounding the spinal cord injury site.[4,7] This absorptive capability was first shown clinically in humans when the omentum was placed in the arms and legs of patients in the treatment of chronic lymphedema.[8] It was later reported in the treatment of hydrocephalus that the omentum had the capacity to absorb one-third of the entire cerebrospinal fluid reservoir.[9]

Of major importance concerning omental activity is the histologic and neuroelectrical evidence that placing the omentum directly on an acutely injured spinal cord results in a minimum of scar tissue production at the site of an SCI along with preservation of somato-sensory evoked potentials. In contrast to this omental protection, studies of control animals without omentum placement on their SCI demonstrated extensive scarring at the site of their SCI and loss of somato-sensory evoked potentials .[4] Other investigators have confirmed these findings.[10,11]

It is believed that the significant importance of the omentum along with its revascularization capabilities is its ability to absorb the mixture of edema fluid and blood at the spinal cord injury site. Absorption of this material after an SCI includes fibrinogen, which is present in the mixture. Fibrinogen is a component in the blood that leaks from capillaries located in the damaged SC, and is the agent that is activated at the SC injury site to form fibrin (scar). The scar that develops from the presence of fibrinogen

results in varying degrees of ischemia within the SCI area because it causes compression on local capillaries and adjacent blood vessels, decreasing blood flow to the injured area within the SCI. It has also been found that when the omentum is placed on an injured cord, not only is scar markedly reduced, but hemorrhagic necrosis and cavity formation within the cord are also markedly decreased. These favorable findings in experimental animals led to improvement in their motor function and neuroelectrical activity, which were findings not seen in control animals.[12]

Because of these observations, it is theorized that the favorable effects of the omentum in treating an SCI are mainly from its ability to absorb a mixture of edema fluid and blood after an SCI. This apparently is a result of a dynamic equilibrium that develops between the accumulation of edema fluid and blood within and around the injured spinal cord and the absorption of this material by the omentum, which becomes firmly adherent after its placement on the underlying spinal cord. This absorptive action decreases the level of fibrinogen, which is present in the mixture of blood and edema fluid. The danger of fibrin production derived from fibrinogen cannot be overemphasized because fibrin (scar) causes progressive ischemia in the area of an SCI and blocks regenerating axons from growing into the area of the spinal cord injury. One can even theorize that such scar development in and around an injured SC can physically obstruct the normally smooth flow pattern of cerebrospinal fluid, resulting over time in abnormal flow characteristics of the CSF, which may lead to a syrinx, as seen in the development of syringomyelia.

Ischemia caused by scar compression of capillaries in the area of SCI is especially harmful during the weeks and months after SCI, when healing of the spinal cord could be occurring, because an adequate blood supply is critical during this period. Scar tissue that compresses SC blood vessels in the area of injury decreases spinal cord blood flow. If one places the omentum on an SCI site, however, the spinal cord blood flow is increased by a mean of 58% as compared with a lower spinal cord blood flow in control animals that had not had omental application.[13] In addition, when the omentum is placed on a totally transected SC that has been reconstructed by an omental-collagen bridge, there is a 3-to-1 increase in blood vessel density counts penetrating into the omental-collagen bridge as compared with collagen-only bridge reconstruction.[14]

The surgical operation to transpose the intact omental pedicle onto a chronically injured spinal cord has been previously described.[15] The procedure involves separation of the omental attachments to the transverse colon and to the proximal attachments to the greater curvature of the stomach, leaving the right gastroepiploic vessels intact within the omental apron. After these maneuvers, the omental apron has its blood supply coming entirely from the right gastric and gastroepiploic vessels. The omental apron is then surgically tailored to create a long pedicle with its arterial and venous connections remaining intact. The omentum is then brought subcutaneously to the injured area of the spinal cord. A laminectomy is performed and the dura opened over the subcutaneous edematous site, with the omentum being laid directly on the spinal cord after removing pieces of arachnoid and scar in the area of the SCI. The omentum is sutured carefully to the cut edges of the dura. This technique of omental placement, when performed in animals subjected to an acute spinal cord injury, has been shown to improve neuroelectrical and functional activity.[16,17]

Omental transposition

There are no studies at present examining whether OT would be effective in improving the clinical results that follow current surgical treatment for an acute SCI. If absorbing edema fluid and blood at the site of SCI is eventually found to be instrumental in improving postsurgical results of such injuries, the potential effectiveness of OT would be quite important.

Magnetic resonance imaging studies of acute SCIs have been instrumental in predicting the possible longterm neurologic outcomes of such injuries.[18] Blood at the site of an SCI, as shown by MRI, is significantly more serious than the presence of edematous fluid at the injury site.[19-21] If a hemorrhagic area located on the spinal cord is less than 4 mm on an MRI examination, the prognosis is relatively favorable.[22] If traumatic edema remains on an MRI 6 weeks after SCI, however, the opportunity for eventual neurologic improvement may be limited.[23] This information supports the idea that the absorption of edema fluid and blood, which limits scar production, could prove to be the source of improved longterm neurologic results after an SCI.

Because the omentum can absorb edema fluid and blood and reduce the production of post-traumatic scar tissue, it also may allow postinjury invasive axons to grow into the area of an SCI. This activity supports the belief of Freeman,[2] who claimed more than half a century ago, "that axons have a relentless compulsion to grow until they participate in the return of function. If axonal ingrowth is blocked by scar tissue," as claimed by Freeman, "axons continue to grow in circles to form neuromata." This is what currently occurs in the evolution of an SCI. Freeman's statements seem prophetic because an intact omentum, when placed on an acutely injured spinal cord, has been shown in the laboratory to decrease scar tissue, resulting in neuroelectrical preservation and functional improve-

ment.[4,7] Only by critical clinical studies, however, will we learn if favorable comparable results can occur in humans who have suffered an SCI.

In conclusion, at present, the major thrust of basic and clinical research directed toward SCI has been aimed at restoration of neurologic activity in chronic SCI patients. This article, however, has focused on improving the longterm neurologic results of acutely injured SCI patients by treating the spinal cord definitively during the acute stage after injury.

The reason for believing that OT could be effective in an SCI is predicated on the ability of the omentum to limit scar tissue and to add angiogenic agents, growth factors, and numerous neurotransmitters which are present in the omentum.[4,7,16]

Pilot studies have measured the concentration of vasoactive neurochemicals in the omentum. These have included vasoactive biogenic amine neurotransmitters (epinephrine, norepinephrine, dopamine, and endogenous opioid β endorphin) in plasma obtained from isolated omental venous drainage and from intact omental tissue.[24] Data from these studies showed a greater concentration of these biologic substances in omental tissue than in peripheral circulation.

Early studies also showed that not only were vasoactive chemicals present in omental tissue, but omental derived neurotrophic factors were also present.[25] A recent study further confirmed the marked expression of neurotrophins that are present in the omentum.[26]

These studies demonstrated that the omentum not only accumulates neurochemical and neurotrophic agents, but also shows the capability of the structure to actually produce these biologic substances. It remains unknown, however, what effect, if any, these biologic substances might exert in the healing process of an acute spinal cord injury.

Of potentially significant importance has been the recent finding that the human omentum incorporates large numbers of stem cells within its tissues.[27] It is not unreasonable to believe that omental stem cells travel directly into an injured spinal cord through vascular connections at the omental-spinal cord interface. A recent development concerning stem cells that might prove to be important in the early and direct treatment of a spinal cord injury is hyperbaric oxygenation. It has been shown that placing a patient in a hyperbaric oxygen chamber for 2 hours at 2 atmospheres of pressure caused a two-fold increase in stem cells in the peripheral circulation. Patients who received hyperbaric oxygen for 20 treatments, however, showed that the stem cell population increased in the peripheral circulation by eight-fold. It is theorized that the result of this stem cell increase, which was stimulated by hyperbaric oxygen, re-

292   **Goldsmith**   Omental Transposition for Acute Spinal Cord Injury   *J Am Coll Surg*

sulted from mobilization of stem cells originating from bone marrow by way of a nitric oxide reaction.[28] This form of treatment for spinal cord injured patients deserves future consideration, especially if stem cells are eventually found to be important in the treatment of the central nervous system.

There are those who would call for an evaluation of OT by initiating controlled clinical studies on acutely injured spinal cord patients. Such studies, however, would be extremely difficult, if not impossible, to carry out because all high-impact spinal cord injuries are different; and obtaining sufficient numbers of experimental and control patients for these studies would be difficult. What might be done is to choose SCI patients who lose complete motor and sensation immediately after injury, which persists over the following hours, because the condition of these patients rarely results in functional recovery. If a significant number of such patients subjected to OT demonstrated functional return, this would be of high clinical importance.

Currently, patients with an SCI have their vertebral column stabilized, with or without spinal fusion, but little if any attention is directed specifically to the injured spinal cord. The time may have come to evaluate a new surgical approach to an SCI using the omentum to improve present day surgical results, which have not appreciably improved over the last half century.

REFERENCES

1. Heimburger RF. Is there hope for return of function in lower extremities paralyzed by spinal cord injury. J Am Coll Surg 2006;202:1001–1004.
2. Freeman LW. Neuronal regeneration in the central nervous system of man. Successful growth of intercostal nerve anastomosis and growth of intercostal nerve-spinal cord implant. J Neurosurg 1961;18:417–423.
3. Nemecek ST, Peter R, Suba P, et al. Longitudinal extension of edema in experimental spinal cord injury. Acta Neurochir 1977;37:7–16.
4. Goldsmith HS, Steward E, Duckett S. Early application of pedicled omentum to the acutely traumatized spinal cord. Paraplegia 1985;23:100–112.
5. Goldsmith HS, Duckett S, Chen WF. Spinal cord revascularization by intact omentum. Am J Surg 1975;129:262–265.
6. Zhang QX, Magovern CJ, Mack CA, et al. Vascular endothelial growth factor is the major angiogenic factor in omentum: mechanisms of the omentum-mediated angiogenesis. J Surg Res 1997;67:147–154.
7. Goldsmith HS. Revascularization and edema absorption of the brain and spinal cord. In: Liebermann-Meffert D, White H, eds. The greater omentum. New York: Springer-Verlag; 1983:189–197.
8. Goldsmith HS, de los Santos R, Beattie EJ. The relief of chronic lymphedema by omental transposition. Ann Surg 1967;166:571–585.

9. Levander B, Zwetnow NW. Bulk flow of CSF through a lumbo-omental pedicled graft in the dog. Acta Neurochir 1978;41:147–155.
10. Goodkin R, Campbell JB. Sequential pathologic changes in spinal cord injury. Surg Forum 1969;20:430–432.
11. Shimada Y. Experimental study on effect of omental transposition in cats with spinal cord injury. No To Shinki 1995;47:863–873.
12. Shimada Y, Nagashima C. Experimental study on effects of omental transposition in cats with spinal cord injury. In: Goldsmith HS, ed. The omentum: Application to brain and spinal cord. Wilton, CT: Forefront Publishing; 2000: 44–60.
13. Goldsmith HS, de la Torre JC. Axonal regeneration after spinal cord transection and reconstruction. Brain Res 1992;589:217–224.
14. de la Torre JC, Goldsmith HS. Collagen-omental graft in experimental spinal cord transection. Acta Neurochir 1990;102:152–163.
15. Goldsmith HS. Omental transposition to the brain and spinal cord. Surg Rounds 1986;9:22–23.
16. Goldsmith HS. Omental transposition to the spinal cord. In: Ostrander LE, Lee BY, eds. The spinal cord injured patient. New York, NY: Demos Publisher; 2002:381–394.
17. Goldsmith HS. Can the standard treatment of acute spinal cord injury be improved? Perhaps the time has come. Neurol Res 2007;29:6–20.
18. Mascalchi M, Dal Posso G, Dini C, et al. Acute spinal cord trauma: Prognostic value of MRI appearance at 0.5T. Clin Radiol 1993;48:100–108.
19. Silberstein M, Tress BM, Hennessy O. Prediction of neurologic outcome in acute spinal cord injury: The role of CT and MRI. Am J Neuroradiol 1992;13:1597–1608.
20. Elrai S, Souei M, Arifa N, et al. MR imaging in spinal cord injury. J Radiol 2006;87:121–126.
21. Andreoli C, Colalacomo MC, Rojas Beccaglia M, et al. MRI in the acute phase of spinal cord traumatic lesions: Relationships between MRI findings and neurological outcome. Radiol Med (Torino) 2005;110:636–645.
22. Boldin C, Raith J, Fankhauser F, et al. Predicting neurologic recovery in cervical spinal cord injury with postoperative MR imaging. Spine 2006;31:554–559.
23. Shepard MJ, Bracken MB. Magnetic resonance imaging and neurological recovery in acute spinal cord injury: Observation from the National Acute Spinal Cord Injury Study 3. Spinal Cord 1999;37:833–837.
24. McIntosh TK, Goldsmith HS. Vasoactive neurochemicals in the omentum: Implication for CNS injury. In: Goldsmith HS, ed. The omentum: research and clinical applications. New York and Heidelberg: Springer-Verlag;1990: 75–84.
25. Siek GC, Marquis JK, Goldsmith HS. Experimental studies of omentum-derived neurotrophic factors. In: The omentum: research and clinical applications. Goldsmith HS, editor. New York and Heidelberg: Springer-Verlag;1990: 85–96.
26. Dujovny M, Ding YH, Ding Y, et al. Current concepts in the expression of neurotrophins in the greater omentum. Neurol Res 2004;26:226–229.
27. Garcia-Gomez I, Goldsmith HS, Angulo J, et al. Angiogenic capacity of human omental stem cells. Neurol Res 2005;27:807–811.
28. Thom SR, Bhopale VM, Velasquez DC, et al. Stem cell mobilization by hyperbaric oxygen. Am J Physiol Heart Circ 2006;290:H1378–H1386.

Appendix 2

COLLECTIVE REVIEW

Omental Transposition in Treatment of Alzheimer Disease

Harry S Goldsmith, MD, FACS

It is now recognized that Alzheimer disease (AD) is one of the most devastating problems confronting the practice of medicine today. This disease has severe social and economic consequences that will only increase greatly in the future. Currently, there are 1,000 new cases of AD diagnosed daily in the United States.[1] When these patients are added to the 4.5 million Americans already diagnosed with AD, coupled with the expected arrival of future millions of "baby boomers," many of whom will get AD, the result in costs to individuals and government will be in the multiple billions of dollars.

BACKGROUND

The neurodegenerative effects of AD have been well-established, but, because the exact cause of AD remains unknown, it is difficult to develop programs to prevent and treat the disease with any degree of precision. What is known is that in the brain of a patient with AD, there are, at any one time, three neuronal states: normally functioning neurons, dead neurons, and neurons that are slowly deteriorating. The goal in prevention and treatment of AD will be to maintain the viability of normal cerebral neurons and improve neuronal function, or at least prevent it from deteriorating.

AD is a disease in which neurons die slowly during the course of many years. The dementia that eventually occurs as a hallmark of the disease begins to manifest itself when there is loss in the critical mass of neurons located in key regions of the brain that are responsible for cognitive function. When these critically located cerebral neurons lose function during the course of time, dementia can eventually result.

ETIOLOGIC CONCEPTS

Amyloid hypothesis

There is a belief among many researchers that a relationship exists between the presence of amyloid plaques within the brain and development of AD. Because the major compo-

Competing Interests Declared: None.

Received May 1, 2007; Revised June 11, 2007; Accepted June 14, 2007.
From the University of Nevada School of Medicine, Reno, NV.
Correspondence address: Harry S Goldsmith, MD, FACS, PO Box 493, Glenbrook, NV 89413.

nent of an amyloid plaque is amyloid-β protein (Aβ), this has led to the belief that the amyloid deposition within these plaques is responsible for development of AD. This hypothesis might, at first glance, appear reasonable, but let us examine some of the features of this concept that make its believability unsettling:

1. Presence of amyloid in Petri-dish preparations can cause destruction of neurons; but there is no evidence that amyloid present in the human brain has ever been found to be neurotoxic.[2]
2. There appears to be no relationship between the number of amyloid plaques in the human brain and the degree of dementia severity seen in AD patients.[3]
3. It has been shown that transgenic mice can produce Aβ deposits in association with cognitive loss. It should be stressed that cognitive loss in these rodents occurs before the Aβ deposits that eventually develop within the brain.[4]
4. Many individuals who exhibit normal cognition before their death are found at autopsy to have abundant numbers of amyloid plaques in their brain,[5] some with numbers comparable with patients with AD dementia.[6]
5. Braak and Braak, in their publications, demonstrated that the earliest neuropathological indication of AD is not the number of senile plaques present in the brain.[7,8]

Despite increasing evidence that amyloid plaques are not the underlying cause of AD, enthusiasm continues to persist that they are the cause of the disease.[9] To lessen the probability that amyloid plaques are detrimental to the brain and are the basis for AD, a recent publication has suggested that amyloid–beta peptide are actually beneficial to neuronal survival.[10]

Cholinergic hypothesis

There remains a belief that cerebral cholinergic deficiency might be the cause of cognitive loss in AD patients. This is the basis for the continuing and widespread use of cholinesterase inhibitors in AD, which are administered in an attempt to maintain sufficient levels of acetylcholine (ACh) within the brain. These agents apparently create their effect by impeding the enzyme cholinesterase from breaking down ACh, which is the neurotransmitter that is essential, but considered deficient, in producing adequate cholinergic transmission in critical areas of the brain involved

ISSN 1072-7515/07/$32.00
doi:10.1016/j.jamcollsurg.2007.06.294

Omental Transposition... Reprinted with permission from the *J Am Coll Surg.* 2007;205(6):800-804.

Abbreviations and Acronyms

Aβ	=	amyloid-β protein
ACh	=	acetylcholine
AD	=	Alzheimer disease
ATP	=	adenosine triphosphate
CBF	=	cerebral blood flow
ChAT	=	choline acetyltransferase
MCI	=	mild cognitive impairment
OT	=	omental transposition

with cognition and memory. Because cholinesterase inhibitors have been shown to exert modest but temporary improvement in AD patients, possibly because of a limited increase in cerebral blood flow (CBF),[2,11] the belief persists that a lowered ACh level in AD might well be the main cause of the disease, and if ACh could be increased, especially in the hippocampal area, the AD patient would benefit. This concept warrants questioning.

Choline acetyltransferase (ChAT) is an enzyme involved in the synthesis of ACh and serves as a specific marker for cholinergic neurons. If a lower level of ACh might be the basis for AD, one would expect concentrations of ChAT to be depressed in AD patients as compared with normal controls. Recent studies of patients with mild cognitive impairment (MCI) and moderate AD found that ChAT levels were no different than levels found in nondemented aging patients. It was also found that ChAT levels were elevated in the frontal cortex and hippocampus in patients with MCI. ChAT levels were found to be reduced only in patients who were at the end stage of their disease.[12] These findings lessen the support that ACh is the underlying cause of Alzheimer's disease.

Cerebral hypoperfusion

It has been well-established that there is a decrease in CBF in AD. It has also been generally accepted over the years that the reason for the decrease in CBF in AD patients is neuronal degeneration, which decreases the need for CBF. There is now increasing information that suggests that AD is not the result of neurodegeneration causing the decrease in CBF, but it is mainly the decrease in CBF, especially during advanced aging, that leads to neurodegeneration in AD.[13,14]

If AD is a result of diminished CBF, there are many conditions that lead to a lowering of CBF, the most important of these is aging, which is a normal phenomenon that occurs in all individuals. In addition to aging as a risk factor for AD, there are many other conditions closely associated with development of AD that have a negative effect maintaining CBF. These risk factors include hypertension, cor-

onary artery disease, cardiac arrhythmias, head trauma, myocardial infarction, arteriosclerosis, hypocholesteremia, diabetes type 2, smoking, obesity, and others.[15,16]

A lowering of CBF leads to inadequate oxygen, glucose, and other biologic substances presented to the brain, which are crucial for neuronal survival. Presence of these biologic agents is especially critical for survival of key neurons that are involved in development of AD. When these specific neurons are chronically deprived of the nutrients that are necessary for their continued survival, a serious disruption occurs in the intracellular energy system within the neuron. The effect of this intraneural disruption severely impacts the mitochondrial apparatus within the cell that is directly involved in production of adenosine triphosphate (ATP), which is the energy source of a cell. When sufficient numbers of critically located neurons are affected by this loss of neuronal energy, the end result is dementia of the AD type.

Dependency on blood flow required for ATP production becomes highly critical if ATP deficiency occurs in neurons located in crucial areas of the brain, such as the hippocampus. When these neurons are deprived of their energy source (ATP) because of decreased CBF, oxidative and endoplasmic stress occurs, which directly affects the intracellular mitochondria that is essential for subsequent production of ATP. Oxidative stress arising in the mitochondria has an unfavorable effect on the endoplasmic reticulum and other locations within neurons, which has a negative effect on intracellular protein metabolism, resulting in intracellular-extracellular β amyloid peptide accumulation.[13,16,17] These findings add credibility to the idea that Aβ production is not the cause of neuronal death in AD, but is a marker indicating cellular injury within a neuron, resulting in decreasing ATP levels caused by a decrease in CBF.

Recent studies have shown the closely associated relationship of decreased CBF and development of AD.[18,19] Phase-contrast MRI was used to measure total CBF flowing to the human brain by calculating the blood volume that passes through the internal carotid and basilar arteries. This study demonstrated a significant decrease in the volume of blood flow that passed through these arteries in AD patients (a mean blood flow of 442 mL/minute) as compared with a mean blood flow of 551 mL/minute in nondemented age-matched subjects (p < 0.001). In a younger age group of normal subjects (median age 29 years), phase-contrast MRI studies showed a substantially higher mean blood flow rate of 742 mL/minute, which passed through their internal carotid and basilar arteries. This study demonstrated the marked decrease in the blood supply that normally flows to the brain of elderly and AD patients in comparison with young individuals. The concept that a decreased CBF level can lead to neuronal death and eventual AD has been present for more than a decade, having been raised by de la Torre in 1993.[20] A more recent article stated simply that "chronic or transient suboptimal brain perfusion can well contribute to the metabolic perturbations that are responsible for the lesions characteristic of AD."[21]

A more recent study (Rotterdam) also showed that CBF velocity was an additional factor implicated in AD development, based on the evaluation of "several thousand demented and nondemented elderly patients."[22] This combination of decreased CBF and diminished CBF velocity would have a negative effect on ischemic-sensitive neurons located in critical areas of the brain, such as the hippocampus. As the volume of blood and its velocity continues to diminish to the brain, widespread neuronal deterioration would be expected to eventually lead to development of AD. Adding to the decreased CBF and CBF velocity that routinely occurs in AD patients are physical changes in the external and internal characteristics of capillaries in the brains of these patients that cause hypoperfusion to cerebral neurons. Histochemical studies have shown that capillaries in AD patients lose their structural configuration as these vessels become twisted and kinked, which markedly affects the microcirculatory flow pattern.[23] Blood flow through an unaffected capillary is normally laminar, but if the capillary shape becomes irregular, as seen in capillary vessels in AD, the blood flow pattern through these vessels reverts from normal linear flow to abnormal disturbed flow. This irregular blood flow movement progressing through abnormally shaped capillaries becomes another factor that decreases CBF to critical neurons within the brain.

In addition to the abnormal laminar flow characteristics, there are changes that occur in the walls of capillaries that also adversely affect CBF. Physical abnormalities that occur within the vessel wall of capillaries of AD patients include basement membrane thickening, endothelial cell compression, pericyte degeneration, and vessel luminal distortion.[16] These physical changes damage the endothelial cells lining the wall of the capillaries, resulting in a compromise of nitric oxide activity that normally occurs within these endothelial cells. Endothelial cells are extremely important in CBF flow because they control vascular dilation, which allows for an increase in CBF. When these endothelial cells lining the capillary walls are adversely affected, the lumen of the capillaries lose their ability to dilate and CBF becomes limited. This endothelial cell alteration, vascular smooth muscle cell atrophy, and distortion of small blood vessels in an AD brain, restrict CBF, resulting in cerebral hypoperfusion, which eventually may prove to be the critical issue in subsequent development of AD pathology.

TREATMENT MODALITY

Great amounts of time and money are currently being spent at many centers throughout the world to find a pharmaceutical method to address the neurologic and cognitive problems associated with AD. Multiple drug studies continue to be evaluated in the quest to find a therapeutic approach to AD. Cholinesterase inhibitors are currently in common use for this purpose, but it is well-known that their clinical effects are of short duration, even in patients who reportedly have responded to the drugs. Additionally, adverse side effects of cholinesterase inhibitors drugs can be considerable.[24]

Despite the continuing belief by some investigators that amyloid plaque and, to a lesser degree, ACh deficiency are the underlying causes of AD, interest continues to increase in the belief that the underlying cause of AD might well prove to be hypoperfusion to the brain.[25-28] Two factors generally accepted in AD etiology are advancing age and various risk factors that are known to decrease CBF. If decreased CBF can eventually prove to be the underlying basis for AD development, strenuous efforts should continue to be directed to devising methods, medical or surgical, to increase CBF and to learn its effect on patients. If decreased CBF is found to be the case, methods to increase blood flow to the brain must take the highest priority.

I am unaware of any pharmaceutical treatment that can increase CBF to a substantial degree for an extended period of time. There is now a surgical procedure that has been proved to be able to add a substantial amount of blood during a protracted period of time to the human brain.[29] Of considerable importance is the fact that the operation has been shown to cause postoperative reversal of symptoms in AD patients.[30-32] This operation, known as omental transposition (OT), is a procedure that deserves critical evaluation, especially for patients with late MCI and early AD patients.

OT is a surgical procedure in which the omentum is surgically lengthened into an extensive intact pedicle within the peritoneal cavity, with its blood supply remaining intact. The omental pedicle is then brought subcutaneously up the chest, neck, and behind the ear. A craniotomy is performed and the dura opened, followed by removing small portions of the pia mater. The omentum is then laid directly on the underlying brain and the craniotomy bone is replaced.[33] Blood vessels have been shown histologically to penetrate directly, vertically, and rapidly from the omentum into the underlying brain within days after the procedure, allowing extracerebral blood and biologic substances derived from the omentum to enter the AD brain.[34,35]

Important biologic agents are present in omental tissue, including neurotransmitters,[36] nerve growth,[37] and angio-

Vol. 205, No. 6, December 2007   **Goldsmith**   Omental Transposition in Treatment of AD   **803**

genic factors,[38] especially vascular endothelial growth factor, which is the most angiogenic substance in the human body, with the greatest concentration of vascular endothelial growth factor being present in omental tissue.[39] Of recent interest is the finding of large numbers of stem cells that are present in human omentum.[40]

A pharmaceutical approach in the treatment of AD would certainly be more acceptable to patients, as opposed to a surgical procedure such as OT. If a patient today shows evidence of advanced MCI or early AD, the possibility of a favorable approach for relief of these conditions by any present-day treatment is quite limited. Unfortunately, no one knows how many years or decades it might take for a reliable pharmaceutical approach to AD to become a reality.

Although not a cure, OT has been shown to attain a favorable cognitive response for several years, with most patients in the late stages of AD. It seems reasonable to believe that if patients were operated earlier in the development of AD, an improved longterm postoperative result would be expected, because more viable neurons would be available for metabolic stabilization. Allowing a patient with AD to function with his family on a day-to-day basis during an extended time period would be a benefit of enormous proportion to family members, and would also be financially beneficial in the care and management of AD patients. Performing a small study involving OT on AD patients in a strictly controlled setting could be limited in number, because only six subjects are necessary for statistical analysis of results.

Based on patients who have undergone OT for AD, it would be expected that several patients in the study would have a favorable neurologic effect because of energizing of deteriorating cerebral neurons that are in the process of dying. OT has already been shown to be helpful in reversing symptoms in AD patients (9 of 25 patients have reversed symptoms, in my personal surgical experience), most of the patients being in the advanced stage of their disease.[32] Unfortunately, none of these AD patients were involved in a randomized or controlled study.

One can expect that there would be AD patients who would choose to undergo OT under strict experimental control if they considered the possibility that the operation might have a favorable effect on their cognitive symptoms. Patients would be informed that the purpose of the operation is to increase blood flow and critical biologic substances into their AD brains, in the hope that the procedure would stabilize their condition and possibly reverse their cognitive symptoms.

Technical aspects of performing OT are not difficult when performed by a well-trained general and neurologic surgeon. As in all new surgical procedures, there are maneuvers that are important, and the team that performs OT should be aware of these maneuvers, so as not to lessen the chance of subsequent neurologic improvement. If the operation is performed by people without experience or awareness of the possible complexity of this operation, as in any operation, poor postoperative results can result. If this occurs, it can lead to the reporting that the operation is difficult, unsafe, and without clinical justification—comments that are unjustified.[41,42]

In conclusion, AD develops from decreased CBF, and OT has the potential to be helpful to an AD patient by adding a substantial amount of CBF and critical biologic agents to their AD brain. Because of the devastating nature of AD to both patient and family, it would appear that a well-controlled study involving a small number of AD patients is not only justified, but appears necessary. A favorable result from such a study could prove very important. Khachaturian recently described the remarkable advances that have been made in the last 20 years in knowledge pertaining to AD.[43] Unfortunately, no comparable advances have been made in the therapeutic area. OT appears worthy of evaluation until pharmacological methods are developed to prevent and treat AD.

REFERENCES

1. Hebert LE, Scherr PA, Bennett DA, Evans DA. Alzheimer disease in the US population: prevalence estimates using the 2000 census. Arch Neurol 2004;61:802–803.
2. de la Torre JC. Is Alzheimer disease a neurodegenerative or a vascular disorder? Data, dogma, and dialectics. Lancet Neurol 2004;3:184–189.
3. Terry RD, Masliah E, Salmon DP, et al. Physical basis of cognitive alterations in Alzheimer's disease: synapse loss is the major correlate of cognitive impairment. Ann Neurol 1991;30:572–580.
4. Hsiao K, Chapman P, Nilsen S. Correlative memory deficits, A-beta elevation and amyloid plaques in transgenic mice. Science 1996;274:99–102.
5. Davis DG, Schmitt FA, Wekstein DR, Markesbery WR. Alzheimer neuropathologic alterations in aged cognitively normal subjects. J Neuropathol Exp Neurol 1999;58:376–388.
6. Arriagada PV, Growdon JH, Hedley-White ET, Hyman B. Neurofibrillar tangles but not senile plaques parallel duration and severity of Alzheimer disease. Neurology 1992;42:631–639.
7. Braak H, Braak E. Age, neurofibrillary changes, A-beta and onset of Alzheimer disease Neurosci Lett 1996;210:87–90.
8. Braak H, Braak E. Frequency of stages of Alzheimer-related lesions in different age categories. Neurobiol Aging 1997;4:351–357.
9. Hardy J, Selkoe DJ. The amyloid hypothesis of Alzheimer's disease: progress and problems on the road to therapeutics. Science 2002;297:353–356.
10. Leigh D, Plant JP, Boyle IF, et al. The production of amyloid-beta peptide is a critical requirement for the viability of central neurons. J Neurosci 2003;23:5531–5535.

11. Nakano S, Asada A, Matsudo H, et al. Donepezil hydrochloride preserves blood flow in patients with Alzheimer disease. J Nucl Med 2001;42:1441–1445.

12. Dekosky ST, Ikonomovic MD. Upregulation of choline acetyltransferase activity in hippocampus and frontal cortex of elderly subjects with mild cognitive impairment. Ann Neurol 2002;51: 145–155.

13. de la Torre JC. How do heart disease and stroke become risk factors in Alzheimer disease? Neurol Res 2006;28:1–8.

14. Johnson KA, Jones K, Holman BL, et al. Preclinical production of Alzheimer disease using SPECT. Neurology 1998;50:1563–1571.

15. Meyer JS, Rauch G, Rauch RA, Haque E. Risk factors for cerebral hypoperfusion, mild cognitive impairment and dementia. Neurobiol Aging 2002;21:161–169.

16. de la Torre JC. Cerebral hypoperfusion, capillary degeneration and development of Alzheimer disease. Alzheimer Dis Assoc Disord 2000;14:573–581.

17. Stieber A, Mourelatos Z, Gonatas NK. In Alzheimer's disease the Golgi apparatus of a population of neurons without neurofibrillary tangles is fragmented and atrophic. Am J Pathol 1996; 148:415–426.

18. Spilt A, Box FMA, van der Geest RJ, et al. Reproducibility of total cerebral blood flow measurements using phase contrast magnetic resonance imaging. J Magn Reson Imaging 2002;16:1–5.

19. Spilt A, Weverling-Rijnsburger AWE, Middelkoop HAM, et al. Late-onset dementia: structural brain damage and total cerebral blood flow. Radiology 2005;236:990–995.

20. de la Torre JC, Mussivand T. Can disturbed brain microcirculation cause Alzheimer disease? Neurol Res 1993;15:156–153.

21. Roher AE, Kokjohn TA, John TA, Beach TG. An association with great implication: vascular pathology and Alzheimer disease. Alzheimer Dis Assoc Disord 2006;20:73–74.

22. Ruitenberg A, Heijer TD, Bakker SLM. Cerebral hypoperfusion and clinical onset of dementia: the Rotterdam study. Ann Neurol 2005;57:789–794.

23. Fisher VW, Siddigia A, Yusufaly Y. Altered abnormalities in selected areas of brains with Alzheimer disease. Acta Neuropathol 1990;79:672–679.

24. de la Torre JC. Alzheimer's disease is a vasocognopathy: a new term to describe its nature. Neurol Res 2004;26:517–524.

25. de la Torre JC. Critically attained threshold of cerebral hypoperfusion: can it cause Alzheimer disease. Ann NY Acad Sci 2000; 903:424–436.

26. Roher AE, Garami Z, Alexandrov AV, et al. Interaction of cardiovascular disease and neurodegeneration: transcranial Doppler ultrasonography and Alzheimer disease. Neurol Res 2006;28: 672–678.

27. Akkawi KA, Borroni B, Agosti C, et al. Volume cerebral blood flow reduction in preclinical stage in Alzheimer disease: evidence from ultrasonography study. J Neurol 2005;252:559–563.

28. Miklossy J. Cerebral hypoperfusion induces cortical watershed neuroinfarcts which may further aggravate cognitive decline in Alzheimer disease. Neurol Res 2003;25:605–610.

29. Goldsmith HS, Bacciu M, Cosso M, et al. Regional cerebral blood flow after omental transposition to the ischemic brain in man: a five-year follow-up study. Acta Neurochir 1990;106:145–152.

30. Goldsmith HS. Role of the omentum in the treatment of Alzheimer disease. Neurol Res 2001;23:555–564.

31. Goldsmith HS. Treatment of Alzheimer disease by transposition of the omentum. Ann NY Acad Sci 2002;977:454–467.

32. Goldsmith HS, Wu W, Zhong J, et al. Omental transposition to the brain as a surgical method for treating Alzheimer disease. Neurol Res 2003;25:625–634.

33. Goldsmith HS. Omental transposition to the brain and spinal cord. Surg Rounds 1986;9:22–33.

34. Goldsmith HS, Chen WF, Duckett S. Brain vascularization by intact omentum. Arch Surg 1973;106:695–698.

35. Pau A, Viale ES, Turtus S. Effect of omental transposition to the brain on the cortical content of norepinephrine, dopamine, 5 hydroxytryptomine and 5-hydroxyindolacetic acid in experimental cerebral ischemia. Acta Neurochir 1980;51:253–257.

36. Goldsmith HS, McIntosh T, Vesina R, Colton T. Vasoactive neurochemicals identified in omentum. Br J Neurosurg 1987; 1:359–364.

37. Sick G, Maquis JK, Goldsmith HS. Experimental studies of omentum-derived neurotrophic factors. In: Goldsmith HS, ed. The omentum—research and clinical applications. New York: Springer-Verlag; 1990:109–116.

38. Goldsmith HS, Griffith A, Kupferman A, Catsinpoolis N. Lipid angiogenic factor from omentum. JAMA 1984;252:2034–2036.

39. Zhang QX, Magovern CJ, Mack CA, et al. Vascular endothelial growth factor is the major angiogenic factor in omentum: mechanism of the omentum-mediated angiogenesis. J Surg Res 1997; 67:147–154.

40. Garcia-Gomez I, Goldsmith HS, Angulo J, et al. Angiogenic capacity of human omental stem cells. Neurol Res 2005;27: 807–811.

41. Clifton GL, Donovan WH, Dimitrijevic MM, et al. Omental transposition in chronic spinal cord injury. Spinal Cord 1996; 34:193–203.

42. Goldsmith HS. Omental transposition in spinal cord injury—a rebuttal. Spinal Cord 1997;35:189–191.

43. Khachaturian ZS. Diagnosis of Alzheimer disease: two decades of progress. Alzheimer's & Dementia 2005;1:93–98.

236

INDEX